Health Care Financial Management for Nurse Managers

Health Care Financial Management for Nurse Managers

Applications in Hospitals, Long-Term Care, Home Care, and Ambulatory Care

Janne Dunham-Taylor, PhD, RN
Chair and Professor
Department of Adult Nursing
East Tennessee State University
Johnson City, TN

Joseph Z. Pinczuk, MHA
Retired CFO

JONES AND BARTLETT PUBLISHERS
Sudbury, Massachusetts
BOSTON   TORONTO   LONDON   SINGAPORE

Jones and Bartlett Publishers
40 Tall Pine Drive
Sudbury, MA 01776
978-443-5000
info@jbpub.com
www.jbpub.com

Jones and Bartlett Publishers
Canada
6339 Ormindale Way
Mississauga, ON L5V 1J2
CANADA

Jones and Bartlett Publishers
International
Barb House, Barb Mews
London W6 7PA
UK

Jones and Bartlett's books and products are available through most bookstores and online booksellers. To contact Jones and Bartlett Publishers directly, call 800-832-0034, fax 978-443-8000, or visit our website www.jbpub.com.

Substantial discounts on bulk quantities of Jones and Bartlett's publications are available to corporations, professional associations, and other qualified organizations. For details and specific discount information, contact the special sales department at Jones and Bartlett via the above contact information or send an email to specialsales@jbpub.com.

Library of Congress Cataloging-in-Publication Data

Dunham-Taylor, Janne.
  Healthcare financial management for nurse managers. Applications in hospitals, long-term care, home care, and ambulatory care / Janne Dunham-Taylor, Jospeh Z. Pinczuk.
      p. cm.
  Includes bibliographical references and index.
  ISBN 0-7637-3475-6 (pbk.)
  1. Nurse administrators. 2. Health facilities—Business management. 3. Health facilities—Finance. I. Pinczuk, Joseph. II. Title.
  RT89.D86 2005
  610.73'068—dc22

                              2004029251

Production Credits
Acquisitions Editor: Kevin Sullivan
Production Director: Amy Rose
Associate Production Editor: Tracey Chapman
Associate Editor: Amy Sibley
Marketing Manager: Emily Ekle
Manufacturing and Inventory Coordinator: Amy Bacus
Composition: Paw Print Media
Cover Design: Kristin E. Ohlin
Printing and Binding: Courier Stoughton
Cover Printing: Courier Stoughton

Printed in the United States of America
09 08 07 06 05   10 9 8 7 6 5 4 3 2 1

Acknowledgments

We would like to thank the other people who made this book possible. First, a big thanks to Mrs. Gina Rose, always there to help—creating tables, searching out appropriate sources for permissions, finding sources on the Internet, and generally supporting the authors in this endeavor. Thanks to both Dr. Joellen Edwards and Dr. Pat Smith, the College of Nursing Administration Team, the Adult Nursing Department faculty, and other nursing faculty for their support and encouragement. Thanks to Mrs. Dru Malcolm and Ms. Billie Sills for their valuable feedback on chapters as the book was being written. Thanks also to Mrs. Karen Deyo, who helped convert files, copy, etc., and to Ms. Lana J. Seal and Ms. Megan Alexander who helped with library work, checking references, and copying.

Dedication

This book is dedicated to the many nursing administration students and nurse administrators who have touched our lives. We learned a lot from you and we salute you.

—JDT & JZP

Thanks to Mom, Dad, and the family for all your support and encouragement in completing this venture.

—JDT

I want to thank Rosemary, my wife and best friend, for encouraging me in this labor of love. It is through her patience and understanding that I was able to complete this project.

—JZP

Contents

2 Using Inpatient Tools to Predict Cost and Measure Performance   87

Louise Gifford, MSN, RN

**3   Ignoring the Patient Classification System—
       Another Way to Staff   117**
*Kathryn W. Wilhoit, MSN, RN, CNAA, FACHE, Jane M. Mustain, MSN, RN,
with Special Recognition to Deborah McInturff, Financial Analyst*

4   Acuity-Based Flexible Nursing Budgets   157

Coy L. Smith, ND, MSN, RN, CNAA, CHE

Part II   Long-Term Care Issues   179

5   Managing Long-Term Care Resources   181

*Frances W. "Billie" Sills, MSN, RN, ARNP, CLNC, and
Susie Hutchings, RN, C, CPHQ*

6   The Resident Assessment Instrument (RAI): The Minimum Data Set (MDS)   219

Steven B. Littlehale, MS, APRN, BC, RN, Cheryl Field, MSN, CRRN, RN, and Diane L. Brown, BC, RN

Preface

Janne and Joe have been working together for years. It all started when the CNO at Joe's hospital invited Janne (an experienced nurse administrator teaching at the local university) to come and work with the nurse managers to enhance their knowledge about budgeting. When Janne met Joe (the CFO) she realized that he was an unusual CFO as he both understood and supported the "care" side of health care. Come to find out he was a former respiratory therapist. Joe thought that Janne's information for the nurse managers was important, and it was evident that the CNO and CFO worked well together.

Then Joe began to regularly come to talk to graduate nursing administration students in Janne's fiscal course. He could clearly explain financial terms, the way the finance department worked, and the future implications of reimbursement and how it would affect the health care organization, nurses, the patients, and community.

Gradually the ideas for this book began to take root and blossom. We knew that we did not want to create the typical financial book that kept finances in a silo. Instead we wanted to present finances in the larger dimension—as a part of a greater whole. We also both felt strongly that regular dialogue and respect between finance and nursing was critical to the success of a health care organization. Our goal was to provide nurse administrators with information so they can be more effective in their roles.

This book has been a labor of love but has been fraught with delays. Janne moved to another state. The original contract was with Aspen and when halfway finished there was an 18-month delay until Jones and Bartlett purchased Aspen's book division. Then when finished, the book was too long, so what started as one book became two—both titles starting with *Health Care Financial Management for Nurse Managers*. The first book is *Health Care Financial Management for Nurse Managers: Merging the Heart with the Dollar* with a broader focus of all that affects finances in an organization. The second book is

Health Care Financial Management for Nurse Managers: Applications in Hospitals, Long-Term Care, Home Care, and Ambulatory Care providing specific financial applications in those settings.

This book is made richer by the many contributors who have shared their expertise on certain subjects. We thank them for all their time, knowledge, and dedication to this book.

We hope that this is both practical and helpful for you. We have tried to provide other wonderful references—but, of course, cannot possibly do justice to the many additional resources available.

Contributors

Diane L. Brown, BC, RN, is the CEO of Brown LTC Consultants and JSC Ink Publishing Co. and received her degree from Stonehill College in Health Care Administration. A publisher and educator with over 30 years of operational experience in healthcare, Ms. Brown is the editor of the Briggs Corporation *MDS v2.0 User's Manual, the SB-MDS User's Manual,* the *Survey Guide for Long Term Care,* and is a co-developer of MDS *Guru*—an MDS e-learning tool. She recently co-authored and published the *Quick Guide to Documentation.* Diane has lectured both nationally and internationally on MDS and other related health care issues. She serves on the Board of Directors of the NASPAC, is an instructor for their MDS Nurse Assessment Coordinator Certification Program, and participates on several panels relating to the development of MDS 3.0.

Beth A. Cherry, MSN, RN, CNA, CMPE, received a Bachelor of Science in Nursing from Capital University in Columbus, Ohio and a Master of Science in Nursing from Case Western Reserve University in Cleveland, Ohio. She is a member of the Medical Group Management Association and the American College of Medical Practice Executives. Ms. Cherry is certified in Nursing Administration from the American Nurse Credentialing Center and is a Certified Medical Practice Executive from the American College of Medical Practice Executives. Her past experience includes staff nursing in Labor and Delivery and high risk Obstetrics. She has been the manager of several Ambulatory practices and was the Director of Ambulatory Operations at MetroHealth Medical Center in Cleveland, Ohio. She has served in the role of Acting Division Administrator for the Division of Medicine at The Cleveland Clinic Foundation, Cleveland, Ohio and is currently the Administrator of the Strongsville and Brunswick Family Health Centers, part of the Division of Regional Medical Practice at the Cleveland Clinic Foundation, a role she has held since 1998.

Karen Cober, MSN, RN, CCRN, received her Associate Degree from Palm Beach Community College, her BSN from East Tennessee State University, and her MSN at the University of Tennessee as a Cardiac Clinical Nurse Specialist. Her primary clinical experience is in Medical and Cardiac Intensive Care Units. Mrs. Cober maintained CCRN credentials and BLS/ACLS instructor status for several years. Her experience includes working with Performance Improvement programs in three hospitals and developing education programs, including critical care cases, for hospital staff and acute care patients. Mrs. Cober transitioned to nursing administration in the acute care setting, and, in 1995, accepted the position as Administrator and Director of the home health, hospice, DME, and Infusion companies of Medical Center HomeCare Services owned and operated by Mountain States Health Alliance in Johnson City, TN. She is a wife and mother, and lives in Morristown, TN. Her hobbies include painting and gardening.

Amy M. Cripps, MSN, BSN, RN, graduated with a baccalaureate degree in nursing from Middle Tennessee State University. She received her Master's degree in nursing from East Tennessee State University. She has worked in various areas including medical/surgical nursing, public health, women's health, and geriatric health. She has held the position of MDS Coordinator for National Healthcare Corporation in Smithville, Tennessee. She intends to pursue her doctoral degree and plans to make education and administration her career focus.

Janne Dunham-Taylor, RN, PhD is currently the Chair of Adult Nursing at East Tennessee State University, teaching nursing administration graduate courses at both master's and doctoral levels. Previously she was a head nurse, nursing supervisor, and director of nursing in a state hospital, a university hospital, and a teaching hospital. She has been an assistant dean and has held two acting dean positions, as well as being a chair, in university settings. She has taught nursing administration courses for 19 years. Her research has been concerned with transformational leadership at the CNO level nationally. She has numerous publications on various nursing administration topics.

Gail Gerding, PhD, RN, is an Assistant Professor at the East Tennessee State University College of Nursing. She has experience as a lecturer on community health at Ohio State University, Columbus, OH; Marian College, Indianapolis, IN; and The University of Michigan, Ann Arbor, MI. She has also been a staff nurse in the medical-surgical area in four hospitals, and was a public health nurse at Franklin County Health Department, Columbus, Ohio. She has authored several publications. Gail originally got her ADN, and went on to get her BSN at Mobile College in Mobile, AL; and her MS and PhD in Nursing at Ohio State University, Columbus, OH.

Louise Gifford, MSN, RN, currently works for Summa Health System in Akron, Ohio on the implementation of computerized physician order entry. Previously, as director of case management, she participated in the system's care coordination team's efforts to improve management of critical care patients and early discharge planning from admission to beyond discharge. She has published articles on implementing change to paper documentation and created workbook tools for summarizing activities for performance improvement. She also developed budget tools for 28 nursing units, including the budget worksheet, staffing to census, and a method to assess risk for each nursing unit using budget statistics. Her 36 years as a nurse include experience in an acute care setting for both adults and pediatrics.

Cheryl Field, MSN, CRRN, RN, is the director of clinical and reimbursement services at LTCQ, Inc., a company committed to improving the quality of care in long-term and post-acute settings by providing information-based clinical management tools and services to providers, payers, suppliers, and consumers. Cheryl has 15 years experience in professional nursing specialization in Medicare management with the onset of PPS. Cheryl has served in many roles including nurse manager, program manager, Medicare nurse specialist, and utilization coordinator. Cheryl has lectured nationally on Restraint Reduction and Restorative Nursing. She has presented at national conferences and association meetings on a variety of topics related to post-acute care.

Susie Hutchings, RN, C, CPHQ, has a bachelor of science in nursing from East Tennessee State University in Johnson City, Tennessee. She is certified in Gerontology, (RN, C), received a license as a nursing home administrator, and is certified as a professional in health care quality (CPHQ). Hutchings has more than 20 years experience in acute and long-term care nursing administration and operations. She has extensive experience in quality assurance, Alzheimer's work, drug utilization, and skilled care programs. She began her nursing career at Unicoi County Memorial Hospital in Erwin, Tennessee, as a staff nurse, progressing to charge nurse, in-service director, and director of quality assurance. In 1984, she joined Life Care Centers of America as a director of nursing and advanced to her present position as Senior Vice-President of Clinical Services. Along the way, she has won many professional honors, including Director of Nursing of the Year in Tennessee in 1989–1990, and the Tennessee Health Care Association's Distinguished Professional Service Award in 1991. Hutchings has authored a number of publications and papers, and has done numerous presentations to national organizations on Alzheimer's disease, conflict management, quality assurance, and staff management. Among her many accomplishments are:

- Development of a facility quality assurance program adopted in many nursing centers throughout the United States.

- Implementation of a facility drug utilization program that received national recognition, including a presentation before the U.S. Special Senate Committee on Aging in Washington, D.C.

Steven B. Littlehale, MS, APRN, BC, RN, is the chief clinical officer at LTCQ, Inc., a company committed to improving the quality of care in long-term and post-acute settings by providing information-based clinical management tools and services to providers, payers, regulators, suppliers, and consumers. He has over 15 years experience in long-term care as a clinician, researcher, educator, and consultant. He previously worked at the Hebrew Rehabilitation Center for the Aged, where he contributed to CMS' MDS v2.0 training materials and lectured internationally on the RAI system. Steven is an invited speaker at several national conferences and association meetings including AHCA, AAHSA, ACHCA, AHLA, and NADONA.

Carol Lee Logan had her first experience in a medical office as receptionist and transcriptionist for an ear, nose, and throat provider in the Upper Michigan Peninsula while her husband was on sabbatical. After the sabbatical, her experience was expanded with another ENT surgeon when she returned to lower Michigan. This latter experience introduced her to the computerization of a medical office. Relocation to East Tennessee gave her the opportunity to further her college education with a BS degree in Computer Science and a minor in Management.

The combination of medical office management and a degree in computer science and management resulted in various management positions in the Department of Family Medicine at East Tennessee State University (1982–1993). The College of Nursing, her current employer, upon opening the first nurse-managed center, contracted with the Department of Family Medicine to consult in the operational procedures of a rural nurse-managed center. This included obtaining federally certified rural health center status.

Deborah K. McInturff is currently the Senior Financial Analyst for Johnson City Medical Center's Nursing Division. Johnson City Medical Center is a part of Mountain States Health Alliance. Debbie began her career in health care in 1975, as a Ward Clerk, and has supported patient care at Johnson City Medical Center in many positions since then, including Ward Clerk Manager, Staffing Secretary, Interim Staffing Manager, Clerical Resource Manager, and Liaison with Information Systems as an Information Specialist.

Jane M. Mustain, MSN, RN, is currently the Nursing Information Manager with Mountain States Health Alliance, and is the Change Management/PI Project Manager with Mountain States Health Alliances' Project: SAFETY*first*. Jane began her career in health care as a Red Cross Junior Volunteer and Emergency Room Secretary. After becoming an RN, she worked with renal transplant patients, became an Acute Care Dialysis Nurse, and then moved into Nursing Education and Organizational Development. She has been a professional nurse for over 24 years.

Joseph Z. Pinczuk, MHA, presently retired, held executive positions overseeing finance, administration, and operations for 29 years. He has a Master's of Professional Management in Hospital Administration from Indiana Northern University and a Bachelors of Business Administration in Accounting from Cleveland State University. He has been a CFO in hospitals ranging in size from 55 beds to serving as the CFO of the Tri-County Hospital Group in Ohio consisting of three hospitals with a total of 254 beds. He also served as CFO of a Continuing Care Retirement Community (CCRC) consisting of 285 resident units, 75 skilled nursing, and 24 assisted living beds. He is a member and had served as a Director on the Board of the Healthcare Financial Management Association (HFMA), NE Ohio Chapter and received the Follmer Bronze, Reeves Silver, and Muncie Gold Awards for his contributions to the organization. A former Adjunct Professor of Nursing, College of Nursing, University of Akron and a co-author of an article "Surviving Capitation," American Journal of Nursing (March 1996).

Frances W. "Billie" Sills, MSN, RN, ARNP, CLNC, received a diploma from St. Mary's School of Nursing in Rochester, MN; a BSN at the University of Miami, Coral Gables, FL; and an MSN as a Clinical Nurse Specialist/Advanced Registered Nurse Practitioner with a double major in administration and education at The University of Alabama. She is a retired Air Force Flight Nurse and has held nursing administrative positions at various settings including a 1200-bed teaching hospital, a 180-bed comprehensive free-standing rehabilitation hospital, and a 120-bed long-term care facility. She has met the challenges, the rewards, and the multiple changes that have occurred in health care over the last couple of decades first hand. She is very active in professional organizations, having held several positions in state nursing associations, Sigma Theta Tau, Association of Rehabilitation Nurses, Case Management Association, and past-president of the American Association of Neuroscience Nurses. She served on the AHA Council for Rehabilitation and Long-Term Care. As an Assistant Professor at the University of Texas, Houston, she was responsible for undergraduate and graduate courses and served as the Director of Student Affairs. She has presented both nationally and internationally on advanced practice, leadership, case management, and gerontology. She presently teaches in the College of Nursing at East Tennessee State University.

Coy L. Smith, ND, MSN, RN, CNAA, CHE, completed the Doctor of Nursing (ND) program at Case Western Reserve University in 1983. He then practiced as an Oncology Certified Nurse (OCN) on a research-based bone marrow transplant unit at University Hospitals of Cleveland. During this time he advanced through the clinical ladder and completed his MSN with a career focus on administration. Moving to Yale-New Haven Hospital he managed a medical, oncology, cardiac telemetry, and bone marrow transplant unit. From 1989 to 1999 he accepted several Director of Nursing roles at The Hospital of St. Raphael in New Haven, where he also became certified in Nursing Administration

Advanced (CNAA). His roles ranged from line to support, covering staff development, quality assurance, shared governance, budget systems, emergency medicine, non-nursing areas, and information systems. While in New Haven he was also appointed to the clinical faculty of Yale School of Nursing and Western Connecticut State University. He is now serving as the Vice President for Patient Care Services at Benedictine Hospital in Kingston, NY.

He has been a member of ANA (ONA, CAN, NYSNA) since 1983; inducted to Sigma Theta Tau in 1985; a member of AONE since 1993, and is also a member of the American College of Healthcare Executives.

Coy's areas of administrative expertise are: Hospital decision support systems, technology, and informatics, finance, nursing retention, patient-centered redesign, staff development, and team building. His area of greatest interest in acute care is the impact of both nursing unit teamwork and the nurse manager on the quality of care delivered.

Areas of research and/or publication have been nursing model of care delivery, nurse satisfaction with model changes, stomatitis, non-pharmacological methods for pain reduction, specialty sleep surfaces, health information technology, variable budgeting, and hospital-acquired pressure ulcers.

Jane K. Walker, MSN, BBA, RN, EMT, received a Baccalaureate in Business Administration from East Tennessee State University (ETSU) in 1990, an ADN from Walter's State Community College in 1993, a BSN from ETSU in 1999, and an MSN in Nursing Administration from ETSU in 2004. She was an emergency room nurse at East Tennessee Children's Hospital from 1993 to 2001 in both staff and charge nurse positions. From 2001 to 2004 she worked as the phone triage/nurse case manager in a pediatric pulmonology practice. Presently, she is an Assistant Professor in nursing at Walter's State Community College and is in the doctoral nursing program at ETSU. She is married with two daughters and three cats. She enjoys leisure reading, swimming, and playing on the computer with her children.

Kathryn W. Wilhoit, MSN, RN, CNAA, FACHE, is currently the Chief Nurse Executive for Mountain States Health Alliance (MSHA), a locally owned and managed nine-hospital healthcare system based in Johnson City, Tennessee. MSHA provides an integrated, comprehensive continuum of care to people in 28 counties in Tennessee, Virginia, Kentucky, and North Carolina. Ms. Wilhoit is a master's prepared nurse with over 27 years of professional nursing experience. She has been a staff nurse, head nurse, director of nursing in a hospital setting, instructor and coordinator of a practical nursing program, director of nursing education in a community hospital, associate administrator of a tertiary care hospital, vice president, and vice president and CNO of a tertiary care, teaching and referral hospital.

PART I

Hospital Issues

If one is working in a hospital setting it is helpful to understand some economic and financial background. Chapter 1 explains hospital classifications, ownership categories, and includes the critical access hospital designation. These classifications, plus current reimbursement changes and the resulting strategic maneuvers, such as mergers, alliances, acquisitions, joint ventures, and other internal strategies, influence the hospital's role and impact on the changing health care environment. Then this chapter turns to a description of important reimbursement issues in hospitals, ambulatory settings, physician practices, and, lastly, with nursing services. Other important matters relating to compliance, quality, accreditation, benchmarking, and risk management are provided. A sample of a Balanced Scorecard is given for hospital-based health care.

Once a nurse manager understands these basics, Chapter 2 focuses on the key elements of the budget process and provides effective budgeting tools for inpatient care. With ever-increasing responsibilities, the role of the nurse manager has expanded. This chapter covers the financial responsibilities in nursing from building the labor and materials/supply budgets, implementing the labor budget plan, and monitoring and analyzing the budgets. This chapter bases the staffing plan and the labor budget on patient classification data.

Chapter 3 covers the difficult staffing-related decisions that a nurse administrator makes when a patient classification system is unavailable. Here, nurse administrators describe a staffing process based on nursing hours per patient day (NHPPD), seeking to answer the question, "Can the NHPPD-based staffing process provide timely and accurate information?" The nurse manager is given information on budgeting, benchmarking, and staff mix determinations. Various calculations are illustrated to determine unit-specific total patient days, daily staffing, nursing hours per patient day (NHPPD) for both budget and targeted goals, and for direct and indirect care hours. This chapter also examines how to measure success, an evaluation of this staffing method, and the Chief Nursing Officer (CNO) evaluation.

Chapter 4 provides labor and non-labor flexible item budgets and assists managers to develop meaningful acuity-based variable budgets. Patient classification acuity levels become the products "produced" on the nursing units. This chapter covers how to set up various budgets and types of expenses in the budget system.

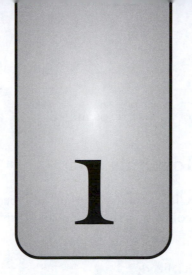

Overview of Hospital-Based Care

Jane K. Walker, MSN, BBA, RN, EMT

That which is, already has been; that which is to be, already is.
Ecclesiastes 3:15

Introduction

The quotation from Ecclesiastes (above) is the perfect way in which to view hospital-based health care. It is interesting to note that we are moving back to providing most health care in the home, where it historically occurred. By understanding that families, mostly the female members of those families, cared for sick loved ones at home in the earliest history of the United States, it is not difficult to notice a certain parallel with the health care system today. The goal today is to "treat 'em and street 'em" back to home care as quickly as possible. This philosophy has become important in an effort to control skyrocketing health care costs. However, to have a greater understanding of the health care arena today, it is imperative that everyone is on the same "page of the hymnal" with respect to hospital-based care.

Classification of Hospitals

Under a large umbrella encompassing all subtypes, there are three basic categories of hospitals according to the American Hospital Association. Hospitals are usually considered:

- General or specialized,

- Teaching or community, and

- For-profit (proprietary), nonprofit, or public (http://www.AHA.org).

General versus Specialty

There were more than 4,800 *general* hospitals in the United States in 2000, according to the Centers for Medicare and Medicaid Services (CMS). General hospitals offer a wide range of services and provide treatment for a wide variety of illnesses (2003). Exhibit 1-1 contains a national map of United States' general hospitals. The more than 1,000 *specialty* hospitals in the year 2000, according to CMS, concentrate on one particular condition, such as rehabilitation or mental illness, or on one type of patient, such as a hospital organized solely for children (Centers for Medicare and Medicaid Services, 2003). This is graphically depicted in Exhibit 1-2.

Teaching versus Community

Teaching hospitals are usually large organizations that are often affiliated with a university or medical school. For example, one teaching hospital is Duke University Medical Center in Durham, North Carolina. This particular hospital is licensed for 1,019 beds (Duke University Health Systems Medical Center Information Systems, 2002). Teaching hospitals not only provide services for patients, but also provide a teaching environment for physicians and other health care professionals. In 2000 there were almost 1,100 teaching hospitals, 22 percent of the total U.S. hospitals. Of these, 90 percent are located in urban areas with an average of 186 beds (American Hospital Association, 2002). According to Blumenthal, "teaching hospitals . . . are committed to maintaining their social missions of research, medical education, and providing care to the poor and uninsured. Needless to say, this places them at a financial disadvantage" (American Hospital Association, p. 1).

Since teaching hospitals carry this added financial burden, Medicare reimburses these institutions at a higher rate than non-teaching hospitals. This increased reimbursement rate is known as the Medicare Direct Graduate Medical Education and Disproportionate Share payment adjustment (American Hospital Association, 2002).

The Balanced Budget Act of 1997 added additional financial woes for teaching facilities by reducing Medicare and Medicaid reimbursements. Medi-

Exhibit 1-1   Short-Term General Hospitals and Critical Access Hospitals (CAHs) 2002, Nonmetropolitan Counties

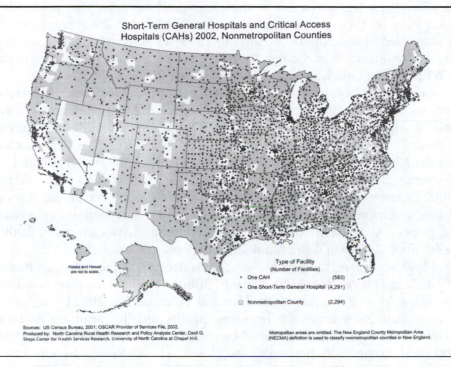

Sources: US Census Bureau, 2001; OSCAR Provider of Services File, 2002. From http://www. shepscenter.unc.edu-research-programs-ruralprogram-mapbook2003-cah2002.pdf.

Exhibit 1-2   Number of Hospitals by Type, 1980–2000

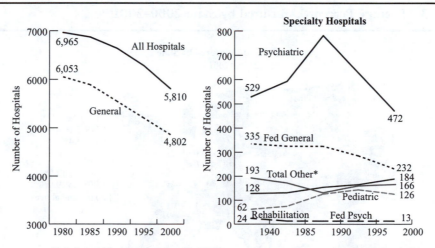

*Includes specialty hospitals such as TB, OB-Gyn; eye, ear, nose and throat; orthopedic and chronic disease.
Source: American Hospital Association, personal communication

Source: American Hospital Association, personal communication.

caid represents about 20 percent of a teaching hospital's costs and pays about 50 cents on the dollar (American Hospital Association Annual Survey, 2000). In addition, there was also a rise in uncompensated care, care that is literally being given away by these teaching facilities. See Exhibit 1-3 for average percentages of uninsured by state in 2000–2001. In 1999, 43 percent of major teaching hospitals were operating in the red. By 2005, that percentage is expected to increase to 61 percent (American Hospital Association, 2002).

Community hospitals are usually smaller, and provide a wide variety of services including routine surgeries and medical care. Most of these are rural hospitals that provide essential services to the communities they serve. An example of this type would be Blue Mountain Hospital in John Day, Oregon, which has less than 25 inpatient beds (Office of Rural Health, Oregon Health and Science University, 2003). According to the Centers for Medicare and Medicaid Services (2002), community hospitals are facilities that are not government owned, that do not specialize in any one type of service, and whose facilities are available to the public. As reported by the American Hospital Association, in 2000 there were about 2,200 rural or community hospitals (2003).

However, decreased reimbursement, as defined by the Balanced Budget Act of 1997, has hit rural hospitals hard. In 2000, 34 percent of rural hospitals were operating at a loss (American Hospital Association, 2002). Because these smaller facilities average 58 beds, no profits usually mean *no* hospital. See Exhibit 1-4 for the distribution of bed size in rural hospitals. Since 1980 over 400 rural, community hospitals have closed. These closings have reached such dire proportions that the Balanced Budget Refinement Act of 1999 was initiated to create financial incentives for these hospitals to remain open. An in-depth discussion of this program can be found later in this chapter under *Critical Access Hospitals.*

Exhibit 1-3   Average Percent Uninsured by State 2000–2001

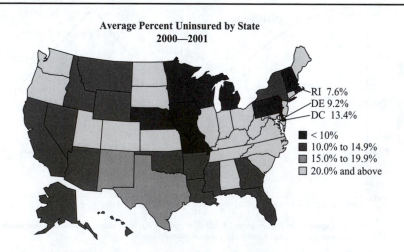

Source: U.S. Census Bureau.

Exhibit 1-4 Distribution of Community Hospitals by Number of Beds

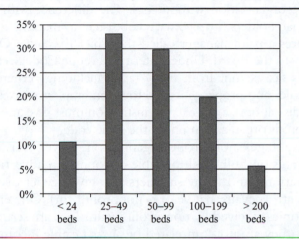

Source: The Lewin Group (2002, June). Analysis of American Hospital Association Annual Survey, 2000. *Trendwatch,* 4 (1).

Ownership—For-Profit, Not-for-Profit, Government

Financially, health care institutions are also organized by ownership. A *for-profit* corporation usually has shareholders (part owners in the hospital) to which the profits are distributed as dividends. This dividend is in return for capital investment in the hospital. However, these dividends are taxable to the hospital corporation when the monies are distributed. Alternatively, the profits may be kept in the hospital as retained earnings, which are not taxable.

In *for-profit* hospitals the shareholders elect a Board of Directors, responsible for the overall management of the hospital. The executive management team is hired (and fired) by the Directors, and is responsible for the operations of the facility (http://www.cob.sjsu.edu/macswa_g/Corporations.rtf).

According to Sackman (n.d.), one of the largest for-profit hospitals, Columbia-HCA, "is buying everything in sight to increase their market concentration. In Texas alone, Columbia now owns 71 of the approximately 500 hospitals in the state: It is the largest private employer in Florida, and the nation's tenth largest employer overall" (p. 1). This chain is based in Nashville, Tennessee.

On a smaller scale, another example of a for-profit hospital would be Edinburg Hospital in Texas. Universal Health Services of King of Prussia, Pennsylvania, purchased this hospital in 1997 from the city health authority. Universal Health Services is a management company that has expertise in managing for-profit hospitals, and has turned this hospital into an effective and efficient organization that is turning a profit (Gilbert, 1997).

If there are no shareholders, then the facility is considered *non-profit* or *voluntary*. The non-profit or voluntary organization is organized under a religious faction, charitable organization, educational organization, or voluntary support, and the goals for the hospital do not include making a profit.

Like for-profit hospitals, ultimate responsibility rests with a Board of Directors that serves the organization without pay. The difference with non-profits is that there are no shareholders (http://www.cob.sjsu.edu/macswa_g/Corporations.rtf). This Board hires a paid manager called the Chief Executive Officer (CEO), who reports directly to the Board. Under Internal Revenue Code Section 501 (c) (3) the organization is tax-exempt from many taxes, including certain Federal and State taxes such as sales and property taxes. However, employee taxes must still be paid. By law, upon dissolution, a tax-exempt institution must give any remaining assets to another non-profit organization under the same code.

Other advantages non-profit organizations have over for-profits include lower postal rates on bulk mail, possible discounts on advertising to other non-profit organizations, and many suppliers also give deeper discounts on supplies (http://www.attorneyalternative.org/nonprofit.htm). One enormous disadvantage is that monies received by non-profit institutions are scrutinized very closely to ensure that they are not "unrelated business taxable income" thereby kicking the hospital into for-profit status.

If an organization is *government owned and operated*, it is supported by taxes paid by the public. The echelon of ownership may be at a local, state, or federal government level. The most unfortunate aspect of government-run facilities is that services are more prone to curtailments with budget cutbacks (American Hospital Association, 2002).

Critical Access Hospitals

An important subtype within the hospital designation is the *Critical Access Hospital*. The critical access hospital designation was created in 1997 by the Balanced Budget Act. The Medicare Rural Hospital Flexibility Program was initiated to act as a safety net to ensure that Medicare beneficiaries would be able to access health care services in smaller, rural communities. According to Busby and Busby (2001), the critical access hospital program is the most important part of this federal initiative to provide federal funding to states to keep the doors of rural, community hospitals open. The program was a necessity given that rural hospitals have experienced revenue decreases due to:

> A *Critical Access Hospital (CAH)* is a rural hospital that meets federally mandated requirements to ensure that critical health care services will be available to Medicare recipients. Designation as a CAH usually ensures higher reimbursement for services provided.

- Shorter length of stays as mandated by new Medicare reimbursement laws;

- Caps on payments by insurance companies (to be discussed in detail later); and

- Residents migrating to larger, more metropolitan hospitals (American Hospital Association, 2002).

The Balanced Budget Refinement Act of 1999 subsequently initiated key criteria for designation as a critical access hospital. Exhibit 1-5 shows details of the criteria required (Busby and Busby, 2001). The Joint Commission on Accreditation of Hospital Organizations (JCAHO) proposed that they become an accrediting body to decide whether criteria are met. On November 21, 2002, "the Centers for Medicare and Medicaid Services (CMS) granted the Joint Commission *deemed status* for the critical access hospital program. The Joint Commission can provide an accreditation survey for the critical access hospital, which will substitute for a Medicare survey" (Christiansen, 2003, p. 18). Once deemed as an appropriate candidate, the JCAHO surveyor notifies CMS (Centers for Medicare and Medicaid Services), and the hospital is converted to a critical access hospital (Christiansen, p. 18). However, it is an option to become accredited by Joint Commission, not mandatory (American Organization of Nurse Executives, 2002).

The primary benefit of becoming a critical access hospital is that it moves hospitals from the *prospective payment system* to a *cost-based reimbursement* for both inpatient and outpatient services (National Conference of State Legislatures, 2002). In other words, the hospital is reimbursed on a higher fee-for-service basis. The hospital would request reimbursement for the entire cost of taking care

Exhibit 1-5   Medicare Rural Health Flexibility Program: Critical Access Hospital Criteria

Eligibility Criteria	Approved Health Plan
Hospital type	Not-for-profit or for-profit
Service limit	Average of 96 hours—patient length of stay
Service limit (size)	15 acute beds (maximum) and 10 swing beds (beds maximum) no more than 25 beds with swing beds
Location criteria	Rural and 35+ mile drive to the hospital or another critical access hospital (15 miles in mountains or area with secondary roads or state certified as a necessary provider
Medicare reimbursement	Cost-based
Required services	Inpatient; laboratory; radiology; some auxiliary and support services may be provided part-time off-site
Emergency Services	Available 24 hours; staff has emergency service training or experience; staff on call and available within 30 minutes
Medical staff	At least one physician (need not be on site); may include mid-level practitioners
Hours of operation	24 hours if occupied; if not occupied, emergency services made available
Networking	Critical access hospital and at least one other hospital; agreement(s) are maintained with network hospital(s) for referral and transfer, transportation services, and communications; and agreement with network hospital, peer review organization, or equivalent for credentialing and quality assurance

Source: Busby, A. and Busby, A. (2001, June). Critical access hospitals: Rural nursing issues. *Journal of Nursing Administration,* 31(6), 302.

of a particular patient and would be reimbursed 100 percent of those costs. Other advantages are noted in Exhibit 1-6 with explanations of each to follow.

Because of the small size and remote location of most rural community hospitals, patients must receive health care regardless of the ability to pay for those services. If hospitals are not paid for services rendered, often these institutions must close. In fact, "an analysis of hospital financial data shows that in 1999 rural hospitals generally had operation losses of 2.9% on Medicare and 10% on Medicaid" (Minge, 2001). From Exhibit 1-7 it is apparent that there are fewer community hospitals with fewer beds treating more patients. Not only are community hospitals treating more patients with less bed space, but according to an American Hospital Workforce Survey from 2001, there are also fewer pharmacists, radiology technicians, billing/coders, laboratory technicians, housekeepers, and maintenance workers available to work in the facilities to take care of the patients that are admitted to the rural facility (United States Department of Health and Human Services, Bureau of Health Professions, 2003).

With each closure brings a further decrease in available hospital beds in these areas. Becoming a critical access hospital provides an alternative to closing since it is possible to increase revenue by increasing reimbursement for services rendered.

Matching community needs to provider capabilities is imperative in rural communities. This decreases the overall financial burden by decreasing the need for transfers to other facilities and specialists. In addition, one criterion for critical access hospital conversion is the employment of at least one physician, specifying that this physician does not have to be on the hospital site. This allows for the "remote supervision of midlevel practitioners" (Busby and Busby, p. 302). *Telemedicine* is also used quite liberally. In fact, "advances in telecommunications technology now allow nurses to care for patients and their families in geographic locations throughout the country" (Hardin and Langford, 2001, p. 243).

> *Telemedicine* is the use of medical information exchanged from one site to another using electronic communications for the health and education of patients or providers and to improve patient care (Centers for Medicare and Medicaid Services, 2003).

According to the American Hospital Association, in recent years telemedicine programs have grown exponentially (see Exhibit 1-8). However, it is important to

---

Exhibit 1-6   Community Hospital Advantages for Converting to a Critical Access Hospital

- Provides an alternative to financially failing rural hospitals;
- Matches community need to provider capabilities;
- Provides regulatory relief to underserved rural communities;
- Lays the foundation for rural health care networks;
- Allows for remote supervision of midlevel practitioners;
- Recognizes that a hospital is essential for community economic viability;
- Establishes a fee-for-service reimbursement rate; and
- Provides for more flexible and accessible emergency services.

Source: Busby, A. & Busby, A. (2001, June). Critical access hospitals: Rural nursing issues. *Journal of Nursing Administration,* 31(6), 304–309.

Exhibit 1-7   Community Hospital Utilization: 1995–1999

	Hospitals	Beds (000)	Admissions (000)	Outpatient visits (000)
1995	5,194	873	30,945	414,345
1996	5,134	862	31,099	439,863
1997	5,057	853	31,577	450,140
1998	5,015	840	31,812	474,193
1999	4,956	830	32,359	495,346

From: Hospital Statistics, 2001. Edition and prior years. Health Forum LLC, an American Hospital Association Company, copyright 2001.

point out that less expensive nurse practitioners would be most capable of meeting the needs of the population utilizing this general rural facility (Kippenbrock, Stacy, Tester, and Richey, 2002). In fact, according to Larkin (2003), "when used correctly, they (nurse practitioners) can improve outcomes, lower costs and make up for reduced residents' hours" (p. 1). These midlevel nurse practitioners would have laboratory, radiological, and other support services available to assist in meeting these needs as required by the listed criteria in Exhibit 1-5.

As stated previously, in an attempt to provide relief to these small community hospitals, the Medicare Rural Hospital Flexibility Program provides higher reimbursement rates on a cost (fee-for-service) basis. Consequently, these facilities have an advantage over the larger urban hospitals that are reimbursed at a prospective payment system rate. The small communities then stay more financially viable with more jobs for residents, as well as for more federal dollars flowing into the area. According to Cordes, "Hospitals are key to the economic health of rural communities. They are major employers . . . and hospital jobs pay well by rural standards.

Exhibit 1-8   Active Telemedicine Programs

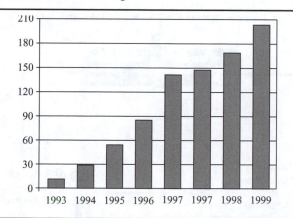

AHA (2002, June). *Challenges facing rural hospitals. Trendwatch* 4(1).

Hospitals attract businesses and residents to rural towns. The goods and services they buy circulate income and generate indirect economic activity, and their local bank deposits create funds to invest in rural businesses and individuals" (1996, p. 2). See Exhibit 1-9 for a representation of this scenario in rural communities.

The critical access hospital must have and maintain a health care network in the rural health care community. Meeting this criterion affords the facility many advantages. This network requirement must include an agreement with one hospital that can accept transfers and referrals if the need arises. Networking can also provide *economies of scale,* "a reduction in cost per unit resulting from increased production, realized through operational efficiencies" (www.investorwords.com). In addition to economies of scale, according to Busby and Busby (2001) "integration of effort with expanded access to information and telecommunications systems" are also advantages when working within a network (p. 302).

Converting to critical access hospital status has one final advantage—an improvement in the overall availability of emergency medical services for the community. Protocols for, training of, and integration of emergency medical services within the community are mandatory. In addition, emergency services within the critical access hospitals must be made available 24 hours per day, 7 days per week, and 365 days per year. All staff must be available within 30 minutes if on call. This is of major importance to community residents who, as Medicare recipients, will be older, thereby having the potential for more serious illnesses and/or accidents.

Critical access hospitals are mostly located in areas that are being dramatically affected by health professional shortages and where the population of Medicare recipients is above average. Exhibit 1-10 shows the location of critical access hospitals as of October 1, 2002.

Exhibit 1-9   Rural Hospitals and Economic Development

Hospitals are key to the economic health of rural communities. They are major employers in rural communities and hospital jobs pay well by rural standards. Hospitals attract businesses and residents to rural towns. The goods and services they buy circulate income and generate indirect economic factivity, and their local bank deposits create funds to invest in rural businesses and individuals.[1]

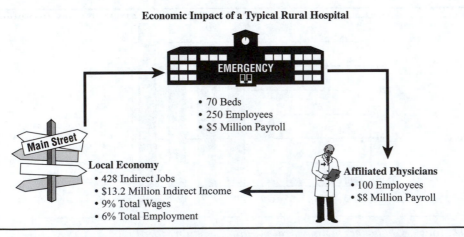

Economic Impact of a Typical Rural Hospital

EMERGENCY

- 70 Beds
- 250 Employees
- $5 Million Payroll

Main Street

Local Economy
- 428 Indirect Jobs
- $13.2 Million Indirect Income
- 9% Total Wages
- 6% Total Employment

Affiliated Physicians
- 100 Employees
- $8 Million Payroll

[1]Cordes, Sam. "Health Care Services and the Rural Economy," The Changing Rural Economy of the Midwest, Chicgao: Federal Reserve Bank of Chicago, 1996.

Exhibit 1-10   Location of Critical Access Hospitals, Current as of October 1, 2002

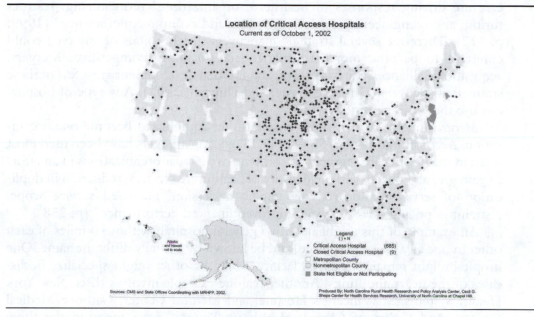

Source: CMS and State Offices Coordinating with MRHFP, 2002. http://www.shepscenter. unc.edu/research_programs/rural_program/maps/cah-updat-oct-01.pdf.

The Medicare Rural Hospital Flexibility Program primarily created the critical access hospital program for hospitals with 15 or fewer inpatient beds. However, there is another program called the Sole Community Hospital (SCH) that also provides assistance for other rural hospitals with 50 or fewer inpatient beds. This program requires that the hospital meet one of the following criteria:

- A location that is more than 35 miles from other like hospitals;

- A location that is less than 35 miles from other like hospitals but because of travel time would make the next closest hospital at least 45 minutes away; or

- Because of weather conditions or local topography, other like hospitals are inaccessible for at least 30 days per year, two out of three years in a row (Healthcare Financing Administration (now CMS), 2001; United States Department of Health and Human Services, 2001).

This Sole Community Hospital program provides adequate Medicare reimbursement and additional funding for technology and infrastructure needs (Centers for Medicare and Medicaid Services, 2003).

The Changing Health Care Environment

In order for hospitals to survive the volatility in the current health care arena, some drastic restructuring has taken place over the last decade or so. According to Brooks, "economic forces in the shape of capitated payments and managed care are driving responses of healthcare organizations' reorganizing, restructuring, and reengineering to decrease waste and economic inefficiency" (1999, p. 112). There are several strategic maneuvers that hospitals of any type could entertain to become more streamlined and/or more competitive. Mergers, acquisitions, alliances, joint ventures, and internal development are a few of these strategic maneuvers (Ginter, Swayne, and Duncan, 2002). Any type of hospital can use these business strategies.

Mergers involve two or more hospitals that combine to become one organization. According to Ginter, Swayne, and Duncan, "mergers have been used most often in the health care segment to combine two similar organizations in an effort to gain greater efficiency in the delivery of health care services, reduction in duplication of services, improved geographic dispersion, increased service scope, restraint in pricing increases, and improved financial performance" (p. 238).

An example of this might be if two general hospitals within 10 miles of each other in one city decide to merge, and be known by a totally different name. One hospital might remain a general facility, while the other might specialize in diseases of the heart and lungs. Another real-life example involves three New York Health Systems: St. Vincent's Hospital and Medical Center, Catholic Medical Centers, and Sisters of Charity Healthcare System. After merging the three became Saint Vincent's Catholic Medical Centers of New York.

Acquisitions involve one hospital purchasing another existing organization, a particular unit, or a product/service of that organization. This is a way for the original organization to rapidly enter a new market. An example is the Community Health Systems hospital chain based in Tennessee, which purchased Western Arizona Regional Medical Centers from Baptist Hospitals and Health Systems based in Phoenix. Community Health Systems gained instant access to the health care market in Arizona. It would have been more than a year with a new construction project to even begin to entice patients to a new facility in an attempt to break into the market in the area (Ginter, Swayne, and Duncan, 2002). The peak of the merger and acquisition activity, in order to realign strategies in the current tumultuous health care arena, was in 1996. According to Ginter, Swayne, and Duncan, 768 hospitals were involved in 235 acquisition or merger deals to restructure into more streamlined health care providers.

Alliances are another means by which a hospital achieves strategic advantage or maintains some stability in the chaotic health care arena. These are contractual agreements that each facility will work closely with the other to fulfill strategic initiatives for both. Federations, consortiums, networks, and systems are all examples of strategic alliances that hospitals could use to restructure, and, hopefully, to reduce some volatility. An example of an alliance would be the West Central Ohio Regional Healthcare Alliance that has a network of allied community hospitals that have a common vision and goals (Ginter, Swayne, and Duncan).

Joint ventures occur when two or more organizations or entities combine resources to accomplish a task that each share as a strategic goal. A large advantage of a joint venture would be to share expenses, risks, and skills with each other. Joint ventures may be contractual agreements, subsidiary corporations, partnerships, or not-for-profit title-holding corporations (Ginter, Swayne, and Duncan, 2002). In recent years, physicians and hospitals have entered into joint ventures for mutual strategic initiatives. For the physician, profits could be increased while decreasing some risks. For the hospital, a referral base is almost guaranteed when the hospital is owned in part by the physician. A recent example is a new Children's Hospital outpatient surgery center in Knoxville, Tennessee, which is owned both by the surgeons and by the hospital.

A final type of strategy in which hospitals might engage to "go with the constantly changing flow" is *internal development*. In this instance, a hospital might expand some service or technology using resources already available within the hospital system to generate new business and/or revenue. One example is that East Tennessee Children's Hospital in Knoxville, Tennessee, developed a primary care practice using internal resources. This occurred at the time TennCare, the state-wide Medicaid program, was initiated in 1993. This internal development was an effort to ensure that children had primary care physicians available to care for them.

Reimbursement Issues

Reimbursement for health care services rendered has changed dramatically over the last two decades in an attempt to control health care costs. According to the Centers for Medicare and Medicaid Services (2003), national health expenditures in the United States in 1965 were almost $41 billion, including both public and private funds. By 2000, that figure had jumped to $1.3 trillion! Medicare spending alone has grown from over $3 billion in 1967 to almost $241 billion in 2001 with 39%, or $93 billion, being spent on inpatient hospitalizations (Centers for Medicare and Medicaid Services, 2002). See Exhibit 1-11 for a representation of Medicare spending over the last 30-plus years.

No wonder all the new regulations from the government exist! Inpatient reimbursement (unless a critical access hospital) changed to a *prospective payment system* (PPS), as enacted by the Amendments to the Social Security Act of 1983. Under this payment system, reimbursement is based on a prospective cost-based payment rate for each hospital stay according to a *diagnosis-related group* (DRG). According to the Centers for Medicare and Medicaid Services, a diagnosis-related group is "a classification system that groups patients according to diagnosis, type of treatment, age, and other relevant criteria. Under the prospective payment system, hospitals are paid a set fee for treating patients in

Exhibit 1-11   Medicare Spending

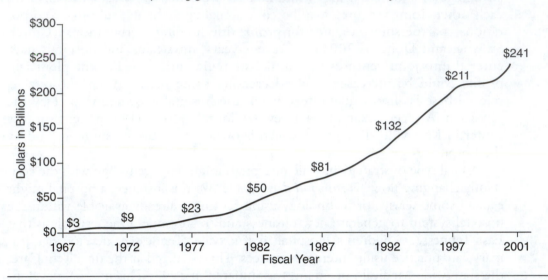

Overall Medicare Spending grew from $3.3 billion in 1967 to nearly $241 billion in 2001.

June 2002 Edition   *Centers for Medicare & Medicaid Services*   Section III.C. Page 3

Note: Overall spending includes benefit dollars, administrative costs, and program integrity costs. Represents Federal spending only.
Source: CMS, Office of the Actuary.

> A *DRG* is a diagnosis-related group that is assigned upon admission to a hospital that determines the flat rate for reimbursement from Medicare, Medicaid, and some larger insurance companies.

a single DRG category, regardless of the actual cost of care for the individual" (2003). Although this was intended to reflect similar amounts of care needed within a diagnostic category, in reality, within a DRG the amount of care varies widely.

When diagnosis-related groups were set up they were not designated to include psychiatric and pediatric diagnoses. Reimbursement of charges pertaining to pediatric and psychiatric medical care is usually on a *per diem* basis. Although this will be discussed in more detail later in the chapter, briefly this means that these particular reimbursements are made on the basis of negotiated prospective payments for **each day** of care, regardless of the resources used. Normal reimbursement under the diagnosis-related group prospective payments is a flat payment regardless of the number of days required for the admission. If this is as clear as mud, please refer to the discussion in the section entitled *Different Strokes for Different Folks* later in this chapter for more detail. Of the diagnoses that are covered by diagnosis-related groups, Exhibit 1-12 lists the top 10 inpatient diagnosis-related groups for fiscal year 2000.

Exhibit 1-12 Top 10 Inpatient DRGs in 2000

1. Heart Failure and Shock
2. Simple Pneumonia, over age 17 with Complications
3. Chronic Obstructive Pulmonary Disease
4. Major Joint and Limb Reattachment Procedures
5. Other Permanent Pacemaker Implants
6. Specific Cerebrovascular Disorders excluding Strokes
7. Psychoses
8. Rehabilitation
9. Esophagitis, Gastroenteritis, and Miscellaneous Digestive Disorders over age 17
10. Gastrointestinal Hemorrhage with Complicating Conditions

Source: Centers for Medicare and Medicaid Services (2002). Top inpatient DRGs for fiscal year 2000. Retrieved July 14, 2003 from http://www.CMS.gov.

This payment, although usually woefully inadequate, is meant to cover an average hospital's operating costs from admission to discharge for that particular diagnostically grouped patient. According to the American Hospital Association, "Medicare and Medicaid reimbursements to hospitals are simply not keeping up with the rising cost of caring" (2003, p. 1). In fact, most institutions would just like to know who is considered "average." This flat rate encourages earlier discharges by attempting to deter "baby-sitting" (i.e., when the patient is medically able to be discharged today but does not have a ride to get home until tomorrow). In addition, most hospitals find it difficult to have a patient physically ready to be discharged in the time allotted according to the diagnosis-related groups. Consequently, hospitals often foot the bill for any inpatient length of stay (LOS) or costs greater than the time or expenses allowed.

Outpatient Reimbursement

Outpatient reimbursement has also drastically changed in response to an overall drive to control health care costs. Since 1980 outpatient services volume has increased by 150%, to generate 35% of total hospital revenue in 2000 (American Hospital Association, 2003). According to the Centers for Medicare and Medicaid Services, in 2001 outpatient spending alone was $20 billion—8% of total Medicare spending (2002). Outpatient services are reimbursed using a uniform *Outpatient Prospective Payment System* (OPPS) called *Ambulatory Payment Classifications* (APCs). This new system went into effect on August 1, 2000 (Centers for Medicare and Medicaid Services, 2003).

Prior to these classifications, facilities were reimbursed on a cost-basis unique to each hospital. As costs were reported, the particular hospital was reimbursed a percentage of those costs.

However, as with inpatient reimbursement from diagnosis-related groups, ambulatory payment classification is a fixed rate of reimbursement. This classification is based on a procedure code from the Current Procedural Terminology (CPT) coder's handbook. Diagnosis codes are still reported, but do not affect reimbursement. Each hospital must decide the different care levels to which a Current Procedural Terminology code is assigned. For example, an emergency department patient visit may be assigned a different Current Procedural Terminology code based upon the intensity of the treatment given. If more support services are used, then the level of care increases, as does the level of reimbursement (Massachusetts College of Emergency Physicians, 2003).

Like inpatient reimbursement by diagnosis-related group, outpatient reimbursement by ambulatory payment classification has items inherent in the reimbursement. These include venipunctures, supplies and equipment, most pharmaceuticals, and surgical dressings. However, intravenous infusions and intramuscular injections receive additional payments as do blood products, some expensive medications, laboratory services, and x-rays. These procedures require a different level/intensity of care (Massachusetts College of Emergency Physicians, 2003). Interestingly, patients in the emergency department (ED) that are in need of a long period of observation to determine appropriate destination (admitted versus discharged to home) cannot be coded higher than if the patient were sent home immediately upon seeing the provider. By disallowing higher charges for observation patients in the emergency department, there is no incentive to observe the patient in the ED (Massachusetts College of Emergency Physicians, 2003).

Inpatient Observation Patients

Inpatient observation patients are an interesting group of patients to discuss with respect to reimbursement and hospital census issues. Medicare developed *strict* guidelines to establish observation status in 1984. To be reimbursed under the observation patient rate, no variance among the guidelines is tolerated (Centers for Medicare and Medicaid Services, 2002). An *observation* to Medicare means any stay within the hospital that is less than 24 hours in duration.

However, originally it was not meant to be a "23-hour admit," which is how some hospitals currently use the observation status. In addition to being less than 24 hours, "observation patient" might mean that the decision for admission still needs to be determined; or that a Medicare patient is admitted as an observation patient because the condition is expected to rapidly improve over the next 23-hour period; or that the diagnosis is unknown and the physician needs time to ascertain the best action for the patient. Exhibit 1-13 illustrates a decision tree that physicians should entertain when contemplating admission versus observation.

Exhibit 1-13   Medicare Decision Tree

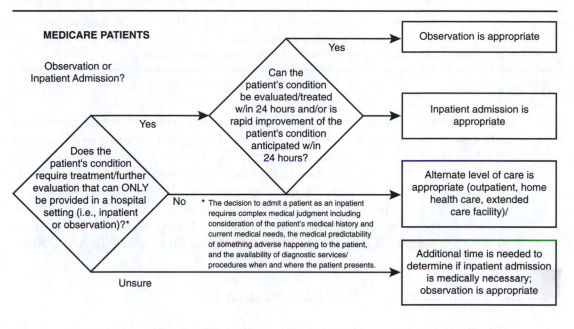

Source: http://www.tmf.org/pepp/prompter_obs_01.pdf.

Observation status cannot be used for any surgical procedures, including routine preoperative and postoperative care, diagnostic testing or interventions, direct admissions, or as a substitute for admission to the hospital (Duke University Medical Center, 2001). This is because Medicare reimbursement for surgical procedures includes care for the usual pre- and post-operative phases of the surgical procedure. The same is true for diagnostic testing. The reimbursement is all-inclusive to avoid double billing (fraud) for the same intervention more than once. If the person needs to be admitted, observation status cannot be used to increase reimbursement, such as to gain another inpatient day, or to decrease the actual inpatient length of stay. Additionally, the patient cannot be placed on observation status based on provider convenience. Exhibit 1-14 provides an example of the type of patient that actually meets the observation status criteria.

Observation Status Fraud

According to Duke University Medical Center, fines could be levied for fraud if guidelines are not strictly followed. Therefore, everyone has to be diligent to ensure that the patient is discharged in 23 hours or less (2001), or is admitted

Exhibit 1-14   Example of the Typical Presentation of an Observation Patient

A 56-year-old female presents to the Emergency Department with diffuse abdominal pain. All initial tests that are completed are negative so a diagnosis cannot be made. Therefore, an observation period is warranted to determine the next appropriate action.

as an inpatient. There are many examples of what constitutes Medicare fraud with observation patients. Two examples are: 1) Surgical procedures are an area in which Medicare fines hospitals liberally for double billing; and 2) Double billing is also an issue with invasive diagnostic procedures, and with outpatient therapeutic services, such as blood administration, which has recovery time already built into the reimbursement from Medicare. (Fraud and abuse are defined in more detail in *Health Care Financial Management for Nurse Managers: Merging the Heart with the Dollar*) Dunham-Taylor and Pinczuk (2006).

Staffing Implications of Observation Patients

Observation patients not only affect reimbursement rates, but also impact the hospital census. Hospitals typically run census tallies for the preceding 24 hours at midnight. For example, on the 30th at midnight, the census is tallied for the previous 24 hours (the 29th) to determine estimated staffing needs for the next 24 hours. However, most observation patients have been discharged by the midnight census, and therefore are never counted in the census. Can you imagine telling that to someone who just received the bill for the observation stay? "Well, Mr. Smith, you counted as a patient for the bill, but not on the census tally. Thus we won't pay the staff that needed to care for you." Does this make sense? Nurse staffing should be based completely on accurate census (the actual number of patients in the hospital at any time during the 24 hours) and patient acuity (how sick patients are). Often the best source of information for more accurate data is a *patient classification system*. See Exhibit 1-15 for a graphic depiction of differences in time of day measurements.

Patient Classification Systems

Patient classification systems are used by nursing departments to capture more accurate patient acuity and census measurement. This data is then used to determine the staffing necessary to provide the needed care. The patient classification system can also be used to heighten reimbursement for the maximum allowable payments. To measure patient acuity, most systems "measure patients' needs for care and care activities," such as assistance with bathing, dressing, drug administration, wound care, documentation, admission and discharge procedures, and other nursing activities (Prescott and Soeken, 1996, p. 14).

Exhibit 1-15 2001 Hospital ER Occupancy Rate at Midnight and at Midday

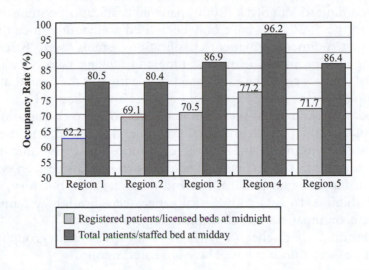

Source: Massachusetts Department of Public Health Ambulance Diversion Survey 2001.

Classification is the ordering of entities into groups or classes on the basis of their similarity, minimizing within-group variance and maximizing between-group variance (Bailey, 1994).

Strategic planning is the ongoing process of looking toward the future, both within the organization and in the external health care environment, to determine where the hospital wants to go and how the hospital wants to get there.

Patient classification systems are useful in several broader organizational arenas such as finance, clinical operations such as staffing and effectiveness of patient plans, strategic planning, and in evaluation measures including quality assurance and benchmarking (CASEMIX Quarterly, 2003). Because most hospitals have census changes that occur almost every minute of every day, these classification systems help frontline personnel make some sense of alterations that can be quite complex and chaotic, and to have more accurate records of services given. These records can be used to compare workloads, or even to compare staffing used for similar patients or units.

Although used before the passage of the Medicare inpatient prospective payment system in the early 1980s, the patient classification system provided an impetus for hospitals to design or to purchase systems that would measure the actual cost of the care given. Based on this cost, hospitals could evaluate whether staffing was reasonable to provide the care, and determine whether the prospective payment (DRG) was enough to cover this cost. The data could also be used to decrease the cost of the care given by decreasing the length of inpatient stays, or by changing the skill mix delivering the care. The need for patient classification systems was further enhanced by the ever-escalating costs of inpatient care, and by the need to prove to the public that the quality of the care was appropriate. (The number of RNs actually caring for patients can be used in the quality determination now that the research is starting to link the number of RNs, or nursing staff, to patient outcomes.)

According to Van Slyck (2000) patient classification systems were first introduced in the 1930s but have only been used abundantly since the early 1980s. These first rudimentary patient classification systems "were based on an industrial engineering model of nurses' time and nursing tasks. It was thought that patients' acuities could be established by identifying the time that it took nurses to complete a task related to patient care" (Van Slyck, p. 61).

Today, we know that there is much more to these classification systems than that! Risks to the patient, the nursing skill level required, and the complexity of the service are as important—maybe even more so—as the time it takes to complete a nursing task (Van Slyck). There are patient classification systems available for both inpatient hospitalizations and outpatient (ambulatory) service utilization. Exhibit 1-16 lists ambulatory patient classification systems. This chapter will focus on inpatient classification systems.

According to Fischer (1995), there are four main groupings of nursing patient classification systems. These are based upon:

- Health conditions,

- Care requirements,

- Treatment characteristics, and

- Outcomes based on critical indicators of care (Hoffman and Wakefield, 1986).

Exhibit 1-16   Ambulatory Patient Classification Systems

Medically Focused

1. International Classification of Health Problems in Primary Care (ICHPPC)
2. Ambulatory Visit Groups (AVG)
3. Ambulatory Patient Groups (APG)
4. Products of Ambulatory Care (PAC)
5. Ambulatory Care Groups (ACG)
6. Ambulatory Service Index (ASI)

Nursing Focused

1. Ambulatory Care Client Classification Instrument (ACCCI)
2. Allocation Resource Identification and Costing System (ARIC)
3. Ambulatory Care Patient Classification Tool (ACPCT)
4. Patient Intensity for Nursing Ambulatory Care (PINAC)

Source: Reprinted from *Nursing Economic$*, 1996, Volume 14, Number 1, pp. 14–21, 33. Reprinted with permission of the publisher, Jannetti Publications, Inc., East Holly Avenue Box 56, Pitman, NJ 08071-0056. Phone (856) 256-2300; Fax (856) 589-7463. (For a sample issue of the journal visit the www.nursingeconomics.net).

There are many different inpatient classification systems since many companies exist that would LOVE to sell their system to your hospital. Exhibit 1-17 enumerates some methods in use. However, a discussion of the two most basic types follows. (There is an entire chapter on patient classification systems in Dunham-Taylor and Pinczuk (2006) *Health Care Financial Management for Nurse Managers: Merging the Heart with the Dollar.*)

Both prototype systems and factor evaluation systems have one particular goal in mind: to assist managers to allocate resources. Prototype systems are based on categorical descriptions. Patients are assigned to the category in which their nursing needs fit best. However, according to Hoffman and Wakefield, these systems have a major disadvantage in that they are purely based on subjective data, i.e., the nurse's objective assessment and the output of critical thinking have no bearing on patient classifications. Validity and reliability are generally a problem with prototype systems.

Factor evaluation systems have specific criteria on which each patient is ranked or scored. These rankings include not only areas of self-care ability, but also requirements for respiratory treatments, oxygen, intravenous fluid administration, or emotional support. According to Hoffman and Wakefield, categories usually include "nutrition, intake and output, vital signs, bath/skin care, ambulation, medications, treatments, teaching, psychosocial, and special considerations (such as hearing loss, visual loss, confusion, infection isolation)" (p. 24). The classification data can also include activities such as documentation of the care, and indicate the time it takes to admit and discharge a patient. Both subjective and objective assessments are therefore important in these scores.

Factor evaluation rankings are then totaled and based on a preset scale; the point total determines that particular patient's classification. Because resource allocation (nursing care and supplies) is the ultimate goal, factor evaluation systems have a time element assigned to each category. This time allocation correlates the score with nursing resources. Thus, individual patient needs are associated with staffing requirements (Hoffman and Wakefield). Reliability and validity can also be better established with factor systems (Ebener, 1985; Giovannetti and Mayer, 1984).

Exhibit 1-17   Inpatient Nursing Classification Systems

---

1. Patient Intensity for Nursing Index (PINI)
2. Population Care Requirements
3. Individual Patient Time Model
4. Inpatient Methodology
5. Mental Health Methodology
6. Emerge Methodology
7. Perinatal Methodology

Source: Reprinted from *Nursing Economic$*, 1996, Volume 14, Number 1, pp. 14–21, 33. Reprinted with permission of the publisher, Jannetti Publications, Inc., East Holly Avenue Box 56, Pitman, NJ 08071-0056. Phone (856) 256-2300; Fax (856) 589-7463. (For a sample issue of the journal visit the www.nursingeconomics.net).

Patient classifications systems benefit various departments in a hospital in various ways. According to Van Slyck (2000) some uses include:

1. A way in which to measure "patient placement and leverage of care progression" (the ability to move to a unit that renders less one-on-one nursing time),

2. Identifying critical pathways (to be discussed later in this chapter) or protocol variances,

3. Correlating patient acuities with necessary staff development,

4. Determination of operating budgets for all inpatient nursing units including both the "average daily census and the average acuity of the patients to be cared for,"

5. Pricing and variability in billing for nursing services,

6. The ability to utilize the data on admissions, discharges, and transfers in order to validate staffing requests,

7. Documentation of actual time spent in patient care activities in order to redesign roles as necessary,

8. Providing information for accurate and precise position descriptions,

9. Better alignment of staff at all levels to more appropriately correlate with patient needs (Van Slyck, pp. 64–65), and

10. Providing data for patient outcomes research (Prescott and Soeken).

It is certainly not difficult to understand why these systems can be so important to a hospital given all the data that can be compiled.

What Things Impact the Bottom Line for Hospitals?

Answering this question is like the Jeopardy® Daily Double Question. Every action, or non-action, within the organization impacts the bottom line, which is part of the theme for this entire book as well as the accompanying book, Dunham-Taylor and Pinczuk (2006) *Health Care Financial Management for Nurse Managers: Merging the Heart with the Dollar.* Turning to finance, there are some major topics we will touch upon here to assure understanding of some financial basics.

Different Strokes for Different Folks

As was previously mentioned, different types of hospitals and the services that are provided within are reimbursed differently. Some of the major types of reimbursement are defined and briefly explained in this section.

Fee-for-Service, or *billed charges reimbursement* is one of the simplest reimbursements to explain. Simply, the hospital is paid what is **charged** for the services they provide. The biggest disadvantage for the health care system is that, although there are usually maximums that will be paid for a particular service, there are no deterrents to how many services are rendered. Therefore, providers are free to order tests regardless of the actual necessity. The biggest advantage is that providers actually can order the services that are needed for a patient without the red tape of managed care approvals and paperwork determining if the service is justified. This system can also contribute to a healthier bottom line for the institution because as long as each price charged covers the actual costs involved in providing the service, a positive income results. This is retrospective reimbursement.

Cost reimbursement involves the hospital getting paid the amount that it **costs** the facility to provide the service to the patient. Historically, Medicare reimbursed under this method. Cost reimbursement is now only used for inpatient psychiatric care and in procedures that involve organ procurement from a donor (Marks, n.d.). This is a very complex method with a multitude of paper trails necessary to determine the exact cost per service per individual hospital. This method is further complicated because each hospital negotiates its own reimbursement amount with the payor. With cost reimbursement, the bottom line should be favorably affected as long as services rendered were charged without fail, and as long as the actual cost associated with the charge is documented. However, there are few incentives for cost control. Like fee-for-service, this is also retrospective reimbursement.

The method currently used by Medicare and Medicaid most often reimburses hospitals for services to Medicare recipients using the *prospective payment model.* This involves diagnosis-related groups (DRGs). As its name implies, this prospective reimbursement model uses a flat fee for each service rendered, regardless of how much it actually costs the facility to render the service. The biggest disadvantage with prospective reimbursement is that the hospital bears the brunt of the financial woes should the actual costs far outweigh the reimbursement received. Therefore, each service must be coded as correctly and completely as possible, and costs must be kept below charges. The biggest advantage to the entire health care system is that usually services are only ordered if necessary. Until 2003, rehabilitation services were excluded from prospective payment reimbursement. However, as of 2003, rehabilitation services are now reimbursed under a prospective payment system called *case-mix groups* (Marks, n.d.).

Capitation is a fourth type of reimbursement. This is also considered a prospective model of payment since the hospital is paid based on the number of people enrolled. This type is used by hospitals that have self-funded insurance through managed care contracts. The greatest disadvantage is that the hospital is paid the same regardless of the amount of services provided. Therefore, a large increase in utilization, especially with services such as admissions, has injurious results on the bottom line. One advantage is that there is a monthly payment based on enrollment.

Per Diem reimbursement means that the payor reimburses the hospital for each day that a patient stays in the hospital. This is a retrospective reimbursement method: the hospital is paid after the patient is discharged. This reimbursement type would most likely have a favorable effect on the hospital bottom line. However, there would be no impetus to discharge the patient as quickly as possible. Many maternal and normal infant health care services are paid on a per diem basis.

Percent of Charges are usually negotiated reimbursements between private payors and the hospital. Since it is **negotiated,** the amount paid varies widely and is quite literally a percent of billed charges. Here it is necessary to ensure a positive bottom line is achieved, that the amount paid closely resembles—is over—the actual cost of services rendered.

For the year 2000, Exhibit 1-18 shows hospital percentages by reimbursement types.

Payor Mix

Payor mix can make or break the bottom line of a health care organization. Payor mix refers to the percentage of each type of insurance (or payor!) that makes payments to the hospital for services rendered. For example, Hospital X might have 45 percent of patients with private health insurance, or commercial health insurance (such as Blue Cross/Blue Shield or John Deere), 35 percent Medicare patients, 18 percent Medicaid patients, 1.5 percent that are self-pay,

Exhibit 1-18   Hospital Managed Care Payment Arrangements, 2000

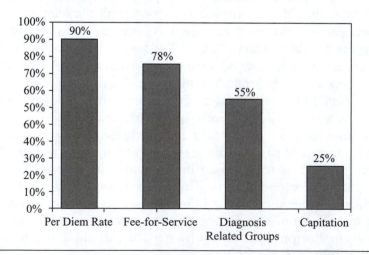

Source: Trends and Indicators in the Changing Health Care Marketplace, 2002, Kaiser Family Foundation.

Exhibit 1-19   Personal Health Care Expenditures by Source of Funds: Selected Calendar Years 1980–2001

Year	Total	Out-of-Pocket Payments	Third-Party Payments							
			Total	Private Health Insurance	Other Private Funds	Public			Medicare[3]	Medicaid[4]
						Total	Federal[2]	State and Local[2]		
					Amount in Billions					
Historical Estimates										
1980	$214.6	$58.2	$156.4	$60.6	$9.2	$86.6	$62.8	$23.8	$36.3	$24.7
1990	609.4	137.3	472.1	203.6	30.6	237.9	174.2	63.7	107.3	69.7
1998	1,009.4	175.2	834.2	341.3	54.8	438.2	335.0	103.2	204.3	160.1
1999	1,064.6	184.4	880.2	365.8	56.8	457.6	347.5	110.1	206.3	174.0
2000	1,137.5	194.7	942.9	397.1	56.3	489.5	371.1	118.4	216.8	189.2
2001	1,236.4	205.5	1,030.9	437.2	56.7	537.0	406.6	130.4	234.5	209.6

Source: CMS, Office of Actuary.

[1]The health spending projections were based on the 2001 version of the National Health Expenditures (NHE) released in January 2003.
[2]Includes Medicaid SCHIP Expansion and SCHIP.
[3]Subset of Federal funds.
[4]Subset of Federal and State and local funds. Includes Medicaid SCHIP Expansion.
[5]Calculation of per capita estimates is inappropriate.
NOTES: Per capita amounts based on July 1 Census resident based population estimates. Numbers and percents may not add to totals because of rounding.

Source: http://www.cms.hhs.gov/statistics/nhe/projections-2002/t5.asp

and the remaining 0.5 percent indigent, or charity, care. This payor mix is more positive than that of Hospital Y that has 55 percent Medicaid, almost no Medicare patients, 44 percent commercial, 0.5 percent indigent, and 0.5 percent self-pay. Hospital Y could be decimated should reimbursement drop significantly from Medicaid. For instance, Tennessee hospitals would desperately like to reduce the number of patients that are covered under the State's Medicaid program, or TennCare, because of low cost reimbursement. Many hospitals in the state have had to close, or shut down services, since the program's inception in 1993 because of historically low reimbursement rates.

Payor mix is directly affected by managed care practices that insurers insist upon having in place before payment will be made. Since the inception of managed care, each payor has certain rules that apply to hospital services (see the section on precertification for examples). If these rules are not followed, the payor, whether commercial, government, or otherwise, is not obligated to pay for the services already rendered. Therefore, it behooves the hospital to play by the rules of all insurers and jump through the hoops to ensure payment. See Exhibit 1-19 to further detail expenditures per payor in 2001.

Impact of Labor Costs on Budgeting

A budget is an estimate of money that is available for the next spending period for a particular area of expense. In this particular section, the focus is on labor costs and how they impact the bottom line. In recent years, labor costs have negatively impacted the bottom line because they have increased so dramatically.

Labor costs quite obviously are a large percentage of a hospital's budget. In fact, research compiled by Price Waterhouse Coopers shows that almost 60 percent of a hospital's budget is tied up in labor costs (Hawthorne, 2003) (see Exhibit 1-20). Labor costs include not only wages, but also employee benefits like vacation time, insurance benefits, Medicare payments, sick time, and any fringe benefits provided (upper level management may be allowed a new car every third year for example). According to Hawthorne, "between 1997 and 2001, hospital wage and benefit increases nearly tripled nationwide, according to the same Price Waterhouse Coopers report" (p. 1).

According to the Center for Studying Health System Change, in a report published in September, 2001, hospitals are absorbing most of the increase in labor costs in an attempt to obtain or keep the much needed labor. There are serious shortages of nurses, radiologists, and pharmacists. When the demand outweighs supply, costs—in the form of salaries—increase in an effort to attract needed health care professionals http://www.premierinc.com/frames, 2001). It can be very difficult to estimate (read: guesstimate) the budget as labor costs increase 3 percent, 4 percent, or even up to 6 percent per year. In addition, the cost of contract labor, or those individuals that are "on lease" to the hospital during a labor crunch, is estimated to increase anywhere from 20–30 percent since their contracts are in such demand http://www.premierinc.com/frames, 2001).

Exhibit 1-20   Percent of Total Hospital Costs by Type of Expense*

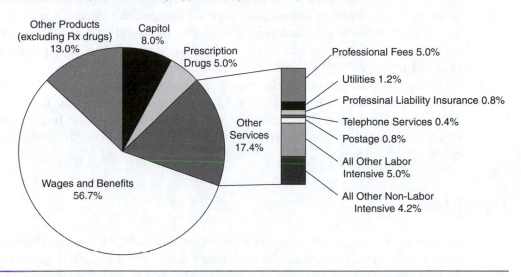

Percent of Total Hospital Costs by Type of Expense*

*Based on CMS Medicare Hospital Market Basket Index weights from 1997.
Source: Centers for Medicare and Medicaid Services (CMS), Office of Actuary: Data from the National Health Statistics Group; *Federal Register,* Medicare Program: Changes to the Hospital Inpatient Prospective Payment Systems and FY 2003 Rates, 67(148), August 1, 2002.

In brief, increasing labor costs can be disastrous for an organization's bottom line. It is imperative that hospital management does its homework to determine trends in the local service area, and plan the budget (guess!) based on this research. Then pray accordingly!

Outsourcing Operational Management Personnel/Improvements

There are hospitals that choose to use other companies that provide either professional management employees, or that provide management advisory services, or both. Companies, such as Quorum Health Resources or Voluntary Hospitals of America, provide these services for hospitals that can pay the price. These companies supply management support services, clinical services, education and training services, and consulting services. Quorum boasts services to over 300 hospitals across 43 states (http://www.Quorum.com) while VHA boasts 2,200 members across 48 states (http://www.VHA.com). One example of a VHA health care system is Cedars-Sinai Health System in Los Angeles, California.

VHA differs from Quorum because VHA is a for-profit cooperative in which members who purchase a VHA product or service earn cash or equity. However, each VHA member is a **community-owned**, or not-for-profit, facility. Therefore, the money or equity earned from the cooperative is used to make the health care system or hospital better for the **community**.

Quorum and VHA assist with strategic initiative design, as well as with daily operations support, such as methods to alleviate the nursing shortage, and how to be one step ahead on compliance issues. Financial management is also offered to improve performance and compliance with managed care contracts. Another service deals with gaps between the hospital organization and physicians by offering to improve physician practice management.

Why use these services? The major advantage is that it alleviates the need to recreate the wheel. Companies like Quorum and VHA already know how to forge rivers that some hospitals may never have had to cross. Improvement is easier and usually less expensive overall, if an organization can avoid learning things the hard way.

Supply Issues

As anyone knows, there is usually power in numbers. Given the thousands of hospitals in the United States, it is no small wonder that hospitals can demand—and receive—price reductions on the supplies used in health care organizations. Using a basic principle of economics, power belongs to the purchaser. One such alliance is Premier, Inc., which is owned by more than 200 hospitals and health care systems in all 50 states (http://www.premiereinc.com). More than 1500 facilities take advantage of the power by purchasing in bulk. Premier, Inc., and other such companies such as VHA (as previously discussed), AllHealth, and Shared Services Healthcare, Inc., can help hospitals control a good portion of the supply train coming into a hospital. This tactic saves resources, including time, effort, and money. Any legal strategy that provides a positive change to the organizational bottom line is well received.

Physician Issues

Trending Toward a Shortage?

According to Coile (2003), hospitals could possibly face a shortage of physicians in the future. He discusses ten factors impacting the future availability of physicians to staff our hospitals. These are:

1. baby boomer retirement,

2. women physicians who work less than a full-time physician schedule,

3. malpractice costs that are sky-rocketing,

4. rising expenses to practice,

5. managed care hassles,

6. decreased reimbursements from Medicare and Medicaid,

7. other alternative professional careers (managed care companies!),

8. collapse of physician practice administrative firms,

9. long daily hours with few days off, and

10. legally mandated medical coverage for all Americans in the future could require more physicians.

To staff our hospitals appropriately, health care organizations must become adept at physician recruitment and retention by somehow decreasing the impact of these ten factors.

Physician Alliances and Contracts

In 2002 physician practices that were not owned by hospitals, called *independent practices*, continued to make more money than practices owned by hospitals. Therefore, there has been a growing trend for hospitals, especially large medical centers, to subsidize physician practices so the physician will practice within a hospital-based practice. These subsidies offset the financial losses that the *hospital-owned practices* are apt to incur (Hoppszallern, 2003). However, if a physician chooses not to take the risk of being truly independent, and does not wish to be hospital-based, there are two other practice patterns from which to chose: *alliances* and *contracts*.

Alliances are "voluntary arrangements between firms involving exchange, sharing, or codevelopment of products, technologies, or services" (Gulati, 1998, p. 29). In other words, two or more entities become allies for one another for "you scratch my back and I'll scratch yours." There are four main types of alliances: 1) independent practitioner associations, 2) physician-hospital organizations, 3) management services organizations, and 4) medical foundations models (Burns, Bazzoli, Dynan, and Wholey, 2000). According to Burns, et al.,

> independent practitioner alliances and physician-hospital organizations constitute vehicles for . . . collaboration and joint contracting with managed care organizations. Other alliances such as management services organizations and medical foundations, serve as vehicles to pursue not only these goals but also to provide physicians with managerial expertise and capital in developing their practices (2000, p. 3).

Refer to Exhibit 1-21 for recent trend information on the types of alliances from 1994 to 2000.

Other Physician Practice Patterns

With the dawning of the managed care revolution came unbelievable changes in physicians' practices. In the past, physicians were allowed to make treatment decisions based on the avenue that might prove to be in the patient's best

Exhibit 1-21   Percentage of Hospitals with Physician Affiliates by Type of Relationship 1994–2000

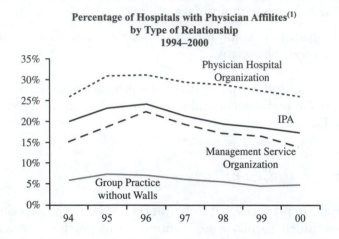

Percentage of Hospitals with Physician Affilites[1]
by Type of Relationship
1994–2000

[1] *A hospital is considered to have a physician relationship if the relationship exists as part of the hospital or a system or network of which the hospital is a part.*

Source: The Lewin Group analysis of American Hospital Association Annual Survey data, 1994–2000 for community hospitals.

interest, regardless of expense. However, with the advent of managed care and attempts at controlling spiraling health care costs, those choices have changed. Currently, payors seem to have the final say as to the medical necessity of an admission or procedure (see *case management* section for further discussion). There have been dramatic changes in physician practice patterns that have affected hospital-based health care.

According to the United States Department of Health and Human Services, a *hospitalist* is a physician who has no actual office practice but instead focuses on the care of patients who have been admitted to the hospital (2002). The concept of a hospitalist started in 1996 and was coined by Wachter and Goldman (2002). The concept came about for several reasons:

> cost pressures on hospitals, physician groups, and managed care organizations; the increased acuity of hospitalized patients, and the accelerated pace of their hospitalizations; the time pressures on primary care physicians in the office; the decreasing inpatient volumes of most primary care physicians; and the evidence that practice makes perfect in other medical fields (Wachter and Goldman, p. 487).

Since 1996 hospitalist programs are becoming more common, and are in fact in many major medical centers across the United States. Examples of hospitals that have hospitalists covering admitted patients include Mayo Clinic, Duke University Medical Center, and UCLA Medical Center (Wachter and Goldman,

2002). According to the American Hospital Association's *Hospital and Health Network*, 15 percent of hospitals employed hospitalists between 1997 and 2002. There are also more hospitalist-only groups with more employed by university and/or medical schools (Darves, p. 22). According to Darves (2003), "nearly 40 percent of hospitalists are employed by hospitals directly, or by hospital-management companies, and about 20 percent by hospitalists-only medical groups. The remaining 40 percent work in multispecialty groups, academic medicine, or as sole contractors, or insurance-company employees" (p. 5).

A major impetus for instituting the hospitalist to attend to patients while in the hospital has been to control costs. According to one hospital's senior vice president, their hospitalists average a savings of about $600 per patient admission over non-hospitalist physicians (http://www.VHA.com). Given this track record, according to VHA and health care experts, the number of hospitalists will quadruple to more than 25,000 in the next decade (2003). According to Goldsmith, he predicts that "hospital practice is going to be a distinct discipline in medicine" (as cited in Weber, 2003, p. 10).

Primary care physicians, who at first were not at all thrilled with the thought of someone else tending to their patients, have now figured out that they, too, can have a real life without spending 60 or more hours working every week between the office and the hospital. In fact, according to Terry, "primary care physicians are increasingly *demanding* that the institutions they're affiliated with start hospitalist programs" (p. 72). However, communication between the primary care physician and the hospitalist is imperative to ensure the quality of the care that patients receive.

Other changes that have become apparent in physician practice patterns are that in the past two decades or so, more physicians are practicing in groups, fewer are practicing alone, and more are practicing as physician employees (see Exhibit 1-22 for a graphic depiction of these statistics). Solo physicians working and running their own offices have become less common in the past twenty years. In fact, according to the American Medical Association (as cited by the Centers for Medicare and Medicaid Services, 2002), there were 18 percent fewer sole practice physicians in 1999 as there were in 1984 (again, see Exhibit 1-22). Perhaps this change is due to more red tape in the way of managed care, employment laws, and higher acuity patients. Additionally, one or two physicians can hardly follow patients in the office, in the hospital, be on-call every night and every weekend, and actually have a life outside of work. Although compensation may be good, physicians would experience burnout quickly at this sole practice pace.

Groups of physicians are sometimes comprised of twenty or more physicians, nurse practitioners, and physician assistants. What better way to keep on-call and rounding time to a minimum? Practicing medicine in a group of physicians ensures that the physicians within the group have a life outside of work. A financial advantage is that all contribute to the clerical costs plus the Internet costs needed for billing. Group practices tend to have lower malpractice insurance rates for the physicians within the group because within the group, physicians can have certain specialties, and they can assist one another when necessary. In addition, larger groups can better weather economic downturns such as decreased Medicaid or Medicare

Exhibit 1-22 The Percentage of Physicians in Differing Practice Arrangements, 1984–1999

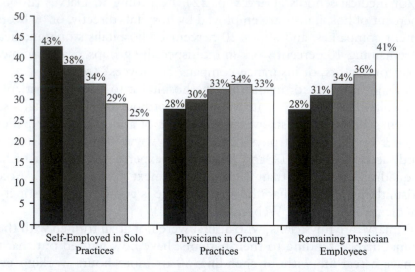

Declines in solo practice physicians are offset by increases in salaried physicians.

*The 1999 data do not include group practice employees in the group practice data, and instead include them in the physician employee column.

Source: AMA Socioeconomic Monitoring System and AMA Physician Masterfile.

reimbursement rates. One of the biggest advantages however, is that larger groups usually have enhanced contracting leverage in contractual discussions with the hospitals in which they practice. Can you imagine how detrimental it would be to a hospital if a group of 15 orthopedists walked out on contract negotiations? These advantages have caused the recent rise in group medical practices. According to Exhibit 1-22, since 1984 physicians practicing in groups has risen about 5 percent.

The final portion of the graph in Exhibit 1-22 portrays a drastic increase in the number of physicians who choose to be physician employees. Since the physician is paid a salary, there is less financial risk to the physician. In addition, the hospital or physician employer absorbs some of the costs for practicing such as licensing fees, malpractice insurance, medical and dental insurance costs, and office staff labor costs. The disadvantage, however, is the loss of autonomy.

Gain Sharing

Gain sharing involves contractual agreements in which all parties signing the contract have mutual benefits and advantages. The concept is relatively simple when an example is used in illustration. Let's say Mr. Z works in a zoo somewhere in the United States. The raw meat supplier that enables the zookeepers to feed the lions strikes a deal with the keeper that feeds the lions on a daily basis. This deal involves monetary rewards to this particular keeper if he can cut the cost of the meat that is necessary to feed the lions. Therefore, in order to meet this expectation, Mr. Z decides not to feed the lions all the raw meat that they need every day. He then gets to keep some of the money that the raw meat supplier saves. Do you see that the only losers here are the lions?

There would be a natural temptation for hospitals and physicians to strike deals in which the end product for each party would be financially beneficial. This is not to say that physicians and/or hospitals would deliberately render less than quality care in order to save money. However, hospitals would favor making these arrangements with physicians in an attempt to increase productivity and decrease costs. In 1992 the Office of the Inspector General issued a Special Advisory Bulletin prohibiting physicians from receiving, and hospitals from paying money, **to reduce or limit care** to Medicare and/or Medicaid patients (Halasa, n.d.). The penalty to the hospital found in violation of this statute? The hospital would pay $2,000 **per patient** involved with the physician payments (http://www.hospitalmanagement.net./informer/management/manage9/). Depending on the time frame in which the violations were occurring, hospitals could face major penalties.

In 1999 the Office of the Inspector General relaxed a bit on the enforcement of this type of arrangement between hospitals and physicians, and allows for limited gain sharing. *Limited gain sharing* pays monetary rewards to physicians who participate in cost-saving, quality-improvement type of organizational programs. However, the following were stipulated as safeguards to limit the potential for gain sharing abuse:

- Quality care reviews must take place,

- Payments are made per capita if and only if the physician group meets expectations (not individual physician performance),

- Performance must be based on time periods of at least one year,

- Hospital profit cannot be used as a criteria to determine performance,

- Affected patients are aware of the plan and cost-saving measures to be taken, and

- Specific cost-saving opportunities must be enumerated by the contract (http://www.hospitalmanagement.net./informer/management/manage9/).

In this way, the Office of the Inspector General has opened the door for incentives to be in place to control rising health care costs without disrupting the quality care rendered to the patients.

Medical Directorships

According to Cardinal (2003, as cited in the Physician Compensation Report) decreased physician and hospital reimbursement rates, and increased medical practice costs have also given physicians the desire to have sources of other income besides their medical practices. Part-time or even full-time *medical directorships* lend physicians the ability to be less dependent on reimbursement from managed care companies and the like for their income. These agreements between the physician and the hospital can be *contractual* or an actual *employment* situation, in which the physician works directly for the hospital. In order to ensure that the directorship position does not break any laws, there are specific recommendations that physicians and hospital administrators should be aware of:

- The contract should be written, with a clear description of the position responsibilities and time expected to be spent fulfilling them.

- Accurate and timely records of duties performed and time logs should be kept up-to-date.

- Compensation for these directorial duties should be at market value only to ensure compliance with the rules of the Internal Revenue Service.

- There should be no relationship between the amount of compensation and actual business that the physician provides for the hospital by patient referrals or other services (Physician Compensation Report, 2003).

- Compensation should be made as a flat fee for medical directorship services, and not based on a percentage of what the physician could have billed for those hours (Report on Medicare Compliance, 2003, September).

These recommendations are meant to keep physicians and hospitals out of hot water with government agencies such as Medicare for inappropriately high compensation, fraud and abuse with regard to *kickbacks* (you scratch my back and I'll scratch yours), and self-referrals (more on this to follow). Documentation is the key to ensuring that the physicians in these roles are providing the services for which they are being paid.

> *Kickbacks* are illegal payments made in return for a referral that results in a transaction or contract (investorwords.com).

I Said Stark, not Stork

The *Stark Law* was passed in January 1995, as Section 1877 under the Social Security Act, but was not actually in effect until January 2001, when the final regulations were released. The law was enacted to make it illegal for physicians, including chiropractors and dentists but excluding nurse practitioners and physician assistants, to make Medicare or Medicaid patient referrals for services to a hospital in which they have a financial interest or relationship. The statute also states that immediate family members of the physician cannot hold financial interest in a facility to which the physician makes a referral for health care services. See http://www.cms.hhs.gov/medicare/currentcodes.pdf for a complete list of included services. Violations are punishable by $15,000 as a civil money penalty (Gosfield, 2003).

It is important to note, however, that there are over 20 exceptions to the Stark Law. Most importantly, according to Gosfield, in order to "qualify for several exceptions . . . a practice must meet all of the elements of the Stark statute's definition of a group practice" (p. 4). Exceptions include in-office ancillary services such as x-rays, referrals to physicians within the referring physician's own group (see the box that follows for an example of this exception), those referrals made for patients within prepaid health plans, office space and equipment rental, physician self-referrals, and instances of physician recruitment.

To ensure compliance with the Stark Law, there are technical elements of each exception to which the hospital and physician should pay close attention. Some of the elements that MUST be in any agreement between a physician and a hospital include:

- A written agreement that is signed by both a hospital administrator and the physician,

- The term of the agreement has to be for at least one year,

- A fair and reasonable price for the office space leased regardless of the number of referrals generated by the physician to the hospital, and

- Compensation for the physician for personal services that would be considered fair market value (McCullough, n.d.).[1]

> Example: Dr. ABC is seeing a pregnant female who has concerns about the likelihood that the baby might have certain hereditary diseases that run in her family. Dr. ABC refers the patient to the group's geneticist for counseling and possible testing. This in-group referral would not violate the Stark Law provided the group was considered "a group" under the Law.

Technological Advances in Physician Practice

With technological advances occurring daily, there is no end to the possibilities and the repercussions for physician practices. Electronic medical records, personal digital assistants, and telemedicine make it faster, more convenient, and easier than ever before to be a physician. Gone are the days of getting a call in the middle of the night and having to drive to the hospital just to look at an x-ray. Now the radiology department can "beam" them straight to the physician wherever he or she might be. Records are now electronic—there is no need to fight over the patient's chart to write an order. Nor is it necessary to physically go to the Medical Records department to sign charts/orders. These can now be signed by electronic signature authentication; it can be done from any computer with Internet access, along with a username and password.

---

[1]For more detailed information on the Stark Law please refer to http://www.cms.hhs.gov/medlearn/refphys.asp.

For example, according to Morrissey (2002) "on the average day, more that 600 physicians tap directly into the latest information available on patients receiving care at Memorial Health's 432-bed teaching hospital in Savannah, Georgia" (p. 1). Soon there will be no reason for a physician to write out a prescription on a piece of paper. Already, physicians can "beam" the prescription directly to the patient's pharmacy of choice with the assistance of a personal digital assistant. Advances such as these are "keepers" according to Kaiser (as cited in Weber, 2003, p. 12), and soon "we'll be able to do everything in the country from a central point."

Nursing Issues

I would indeed be a poor excuse for a nurse if I did not at least mention some issues that are a very real part of nursing practice today. The influx of students interested in nursing as a career has been historically cyclical in nature. Some years the nursing schools around the country are overwhelmed with applicants; other years the class seats go empty. Recently however, the shortage of nurses has reached desperate heights, and hospitals are offering unbelievable incentives for nurses to work at their facility. The following is some discussion of this phenomenon.

Career Choices

In years past the career paths that were available for women were limited. Homemaker, teacher, or nurse was pretty much the whole kit and kaboodle. However, as women's rights became more prominent and women became more educated, these career paths faced competition. Careers that offered more money, more prestige, better working hours, and fewer legal and health risks, won over many women who might have entered into nursing otherwise. For this reason, the nursing shortage might not be so cyclical anymore. It could very well be here to stay.

Man is a peculiar animal. He can only read the writing on the wall when his back is up against it.

Stevenson, A., as cited in *American Organization of Nurse Executives* (2003). Health work environments: Striving for excellence, Volume II, 4.

Some Stats and Contributing Factors

The average age of a staff nurse in the year 2000 was 43.3 years according to the American Association of Colleges of Nursing (2003). The trend is for this average to increase as the numbers of baby-boomer nurses outweigh younger nurses starting into the profession. Those sitting for the national licensing exam for nurses, the NCLEX-RN®, have decreased 31.3 percent from 1995 to 2002 (National Council of State Boards of Nursing, as cited in the American Association of Colleges of Nursing, 2003). When the U.S. Bureau of Labor Statistics has estimated that by 2010 more than one million new and replacement nurses will be needed (Ibid), it is no small wonder that nurses are feeling the weight of "overworked and underpaid."

I once had a t-shirt that had the top 10 reasons to become a nurse. All of them were poking fun at some of the issues that arise with respect to the reasons nursing is not so popular anymore. Some of them included the joy of spending all of your holidays with your friends (at work!), 'tis better to give than receive (shots, enemas, you get the picture), and the ability to purchase support hose in bulk. The odd hours, the sometimes thankless tasks (bedpan duty!), and putting up with the doctors (sorry!) all make for such a *wonderful* working environment. However, nurses love the profession, not for all these, but merely for the human contact and the ability to show compassion and make just one person's life more comfortable.

Some more scholarly reasons that nurses are in short supply are:

- Up until recently nursing schools were experiencing a decline in enrollments,

- Nursing schools are experiencing a shortage of faculty to be able to adequately supply instructors for those who do enroll,

- More nurses are either getting out of the profession by quitting (job burnout or dissatisfaction), or retiring, than are entering, and

- More nurses are needed to care for the aging population (American Association of Colleges of Nursing, 2003).

Impact on Patient Care

When there are an insufficient number of nurses in a particular hospital, that hospital must face the inevitable choice of deciding between quality care and closing patient beds. Patients deserve quality care but also deserve access to health care when required. This is a difficult choice to make for anyone who only wants to take care of people.

The impact that a lack of nurses has on those who need them can really be summed up in a few succinct words: less than acceptable outcomes (Aiken, Clarke, Sloane, Sochalski, and Silber, 2002). The potential for more medical errors, higher mortality rates, less safe care, less hand-holding, less compassion, less patient advocacy, and overall inability to provide for our patients, makes for a terrible situation in which we find ourselves.

Magnet Hospital Program

The Magnet Recognition Program is a program that is sponsored by the American Nurses Credentialing Center. The beginning of this program stemmed from a research study that occurred in 1980 in an effort to find the reasons why some hospitals could recruit and retain nurses far better than others. These hospitals were found to have "Forces of Magnetism" that made the hospitals better places in which to work. These forces include:

- High quality nursing leadership that expect strong, professional behavior from the nursing staff. These nursing leaders also were easily accessible and apparently believed in the "management by walking around" principle,

- An organizational structure that is flat and decentralized to facilitate open communication at all levels,

- Nursing management that believes in a participative management style,

- Competitive salaries and benefits with policies and programs that the nursing staff actually *asks* to attend,

- Professional model of nursing care in which the nursing staff are held accountable for their actions and are allowed to function autonomously,

- Quality care that is actually a goal rather than a buzzword,

- Staff nurses are heavily involved in quality improvement strategies (see section on Quality for details),

- Resources for the staff nurse are readily available,

- The hospital and the nursing staff are considered partners in the community,

- Teaching patients and other staff members is a major focus,

- Staff nurses are seen as irreplaceable assets to the facility,

- A collegial bond exists in which physicians and nurses are care partners, not adversaries, and

- An on-going commitment to the professional development of all nursing staff employed by the facility (Monarch, 2003).

Would it not be amazing if we could all work in this Nurses' Heaven Hospital located somewhere in Utopia??? It is my belief that the nursing shortage would soon disappear if there were many more hospitals that had Magnet status.

Working with the Number Crunchers

The financial wizards of any hospital organization face an uphill battle in most health care organizations today. With decreasing reimbursements, increasing red tape, and higher costs, a positive bottom line and a positive outlook for the organization are hard to maintain. However, it is one of the goals of this text to bring the number crunchers and patient care employees closer together, so that all working within a particular hospital have the same goal: *excellent patient care at a reasonable cost to the organization.*

Nurses and financiers have difficulty actually understanding each other because they each come from totally different backgrounds. Finance people think in numbers and the *financial outcome* for the organization, whereas nurses and patient care folks think in *patient outcomes.* This is like comparing apples to oranges. Well, it is time to at least talk in the same fruit family . . . say, a Granny Smith apple to a Macintosh apple.

Since financial people are primarily numbers-driven, those in patient care **must** consider the financial impact of patient outcomes. How will better clinical outcomes help the organization meet the targeted revenues for the particular period? Nurses will get what they want (what is best for the patient and achieve the best possible patient outcomes) from the finance people (who are concerned with money) when every requested improvement is tied in some way to the bottom line—how will it impact the organization?

For example, look at staffing issues. Nurses request increases in the staffing ratios that are set by the organization in hopes of better handling the increase in volume or patient acuity. Ask yourself: is there actually a historical increase in volume and/or acuity, or is it only a recent trend? Nurses must look at day-to-day and week-to-week trends to adjust for small increases or decreases in workload. However, the number crunchers must think in averages. Finance looks at the data over several months, if not years, to determine a trend before agreeing to change staffing requirements. Therefore, nurses need to relate a request to the bottom line and average over time to get their requests heard.

Another difference between nurses and finance people is that finance people are taught to look at the entire system in which the hospital functions. This includes multiple levels: organizational, local, regional, and in some cases a national level. Nurses at the patient's bedside, however, are like horses with blinders on: they look only at that which is right in front of them. Patients do not really care about how the hospital is fairing financially with respect to its neighboring facilities when they are sick and in need of hospitalization. Nurses are taught to be patient advocates from day one of nursing education.

Nurses should think more frequently of the effect that events occurring inside their microcosm have on the entire health care industry. Number crunchers in turn should move away from strictly numbers and learn to become patient advocates as well as advocates for the organization. Great patient satisfaction scores will bring a great bottom line. The only way for nurses and number crunchers to work together is to meet on middle ground.

Case Management

Case Management is one of many new functions to keep costs down in a health care system that is becoming more complex, chaotic, and expensive. After implementing prospective payment for inpatients, costs continued to rise. The Centers for Medicare and Medicaid Services (CMS) therefore initiated *managed care* in another attempt to hold down health care costs. Managed care "emerged as control shifted from the provider to the purchaser (i.e., health maintenance organizations and preferred provider organizations) of health services" (Cohen and Cesta, 2001, p. 25). According to Powell (2000), "managed care was the natural response to a healthcare system of waste and expanding, expensive technology" (p. 2).

Managed care is "a set of techniques ... used to manage health-care costs by influencing patient care decision-making through case-by-case assessment of the appropriateness of care prior to its provision" (Powell, p. 3).

Boles and Neumann (1999) believe that the "basic concept of managed care is to maximize the health status of the population," i.e., with a focus on health maintenance at the highest level possible for a particular disease process (p. 5).

However, it is important to remember that managed care is, generally, a **systems-oriented** approach. Managed care is an attempt by purchasers, mainly insurance companies, to force providers in the health care system to cut costs. If costs go down for the insurance company, then profits go up. An example of managed care is when a primary care physician in a health maintenance organization, or preferred provider organization, is made the gatekeeper to available services and specialties for better cost control. Here a patient cannot go directly for specialty service. Rather, the gatekeeper must determine that the specialty service is needed before the patient can proceed and payment will be made. However, managed care did nothing to actually alleviate the confusion and chaos for the **people** trying to wade through the quagmire that has become the health care system as a whole. Enter *case management*. Case management is an attempt to assist people to negotiate the mazes that seem to be so common with managed health care.

Case management is the "process of coordinating patient care across the continuum to assure optimal quality outcomes, patient satisfaction, and appropriate use of resources" (Cohen and Cesta, p. 74).

Case management was first introduced in North America after World War II as a way to coordinate efforts with psychiatric patients that were discharged from inpatient facilities. By the early 1960s, case management was used within long-term care in an effort to control costs. By the 1980s—the era of managed care and the Prospective Payment System—case management moved further into the health care system in an attempt to make more services available to more people, while also managing to control costs (Lee, Mackenzie, Dudley-Brown, and Chin, 1998, p. 933). Not such a short order to fulfill! There are two main ways case management is practiced. One way is an "essential part of care-giving activities"; the other is one where "some payers have been superimposed on the provider system as a mechanism to control costs" (Billows, 1997, p. 526).

Case Management Types

Case management can focus on different populations of patients within the health care community. For instance, *social case management* focuses on the long-term care needs of the elderly. Here the case manager coordinates services to assist the elderly in maintaining independence. One example is the Congregate Housing Services Program in which non-health related services, such as light housekeeping, personal care, meals and/or transportation are coordinated for elderly living in low-income housing (Cohen and Cesta, 2001).

Primary care case management allows the patient's primary physician to be the gatekeeper under a medical model of care. The goal focuses mainly on cost-effectiveness, and emphasizes patient outcomes. A major disadvantage of this type is that no real patient advocacy exists (Cohen and Cesta).

Medical-social case management is a third type of case management. Anyone can function in this capacity according to Cohen and Cesta (2001). This type, like social case management, focuses on long-term care and the elderly, but like primary care case management, the goal is to decrease costs by avoiding hospitalization. Coordination of both medical and social services on a pre-paid basis is the hallmark of this type.

Private case management is for those people who can afford to pay for services outside of publicly funded programs. These case managers focus strictly on what is best for the patient/client. Individualized services are offered by private firms that are usually for-profit, and independently owned and operated (Cohen and Cesta).

The final type, which is discussed in the most detail, is *nursing case management*. Nursing case management models utilize many methods by which to reach a common goal. The common goal, inherent to all nursing models, is the "coordination and integration of *outcomes* and cost" (Cohen and Cesta, p. 15). See Exhibit 1-23 for a listing of different types of case management.

There are two main divisions within nursing case management: within-the-walls case managers primarily coordinate inpatient issues, while beyond-the-walls case managers serve outpatients. We will discuss hospital-based case management here although often the inpatient case manager needs to work with the outpatient case manager as their work frequently overlaps.

Outcomes are the standards of care that determine the goals of patient care. According to Powell (2000, p. 449) an outcome is "the result of a measurable goal." For example, a 72-year-old man comes in for bypass surgery; a goal would be that he would recognize danger signs of clot formation. The outcome is that he can verbalize those danger signs at or before discharge.

Within-the-walls nursing case management focuses on patients within the confines of the hospital. The advantages of being within those confines are that specialized services and resources are available for both the provider and the recipient of case management services. Various methods are used by staff and physicians to monitor and achieve the greatest efficiency of care within the hospital. Examples of methods used

Exhibit 1-23   Types of Case Management

- Nursing case management
- Social case management
- Primary case management
- Medical-social case management
- Private case management

Source: Reprinted from *Nursing Case Management: From Essentials to Advanced Practice Applications*, 3rd ed., Cohen, E. and Cesta, T., 2001, with permission of Elsevier.

include: critical pathways, benchmarking, and outcomes measurements, which will all be discussed in more detail shortly. These methods allow the case manager to more easily achieve the goal of cost-effective care (Cohen and Cesta, 2001).

Since nurse case managers work to coordinate patient care—which ultimately saves money because patients are more apt to receive needed care on a timely basis—the assumption is that patients with complex medical problems need assistance in efficiently and effectively navigating the maze of the health care system. The case manager is thus acting in the patient's best interest and is, therefore, a true patient advocate (Lee et al., 1998). However, as any person working in this role will attest, often there is a struggle for case managers to act in the patient's best interest **and** to effectively control costs without fail. One way in which case managers can assist nurses and physicians in controlling length of stay, thereby increasing reimbursement, is through utilization of critical pathways.

Critical Pathways

Many hospitals use *critical pathways* to control the length of an inpatient stay. These pathways are like maps to keep everyone involved in that particular patient's case on the same page with the same goals. According to Rohrbach, critical pathways are the "pursuit of best practice . . . through evidence-based medicine for a particular illness" (1999, p. 12). According to Cooke and Brodrick (1997), critical pathways were introduced as a way "to enhance managed care . . . to significantly improve multidisciplinary communication and coordination of patient activities in addition to controlling costs" (p. 365). Zander (Cooke and Brodrick, 1997, p. 365) first introduced critical pathways to acute care nursing in 1985 as a tool to specifically assist in controlling health care costs. Pathways have since evolved to adapt to a more complex and chaotic health care system.

According to Renholm, Leino-Kilpi, and Suominem, a critical pathway "is a treatment regimen including time-dependent functions used to standardize the care-process throughout the treatment process" (2002, p. 196). Critical

A critical pathway "identifies a particular progression of events . . . in which each step in the pathway process must be completed in sequence before one proceeds with the next step" (Cooke and Brodrick, 1997, p. 365).

pathways assist nursing and medicine to meet the length-of-stay goals that are set by Medicare diagnosis-related groups (DRG) or Ambulatory Patient Classification (APC) reimbursement. Hospitals may use different terms for this concept, such as "clinical pathway, clinical path, critical path, clinical protocol, care map, and care track" (Renholm et al., 2002, p. 196). Powell (2000) adds two more variations—progress pathways and progress maps. These are all different names for the same concept with the same goal: to reduce length of stay thereby reducing total cost. Other goals include encouraging more efficient and effective use of resources, and giving a better quality care that is also more efficient and effective. See Exhibits 1-24 and 1-25 for examples of critical pathways.

Nurse case managers measure the effectiveness of their efforts in the hospital setting through measuring patient *outcomes*. According to current literature critical pathways can lead to significant improvements in these patient outcomes (Powell, 2000; Rohrbach, 1999; Kowal and Delaney, 1996; Kirk, Michael, Markowsky, Restino, and Zarowitz, 1996). Before we can discuss outcomes, however, we must first discuss variances.

Variances in Critical Pathways

A variance refers to any deviation from the care plan or map that was established at the time that the patient was admitted. These deviations can be positive or negative. Think of a negative variance from a critical path as a detour that the driver (patient) must take because of some unexpected road construction (health complication). These variances usually involve a time delay in the original plan (Cooke and Brodrick, 1997).

A *variance* is any deviation from the pathway care plan.

The multidisciplinary health care team must "improvise and overcome" the problem, thus developing a new plan, or path, by which the original outcome or goal might still be reached. Adjusting the critical pathway to undertake the variance leads to a more coordinated, holistic approach that will still likely lead to outcomes based upon best-practice evidence.

Positive variances are those in which the patient was able to reach the goals of care more quickly, or more efficiently, than expected (Cooke and Brodrick, 1997). For example, if a patient could be discharged on day two of the critical pathway instead of day three because the patient improved more quickly than expected, a positive variance occurred.

Zander has identified three categories that might be the root causes of variances, whether positive or negative in nature. These include: a) flaws in the processes of the institution, b) variances caused by the provider, and 3) unexpected

Exhibit 1-24   Clinical Pathway for Wheezing

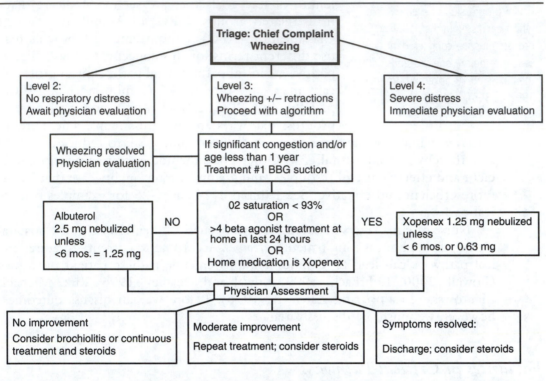

ASTHMA/WHEEZING HISTORY	
Onset of flare up (days):	
Number of Albuterol/Xopenex Rx in the past 24 hrs: _____	Response to Albuterol/Xopenex: ☐ Good ☐ Poor ☐ None
Cough: None: ☐ Mild ☐ Mod ☐ Severe	Post tussive emesis ☐ Yes ☐ No
Retractions: ☐ Yes ☐ No	Wheezing ☐ Yes ☐ No
In the past two nights has the patient awakened due to cough or difficulty breathing: ☐ Yes ☐ No	
How many times does your child wake up at night due to coughing during a typical week? _____	
In a typical week how many Albuterol/Xopenex treatments are given for symptom relief? _____	
Hospitalizations for asthma in past year: _____	ER visits for asthma in past year: _____
_____ ICU Admissions	
Number of oral steroid treatments for asthma in past year: _____ When were they last used? _____	
Followed by Specialist: ☐ Yes ☐ No	Unscheduled M.D. visits in past year for asthma: _____
Last visit to specialist:	RT Signature:
Name of specialist: _____ months ago	Historian Signature:

Exhibit 1-25   Fox Chase Network Community Hospitals Clinical Pathway: Pain Management

L.O.S. = 5 DAYS

	DAY 1	DAY 2	DAY 3	DAY 4	DAY 5
ASSESSMENT EVALUATION	*Initial Nursing Assessment *Initial Pain Assessment *Patient verbalizes and defines acceptable level of pain. *Review Home Meds *Evaluate interventions meds at regular timed intervals. *Report of new pain, 30 min after med. administration *Assess route of pain med	*Re-evaluate pain control *Re-evaluate medication *Utilize ongoing assessment tool *Re-evaluate appropriate route of pain med. for home care on daily basis	→		→
DIET	*As tolerated				
DIAGNOSTIC TESTS	As Indicated: *CBC *Chem Panel *Bone Scan *CT Scan *MRI *X-Ray	*Evaluate and reorder as needed	→		→
CONSULTS	If indicated: *Pain Mgt.-MD, Pain Team *Social Service *Dietary *Physical Medicine *Surgical *Medical Oncology *Radiation *Pastoral Care	*Check completion of consults			

Source: Reprinted with permission by the Association of Community Cancer Centers © 1998 (www.accc-cancer.org) and the Fox Chase Network Community Hospitals.

Exhibit 1-25   Fox Chase Network Community Hospitals Clinical Pathway: Pain Management *(continued)*

Page 2

	DAY 1	DAY 2	DAY 3	DAY 4	DAY 5
PATIENT/STAFF ACTIVITIES Cutaneous Stimulation Exercise Repositioning Immobilization Relaxation & Imagery Cognitive Distraction Patient Education Psychotherapy Support Groups	*Define non-pharmacological therapies *Evaluate and establish ADL skill level and endurance level *ROM	*Identify specific interventions strategies		*Complete instruction in use of strategies and interventions	
MEDICATIONS AND I.V. FLUIDS	*Administer as Ordered: *Consider: *I.V.'s *Analgesics *Opioids *Adjuvant Nsaids *Antiemetics *Bowel Management *Anti-Anxiety *Sleepers	*Identify specific treatment/ strategies utilized	*Evaluate treatment		
INTERVENTIONS TREATMENT	* Administration of meds *VSS q 8 hrs. or as indicated *I + O *Safety Precautions *Skin Prevention				
PATIENT/FAMILY SIGNIFICANT OTHER EDUCATION	*Assess readiness to learn *Assess understanding of disease process and treatment plan *Assess ability to utilize pain assessment tool *Patient receives	*Patient able to communicate pain status	*Pt/family verbalizes scheduling of meds/side effects/management	*Patient able to state side effects and myths *Patient able to state plan of care including discharge	*Provide written plan of care for home.

Source: Reprinted with permission by the Association of Community Cancer Centers © 1998 (www.accc-cancer.org) and the Fox Chase Network Community Hospitals.

Exhibit 1-25   Fox Chase Network Community Hospitals Clinical Pathway: Pain Management (*continued*)

Page 3

	DAY 1	DAY 2	DAY 3	DAY 4	DAY 5
PSYCHOSOCIAL	Assess *Psychosocial *Social *Cultural *Spiritual needs	*Intervention as needed *Check completion of consults	→		
DISCHARGE PLANS	*Identify Social Service/Home Care needs *Make Appropriate referrals *Assess Insurance approved for pain management, route, treatment plan and care giver needs	*Check completion of consults	→		
OUTCOMES	*Patient verbalizes reduced or alleviation of pain as per: *Pain assessment scale *Physical signs/symptoms	*All referrals consults scheduled or completed	*Patient states resources available to assist with pain control		*Patient verbalizes objective of level of pain. Scale 1 to 10 *Patient demonstrates skills required to manage pain

Source: Reprinted with permission by the Association of Community Cancer Centers © 1998 (www.accc-cancer.org) and the Fox Chase Network Community Hospitals.

changes or occurrences with the patient (Cooke and Brodrick, 1997). Examples of each are in the box below.

Problems with Institutional Processes	Problems with the Provider	Problems with the Patient
1. Consults not reported.	1. Consults not received.	1. Pain during consulting physician visit.
2. Equipment not available.	2. Equipment not ordered.	2. Unable to tolerate or understand equipment or test.
3. Test scheduled incorrectly.	3. Test not ordered correctly.	3. Preparation for test not followed (i.e., ate lunch when not allowed to).

When variances occur, a variance analysis should be conducted to analyze what happened. This systematic analysis provides a constant feedback loop that may ascertain weaknesses (or strengths) in the critical pathway. These feedback loops are the groundwork for continuous quality improvement (CQI) programs. Do you see how case management, critical pathways, and variance analysis are all interrelated? Nursing case management usually involves critical pathways that involve variance analysis in order to maintain appropriate pathways. This in turn provides data for *outcomes research and management*.

Outcomes Research and Management

Outcomes management, according to Rohrbach, is the "continuous evaluation of outcomes and comparison to a set standard for the purpose of improving clinical results and processes" (p. 14). *Outcomes research* ascertains that a particular mode of treatment is more effective for a certain patient population. This result could entirely change what is considered best practice for that patient population.

An example: In nursing school, especially in the beginning, the concept that is stressed first and foremost is **HAND WASHING** and something called universal or standard precautions. Well, for those that might not yet be familiar with this, it is simply being on guard and protecting yourself from anything wet that might come from a patient, i.e., blood, urine, or sweat. One favorite story of nursing educators everywhere is where the world of medicine was before the advent of hand washing in between patients. Early outcomes research results, comparing hand washing to no hand washing between patients, found that the patients contracted fewer illnesses when medical personnel washed their hands between patients. Outcomes research changed practice. It changed the way in which medical and nursing personnel protect both themselves and their patient populations from infections. Show me a nurse or doctor who is not seriously into hand washing, and I will show you one who has missed the boat. This becomes a **MAJOR** safety issue.

It is important that the clinical pathway reflect current outcome research results. This is a tall order, as it requires clinicians to pay attention to research that is being reported and not just the day-to-day world of taking care of patients. Conversely, it is just as important not to be so outcome focused that the daily processes are forgotten! It is a definitely a fine line to walk.

Utilization Management—Precertification, Utilization Review, Discharge Planning, and Retrospective Review

Utilization management (UM) is the fine art of the nurse case manager examining how health care services are used. It is the culmination of everything "case management" has worked to achieve. Utilization management both saves money and attempts to ensure that everyone involved in the patient's care will get reimbursed at the highest possible amount for services rendered. In addition, it is also an attempt to identify fraudulent activities, such as overcharging, double billing, or charging for services not rendered. Utilization management answers the increasingly important question: Is a proposed medical service necessary? All levels of the health care continuum practice utilization management, including hospitals, outpatient service providers, private physician providers, managed care organizations, and even Medicare and Medicaid.

In hospital utilization management there are four areas discussed: *precertification, utilization review, discharge planning,* and *retrospective review.* See Exhibit 1-26, which depicts the components of utilization management.

Exhibit 1-26   Components of Utilization Management

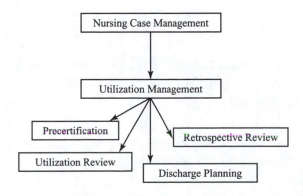

Precertification

Precertification, preadmission review, or prospective review is the act of gaining approval for the health care services that have yet to be rendered (Powell, 2000; Managed Care Concepts, 2002). This is a major attempt to ensure that hospital admission is required for the particular health event occurring with the patient. Most insurance companies require a "precert" for a hospital admission to determine if their criteria for *medical necessity* have been met. This can result in fewer admissions and fewer inpatient hospital days, thereby decreasing overall costs. This, in short, is the act of asking permission for the patient to be admitted to the hospital on a non-urgent basis.

However, obtaining precertification *DOES NOT* guarantee payment for those services. It is merely getting permission for the admission based on the medical facts as presented at the time of the precertification. Note that the patient's physician has the ultimate responsibility for the safety and health of the patient. Therefore, the denial of authorization for services should in no way be construed as an absolute denial if the physician deems admission is medically necessary. In this case the physician and the hospital might choose to appeal the decision, or to fight further with the payor, and to insist that the proposed care *IS* necessary. If the payor still chooses not to pay, the end result is that the physician and hospital might choose to take care of the patient anyway. In this case the physician and hospital probably will not get paid!

Most insurance companies also require precertification for emergency admissions. The hospital is given 24 hours (or the next business day if on the weekends) to notify the insurance company of the admission. This ensures that the patient's needs will be given top priority.

Utilization Review

Utilization review (UR), or concurrent review, occurs during an inpatient stay at the hospital. Often, UR is done when the patient must remain in the hospital longer than was originally precertified. The medical services planned are "evaluated for efficiency, appropriateness, and necessity" (Powell, p. 508). Utilization review also screens for complex issues that should be monitored more closely by

---

The criteria for *medical necessity* include:

1. Is the plan of treatment considered normal for the diagnosis?
2. Are there other less expensive alternative treatments?
3. Could the treatment plan be initiated and maintained as an outpatient?

Source: Managed Care Concepts. (2002). Precertification, utilization review, discharge planning. Retrieved September 22, 2003 from http://www.managedcareconcepts.com.

the nurse case manager, such as custody issues in the case that the patient is a minor. It also ensures that the insurance company is aware of the patient's requirements and that *discharge planning* is still moving forward (Powell, 2000).

Discharge Planning

Discharge planning is one of the most important functions of the nurse case manager, as well as an important component of critical pathways. Each patient must be screened to determine if there is a need for detailed coordination of health care services upon discharge from the hospital. Not all patients will have this requirement. However, for those that do, adverse consequences might occur if these services, and any social issues, are not adequately addressed during the hospital stay. According to Erwin (1999), "recent studies have shown that careful discharge planning, along with good follow-up contact, can significantly improve patients' health upon discharge while decreasing healthcare and social costs" (p. 1).

At the foundation of discharge planning is the caveat that it starts at, or very close to, admission to the facility. This ensures that the nurse case manager is familiar with: 1) the particular patient and family needs, 2) the critical pathway that has been developed to address the health issues for the patient, and 3) the insurance requirements peculiar to each policy upon discharge. Discharge planning needs to start immediately so no unnecessary delays occur when the patient is ready for discharge. If a patient has been assigned a diagnosis-related group (DRG) at admission, with the subsequent flat-rate payment as mandated by Medicare or other insurances, early discharge planning may assist in controlling the length of stay.

Discharge planning, as well as case management and clinical pathways, is most effective when a collaborative process occurs between members of the health care team. In fact, if team meetings involving the physician, the primary caretaker, home health workers, the nurse case manager, the social worker, and other health care team members can occur, *discharge planning* is more likely to achieve continuity of care both within the hospital as well as outside in the community once the patient is discharged.

Another aspect of discharge planning involves a careful review of the insurance requirements so that the insurance criteria can be met before discharge. For example, *levels of care* are assigned to each patient that refer to the stability of the patient at the time of discharge (Powell, 2000). The stability and placement for follow-up care must match. If a level of care is given to a patient and the criteria for that level is not met, the insurance company may deny any benefits payable for the services to be rendered. Some examples of levels of care are listed in Exhibit 1-27.

An example might be helpful in making sure this crucial point is well understood. Let's say that a patient that has been admitted for open-heart surgery is following the critical pathway without any deviations. The nurse case manager, having followed this patient from the beginning of the admission, is familiar with

Exhibit 1-27   Levels of Care Assignments Upon Discharge

A. Acute Care Levels

1. Acute care hospitals (transfers to other facilities)
2. Inpatient Rehabilitation hospitals
3. Transitional hospitals from one level to a lower one

B. Post-acute Care Levels

1. Skilled nursing facilities/units
2. Intermediate care facilities/units
3. Assisted living or custodial care
4. Hospice
5. Rehabilitation units not considered acute care
6. Home health services
7. Specialty pharmacy services

Source: Powell, S. K. *Case management: A practical guide to success in managed care.* Baltimore, MD: Lippincott, Williams, and Wilkins. (2000). pp. 359–386.

the social situation and insurance requirements. There is only one person available to assist this patient upon discharge from the hospital, so the nurse case manager attempts to obtain a bed for this post open-heart patient at a transitional care facility. These hospitals usually take patients that need care just below the intensive care unit level for an extended period of time. This would require that the patient in our example have an acute care *level of care* of three. (See Exhibit 1-27.)

However, the insurance company denies transitional care coverage for this patient because the requirements for that *level of care* have not been met. These requirements may include patients who are ventilator dependent, those who are in need of nutrition intravenously, extensive wound care, intravenous therapies, extensive burn care, hemodialysis, pre-hospice patients for pain control, and those recovering from a coma (Powell, 2000). Since our post open-heart patient has none of these issues, he clearly does not meet the requirements for this level of care.

However, a post-acute level of care of a five or six would be more appropriate. It includes home health and/or rehabilitation services if necessary (which in this example are probably not going to be necessary).

To make matters more confusing, different facilities may have their own set of discharge criteria that must be met! Fortunately, since Medicare is the largest supplier of medical coverage in the United States, most facilities and insurance companies use Medicare's criteria in order to determine the appropriate level of care assignments for patients (Powell, 2000).

As the nurse case manager plans for discharge, prior authorization from the insurance company *must* be obtained. In addition, utilization of services need to be reviewed prior to discharging a patient. If this is not done, the patient may not be eligible for continued services and that payment for such services will not occur. An example of the need for prior authorization would be if a patient were referred to cardiac rehabilitation services following the open-heart surgery from the previous example. If the company providing the rehabilitation services does not ensure that the patient's insurance company is made aware of the services to be rendered, **and** that the insurance company has approved the services and deemed appropriate care, reimbursement for the rehabilitation services will probably be denied!

Retrospective Review

According to Aetna, the purposes behind *retrospective review* are to:

- Analyze any potential quality and/or utilization issues (how to make processes better),

- Initiate appropriate follow-up action, based on quality or utilization issues (how to fix mistakes to keep them from re-occurring),

- Review initial requests for certification made after discharge or after the provision of service (in an attempt to get coverage for services already rendered), and to

- Analyze submitted documentation to determine the rationale behind the failure to follow patient management utilization guidelines (why did we not follow the rules in the first place?) (Aetna, 2003, p. 1).

Retrospective review seems to rarely work. If the original guidelines were not followed to the letter, the insurance company will deny coverage.

Compliance, Quality, Evaluation, Accreditation, and Risk Management Issues

Compliance and Risk Management

Risk management is the proactive way to avoid 'the possibility of loss, injury, disadvantage or destruction' (Simmons, 1998, p. 2). I particularly like this definition because risks are about the **possible** negative outcomes to a certain event or action. From a hospital perspective, the worst possible risk is to human life and/or limb. Duke University is a good example. What risks did they take by giving the teenager who got the wrong heart another one? It could have had a wonderful outcome, but to do nothing would surely have resulted in her death. The administrators and medical staff at Duke decided to attempt another transplant to try to save her life. Risk management is all about avoiding bad outcomes; should they occur, risk management is then about damage control and limiting liability. Sad but true since health care is, after all, a business.

> Risk management is the "sum of all proactive activities . . . intended to accommodate the possibility of failures" (Simmons, C. W. (1998). Risk Management (Managing Standards). Retrieved October 1, 2003 from http://sparc.airtime.co.uk/users/wysywig/risk_1.htm#INTRO.)

Some risk management terminology used to describe adverse events are: adverse patient occurrence, potentially compensable event (if sued the hospital might actually have to pay damages), incident, variance, sentinel event, and occurrence or incident report (Powell, 2000). It would be wise for both nursing and business personnel to familiarize themselves with ways in which to minimize risks to both the hospital and to themselves.

> "A *sentinel event* is an unexpected occurrence involving death or serious physical or psychological injury, or the risk thereof. Serious injury specifically includes loss of limb or function. The phrase, 'or risk thereof' includes any process variation for which a recurrence would carry a significant chance of a serious adverse outcome" (www.jcaho.org/sentinel).

Compliance for a medical facility involves meeting many outside regulatory requirements. An increased level of compliance should lead to lower risks for the hospital. Federal government agencies, such as the Centers for Medicare and Medicaid Services, base the amount of federal money that the facility receives on compliance with mandates from Medicare and Medicaid. Other agencies that mandate policies and regulations include the Equal Employment Opportunity Commission, the Occupational Safety and Health Administration, the Social Security Administration, and the Department of Labor.

Other regulations with which a hospital might need to be in compliance include accreditation bodies, i.e., Joint Commission for the Accreditation of Health Organizations, state and local employment laws, union by-laws if the hospital is unionized, and those by-laws as set forth by the hospital's own Board of Directors. Remember that the hospital should be less at risk for the possibility of "loss, injury, disadvantage, or destruction" if in compliance with all regulatory bodies that are involved at the hospital level (Simmons, 1998, p. 2).

Performance Evaluation and Improvement Measures

In any health care organization, some method of *performance evaluation*, sometimes called control, must be used to determine how well goals for that organization are being accomplished. Performance evaluation is one of the major tasks for any manager within the organization. This is a cyclical process that, after standards have been set, looks at measuring performance so that deviations from the standards can be discovered and corrected. Two performance evaluation measures presently used are *Benchmarking* and the *Balanced Scorecard*.

Adverse event—An untoward, undesirable, and usually unanticipated event, such as death of a patient, an employee, or a visitor in a health care organization. Incidents such as patient falls or improper administration of medications are also considered *adverse patient occurrences* even if there is no permanent effect on the patient.

Potentially compensable event—EXAMPLES: Drug errors which cause irreparable harm to a patient, amputating the wrong body part, or a less obvious incident such as mopping the floor and neglecting to put a "wet floor" sign warning of the potential hazard.

Incident—any unusual problem, incident, or other situation that is likely to lead to undesirable effects or that varies from established policies and procedures or practices.

Variance—The difference between results obtained and those expected. The sources of a variance in a process over time can be grouped into two major classes: common causes and special causes. Excessive variances frequently lead to waste and loss, such as the occurrence of undesirable patient health outcomes and increased cost of health services. *Common-cause variances* are due to the process itself and are produced by interactions of variables of that process, not a disturbance in the process. It can be removed only by making basic changes in the process. *Special-cause variances* are the difference in performance results from assignable causes. Special-cause variances are intermittent, unpredictable, and unstable. It is not inherently present in a system; rather, it arises from causes that are not part of the system as designed.

(Obtained 12/23/04 from the Joint Commission on the Accreditation of Health Care Organizations at http://www.jcaho.org/accredited+organizations/hospitals/sentinel+events/glossary.htm.)

What Is Benchmarking?

Benchmarking is the "continuous process of measuring products, services, and activities against the best levels of performance" (Baker and Baker, 2000, p. 118). It may be used as an evaluation tool to solve specific problems within a hospital, or as a continuous route to obtain total quality management (TQM). According to Thomas Cartin (1999), benchmarking may serve several purposes. These include: to analyze the organizational strengths and weaknesses of work processes and the overall strategic plan, to know who is "the best of the best" of the existing competition and to discover and adapt those "best" practices, and, finally, to become superior and be the new benchmark. In benchmarking, the performance best practices used for comparison within the process may be internal or external, national, regional, or local.

Some of the benefits to initiating a benchmarking program include:

- The motivation to remain or to become the best hospital in the field,
- It is easier to initiate change when it is evident that someone else does something better, and
- It can set a new standard within the hospital that may be long overdue.

> *"He who exercises no forethought but makes light of his opponents*
> *is sure to be captured by them."*
>
> ---
>
> *Source:* Sun Tzu, 4th century B.C. from Camp, R. (1995). *Business Process Benchmarking.* Milwaukee: ASQC, Quality Press.

Adopting those practices that have proven to make another hospital more successful can be an easier way to approach major change.

In order to apply the principles of benchmarking to improve performance within a hospital, there are four continuous steps in the process that must be followed:

1. The organization must understand its own daily processes.

2. The organization must be able to fairly analyze the processes of others.

3. The organization must be willing to realistically compare itself to others.

4. The organization must be willing and able to implement steps to close any performance gaps between it and others (*Introduction to Benchmarking*, 2002).

Although a seemingly straightforward concept and process, benchmarking cannot be successful unless it is treated as a time-consuming, perpetual improvement process. The hospital must be committed to this four-step process that continuously moves from planning, to analyzing, integrating, and implementing (Cartin, 1999). See Exhibit 1-28 for further detail of these four steps in their entirety.

With this continued diligence, benchmarking one's performance against leaders in the hospital arena "can afford the organization more efficient and effective processes, better and faster decision making, better products, more efficient and effective marketing, and smarter people" (APQC 1285, 2001, p. 1).

One problem with benchmarking is that it is easy to believe that one is comparing the same things when it is possible that this is not the case. For instance, even though two different companies benchmark total full time employees or FTEs, it is possible that one company counts temporary employees while the other excludes temporary employees.

Benchmarking in Hospital-Based Health Care

Benchmarking has been utilized in non-health care organizations for several decades in one form or another. However, it has only been recently adopted and used by the health care industry. Benchmarking in health care services is "aimed at achieving efficiency, cost effectiveness, and quality," without adversely affecting patient care outcomes (Anderson-Miles, 1994, p. 1). According to a study completed in 1999 by HCIA-Sachs in Baltimore, Maryland, it is esti-

Exhibit 1-28   Eleven-step benchmarking process

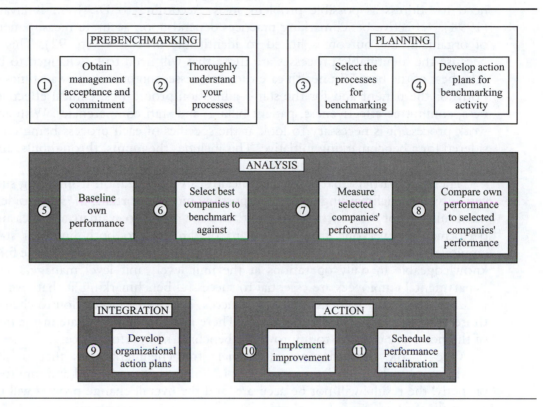

Source: Cartin, T. (1999).

mated that "$26.3 billion in hospital expenses could be cut if all US hospitals performed as well as the top 100 hospitals" (Ramsey, Ormsby, and Marsh, 2000, p. 1).

Ongoing health care reform is a prime motivator to make health care delivery sleeker and less costly. To seize the opportunity to adapt and respond quickly to changes, health care organizations need to compare themselves to others who are the best at health care delivery whether they are cross-country, or cross-town, benchmarking partners. These partners "should face similar challenges and problems" within their scope of healthcare delivery (Anderson-Miles, p. 4).

Based on an extensive literature review concerning benchmarking in health care, it is apparent that benchmarking as a performance evaluation tool or measurement is applicable in all areas of the health care field. Health care accounting, human resources, behavioral health, outpatient surgery, pharmacy, acute care, long-term care, and rehabilitation services are just a few of the service lines that benefit from the benchmarking process (Czarnecki, 1994; Gift, Stoddart, and Wilson, 1994; Hyatt, 2001; United States Department of Health and Human Services, 2001; Ramsey, Ormsby, and Marsh, 2000; Senn, 1998; Hollreiser, 1997; Balicki, Kelly, and Miller, 1995).

There are key issues that each hospital proposing a benchmarking project will need to address as possible problem areas. According to Dr. John Bullivant (1994), "effective benchmarking practices depend upon accurate measurement of organizational outcomes linked to identifiable processes" (p. 92). This is because the identifiable processes are those that will need to be changed to be "the best of the best." In health care these processes might include wait times—both for the patient and for the staff—admission procedures, clinical effectiveness, committee effectiveness, patient billing, and staff competencies. With any work process, it is necessary to look at the specifics of each process being considered for a benchmarking initiative. This includes the inputs, throughputs, and outputs of each process as potential culprits of being the problem.

There are barriers that can keep a health care organization from being successful with benchmarking. First, and possibly most important, *all* stakeholders must fully accept the benchmarking initiative as a means to evaluate and measure performance. Everyone from the board of directors to both line and staff employees must adhere. Because upper level management teams may not be fully knowledgeable in daily operations at the unit level, unit level managers and departmental employees are essential to successful benchmarking at that level.

Another barrier to benchmarking's success is a lack of motivation to change those processes identified by the results. There *must* be an immediate instigation of the necessary changes to improve the benchmarked performance.

One of the most detrimental barriers to benchmarking is that of the "garbage in, garbage out" scenario. That is, if data is not collected and inputted properly, the results will not be accurate, and the overall change process will be adversely affected.

A fourth possible addition to the list of barriers, although certainly not the last, is that of a lack of teamwork. When institutional processes are being benchmarked, everyone within the health care organization needs to remember that all departments are linked together to form the whole. For example, if wait times in the emergency department are identified as the process that needs improvement, then all ancillary departments such as radiology and laboratory need to realize that they also will need to be involved in the change process to improve the overall wait time for the emergency department (Cappozzalo, Hlywak, Kenny, and Krivenko, 1994).

Thus hospitals can, and should, use benchmarking as "an important tool that aids in strategic planning, especially when it offers a national glimpse of others in the industry" (Hyatt, 2001, p. 3). It is necessary however, to begin to think "out of the box" to fully capitalize on the benefits that benchmarking can provide for the industry as a whole.

What Is the Balanced Scorecard?

In the rapidly changing, highly competitive health care arena of today, hospital leaders are finding that the historical approach to measuring performance is insufficient. These measures included financial analyses such as *profit margins* and basic ratios such as those to determine *liquidity* and *return on total assets* (Baker and Baker, 2000). Substituted more recently is the performance evaluation method called the *Balanced Scorecard*. This method was originally co-authored by Robert S. Kaplan and David Norton in an article in 1992 entitled, "The Balanced Scorecard: Measures That Drive Performance," in the *Harvard Business Review* (Robinson, 2000).

> The Balanced Scorecard translates a company's mission and strategy into tangible objectives and measures.
>
> ――
>
> *Source:* isds.bus.lsu.edu/cvoc/learn/bpr/cprojects/spring1998/bsm/page2.html.

According to Kaplan and Norton, financial measures are "lag indicators; they report on outcomes, the consequences of past actions" (2001, p. 3). The balanced scorecard aims to look more to the future using a broader scope in strategic planning, by "considering the impact on finances, customers, internal processes, and employee learning" (Robinson, 2000, p. 23). Included within the broader scope are "both financial and non-financial measures, internal improvements, past outcomes, and ongoing requirements as indications of future performance" (Robinson, 2000, p. 1). Hence, the tool is used to "balance" and to evaluate financial measures with other, more customer- and employee-oriented measures of performance so important in the hospital setting (Nickols, 2000). In this way, it would be possible for all levels of management to be aware of how specific departmental goals affect the overall organizational goals and objectives.

Profit margin is the "bottom line" for a hospital. A positive profit margin means that the hospital had revenues that were greater than expenses.

Liquidity is the ability of the hospital to cover current expenditures.

Return on total assets is a broad measure of how well the hospital is performing financially.

To be successful with the Balanced Scorecard, the hospital must realize that "no organization has ever measured itself into excellence" (Brimson, 2002, p. 2). This means that the organization cannot simply use the scorecard as an evaluation and performance measurement tool, but also must be prepared to *change* based on the results of the measurement process. In addition, processes must be improved to adequately increase the likelihood of organizational success.

According to Brimson, with the Balanced Scorecard, the leaders of the hospital must realize that performance control and measurement is an *ongoing* process. There are tasks that must be accomplished before the tool can be effectively used:

1. The organization must determine short and long-term goals and objectives in strategic planning as well as include the processes necessary to achieve those goals and objectives.

2. Next, key performance indicators must be decided upon as a means to measure the effectiveness of the processes necessary to achieve strategic planning goals and objectives.

3. Lastly, the organization must ensure that all departments and managers have appropriate goals that directly reflect those contained within the strategic plan (Young, 1998).

> The Balanced Scorecard is not a controlling system. It is a communication, informing and learning system.
>
> ---
>
> *Source:* isds.bus.lsu.edu/cvoc/learn/bpr/cprojects/spring1998/bsm/page2.html.

Like benchmarking, putting the Balanced Scorecard into motion is a time-consuming, ongoing process to which everyone within the organization must commit for it to be successful. In addition, according to Kaplan and Norton (2001), the organizations that have been successful in implementing the Balanced Scorecard have also been able to tie incentive compensation for teams directly into the hospital goals and objectives contained within the Balanced Scorecard. Therefore, compensation is directly proportional to the amount of motivation a team has to successfully implement the changes as defined by the Balanced Scorecard. The strategies contained within the initiative then become more of a continual, repetitive process.

The Balanced Scorecard in Hospital-Based Health Care

Since its inception by Kaplan and Norton in 1992, the Balanced Scorecard has been adopted as an evaluation and performance management tool by industries across the board. This includes some healthcare agencies. However, it is a tool still within its infancy, especially in health care, and, therefore, literature expounding on its use is not widespread.

Like benchmarking, there are prime motivators behind the use of the Balanced Scorecard as a tool within the health care industry. These include "mounting pressures to reduce costs, and a desire to maintain or improve the quality of care" (Baker, Brooks, Anderson, Brown, Mckilltop, Murray, and Pink, 1998, p. 1). Baker et al. advocate that performance measures, such as the Balanced Scorecard, are only useful when they compare processes that can, and are, changed to improve patient outcomes.

The original four measures of customer satisfaction, internal processes, learning and growth, and the financial bottom line have been adapted by some health care organizations, see Exhibit 1-29 for an example from Montefiore Hospital. They have included other measurements, such as the societal perspective to "reflect community issues," such as investing in information technology

Exhibit 1-29   Montefiore Hospital's Balanced Scorecard

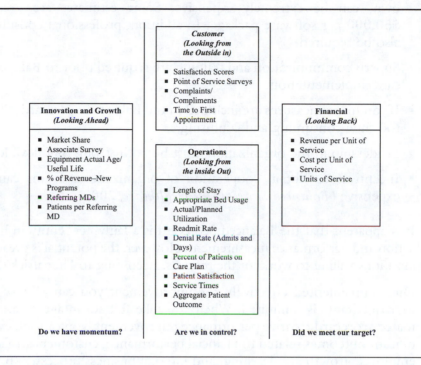

Source: Cartin, T. (1999).

(*Balanced Scorecard in Healthcare*, p. 1). Balanced Scorecard measures, much like benchmarking, must have the unfailing commitment of the entire organization to be successful. In addition, the evaluation and performance measurement process must be linked with the overall strategic goals and objectives for the organization.

There are several pros and cons of implementing a Balanced Scorecard in a health care facility. The pros are as follows:

- It forces a multidisciplinary team approach in order to be successful.

- It forces the entire health care organization to move in one unified direction toward the same strategic goals and objectives.

- The successful Balanced Scorecard ensures that the organizational strategies are well known throughout the organization.

The cons of utilizing the Balanced Scorecard within a health care organization are very important as well, because the organization cannot successfully implement it if any of these factors are present. The cons are:

- The long-existing business model can be difficult for top business executives to relinquish.

- Motivation within the organization is mandatory.

- The Balanced Scorecard software, if one does not use and design one's own, can be extremely expensive. Some estimates are greater than $50,000 per software package. In addition, professional consultants may also be required.

- Superb communication and training are required prior to Balanced Scorecard implementation.

- If too many measures are included in the Balanced Scorecard, they can be too time consuming and confusing.

- Leadership in the organization must be both strong *and* flexible.

- Incentives to obtain cooperation of organizational teams can be very expensive (*Balanced Scorecard in Healthcare*, 2000).

It is apparent that the Balanced Scorecard is a fairly new entity in health care evaluation and performance measurement. However, the potential is great for those organizations willing to work for the rewards. According to Fitzpatrick (2002):

> Once implemented effectively, the improvement you can achieve in all four quadrants is unlimited. When you take full advantage of an automated scorecard to drive performance improvement, you can achieve significant outcomes related to financial performance, customer satisfaction, employee growth and learning, and internal business processes (p. 37).

Successful implementation of this measure can achieve wonderful outcomes.

Other Evaluation Measures—Quality (TQM, CQI, QI, and QA)

Quality is one of the buzzwords that has hit hospital-based health care. Quality has long since been a focus in production and manufacturing, most specifically in Japan (Powell, 2000). How can we measure quality in a nontangible service area such as hospital-based health care? As stated in Chapter 2, quality is an elusive idea that can present somewhat of a perception problem. What I mean to say is that quality to the hospital powers-that-be might not be quality to the patient. There are several means of evaluating quality improvements in an attempt to obtain quality health care. Although there are reams of material available on this one topic, the basic concepts are presented in this chapter. The following website is a great resource: http://www.skyenet.net.

Total Quality Management (TQI), or *Continuous Quality Improvement (CQI)* is an umbrella concept that encompasses many other entities within the quest to achieve quality. One entity within the quality rubric is the risk management activities. Risk and quality are inversely proportional; meaning when quality increases, risk should decrease. The quest for quality in the United States manufacturing industry began as a way to reach the level of competition that was

Total Quality Management =

Organizational Development + Human Resources Development

In order for TQM to be successful, the mission, goals, values, plans, and patterns of the hospital must interconnect with the maximum performance of leadership, personnel, and ownership to obtain high quality organizational performance. *Source:* Green, L. E. (1999). A simplified TQM model. Retrieved September 25, 2003 from http://www.skyenet.net/leg/legindex.htm.

coming from Japan since before the 1960s. In the past decade or so, health care has caught the craze because of skyrocketing costs, more educated consumers, and more competition for patients.

According to the American Society for Quality, *total quality management* (TQM), is a "management approach centered on quality, based on organization-wide participation, and aimed at long-term success through customer satisfaction" (http://www.ASQ.org). It is a proactive, ongoing process used to increase the satisfaction of those patients that have dealings with your hospital. According to Mazur, it is the "**Total** organization using **Quality** principles for the **Management** of its processes" (2003, p. 1). Both internal customers, such as patients and employees in other departments, and external customers such as shareholders or regulatory bodies, are the main focus with this approach. Imperative to this approach is that everyone in the organization must participate by crossing functional boundaries.

Increased competition in the health care industry has been a major impetus for the eternal hunt for ways to improve the hospital's processes. Patient satisfaction with the health care services provided definitely affects the financial bottom line of any hospital. Greater profit leads to organizational stability and employee job security. Therefore quality health care services and improved customer satisfaction lead to improved profitability. Exhibit 1-30 illustrates how quality contributes to profitability.

Springing forth from this management approach are ways to ensure that organization goals for quality are being met. Enter *quality improvement* and *quality assurance*. Quality improvement involves projects that the organization undertakes in an effort to streamline and to improve quality. Quality assurance is described as the particular route that the organization checks to ensure the processes and services are improved.

Both of these concepts encompass the *PDCA* of *total quality management.* These letters stand for:

P–PLAN
D–DO
C–CHECK
A–ACT

Exhibit 1-30   Quality's Contribution to a Profitability

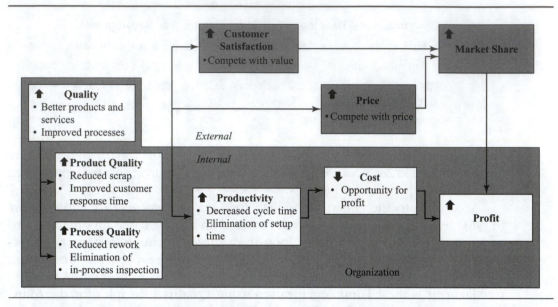

Source: The American Society for Quality (n.d). Retrieved from http://www.ASQ.org.

This cycle is known as the Deming Cycle or the Shewart Cycle. It is called a cycle because a quality improvement project never really ends, hence the words *continuous* quality improvement. According to *The Quality Toolbox* from the American Society for Quality, when starting a project to improve some process, service, or function within the hospital, it is imperative that the opportunity is recognized and the change is **Planned**. No one likes surprises in the workplace, especially ones that involve daily responsibilities and patient outcomes. Next, the change is tested out on a small scale. It is **Done** this way to ensure the least amount of impact should it not go well. The third stage, **Check**, is where the tested change is reviewed; results are analyzed, and any important information is internalized that was gleaned from the change process. The **Act** involves using the information in the Check stage to take action. If the test was successful, the action would be to initiate the changes on a larger scale. If the test was not successful, then the action would be to initiate a different tactic to facilitate further changes that might be successful in the future.

This *Plan-Do-Check-Act* cycle can be useful in many different situations besides starting a quality improvement process. For instance, another use is in data collection for root cause analyses of identified problems such as sentinel events. Many accrediting agencies use this system to judge whether or not a health care organization has made appropriate adjustments to avoid repeated events in the future. An example of its use by the Joint Commission on the Accreditation of Hospital Organizations (JCAHO) is shown in Exhibit 1-31.

Exhibit 1-31   A Framework for a Root Cause Analysis and Action Plan In Response to a Sentinel Event

Level of Analysis		Questions	Findings	Root Cause?	Ask "Why?"	Take Action
What happened?	Sentinel Event	What are the details of the event? (Brief description)				
		When did the event occur? (Date, day of week, time)				
		What area/service was impacted?				
Why did it happen?	The process or activity in which the event occurred.	What are the steps in the process, as designed? (A flow diagram may be helpful here)				
What were the most proximate factors?		What steps were involved in (contributed to) the event?				
(Typically "special cause" variation)	Human factors	What human factors were relevant to the outcome?				
	Equipment factors	How did the equipment performance affect the outcome?				
	Controllable environmental factors	What factors directly affected the outcome?				
	Uncontrollable external factors	Are they truly beyond the organization's control?				
	Other	Are there any other factors that have directly influenced this outcome?				
		What other areas or services are impacted				

Source: © Joint Commission on Accreditation of Healthcare Organizations, 2005. Reprinted with permission.

Exhibit 1-31   A Framework for a Root Cause Analysis and Action Plan In Response to a Sentinel Event *(continued)*

This template is provided as an aid in organizing the steps in a root cause analysis. Not all possibilities and questions will apply in every case, and there may be others that will emerge in the course of the analysis. However, all possibilities and questions should be fully considered in your quest for "root cause" and risk reduction.

As an aid to avoiding "loose ends," the three columns on the right are provided to be checked off for later reference:

- "Root cause?" should be answered "yes" of "No" for each finding. A root cause is typically a finding related to a process or system that has a potential for redesign to reduce risk. If a particular finding that is relevant to the event is not a root cause, be sure that it is addressed later in the analysis with a "Why?" question. Each finding that is identified as a root cause should be considered for an action and addressed in the action plan.

- "Ask 'Why?'" should be checked off whenever it is reasonable to ask why the particular finding occurred (or didn't occur when it should have) – in other words, to drill down further. Each item checked in this column should be addressed later in the analysis with a "Why?" question. It is expected that any significant findings that are not identified as root causes themselves have "roots".

- "Take action?" should be checked for any finding that can reasonably be considered for a risk reduction strategy. Each item checked in this column should be addressed later in the action plan. It will be helpful to write the number of the associated Action Item on page 3 in the "Take Action?" column for each of the findings that requires an action.

Level of Analysis	Questions	Findings	Root Cause?	Ask "Why?"	Take Action
Human Resources issues	To what degree are staff properly qualified and currently competent for their responsibilities?				
	How did actual staffing compare with ideal levels?				
	What are the plans for dealing with contingencies that would tend to reduce effective staffing levels?				
Why did that happen? What systems and processes underlie those proximate factors? (Common cause variation here may lead to special cause variation in dependent processes)					

Source: © Joint Commission on Accreditation of Healthcare Organizations, 2005. Reprinted with permission.

Exhibit 1-31   A Framework for a Root Cause Analysis and Action Plan In Response to a Sentinel Event *(continued)*

Level of Analysis		Questions	Findings	Root Cause?	Ask "Why?"	Take Action
		To what degree is staff performance in the operant process(es) addressed?				
	Information management issues	How can orientation and in-service training be improved?				
		To what degree is all necessary information available when needed? Accurate? Complete? Unambiguous?				
		To what degree is communication among participants adequate?				
	Environmental management issues	To what degree was the physical environment appropriate for the processes being carried out?				
		What systems are in place to identify environmental risks?				
		What emergency and failure-mode responses have been planned and tested?				
	Leadership issues: - Corporate culture	To what degree is the culture conducive to risk identification and reduction?				
	- Encouragement of communication	What are the barriers to communication of potential risk factors?				

Source: © Joint Commission on Accreditation of Healthcare Organizations, 2005. Reprinted with permission.

Exhibit 1-31   A Framework for a Root Cause Analysis and Action Plan In Response to a Sentinel Event *(continued)*

	Risk Reduction Strategies	Measures of Effectiveness
- Clear communication of priorities		
To what degree is the prevention of adverse outcomes communicated as a high priority? How?		
Uncontrollable factors		
What can be done to protect against the effects of these uncontrollable factors?		

Action Plan

For each of the findings identified in the analysis as needing an action, indicate the planned action expected, implementation date and associated measure of effectiveness. OR. …

If after consideration of such a finding, a decision is made not to implement an associated risk reduction strategy, indicate the rationale for not taking action at this time.

Check to be sure that the selected measure will provide data that will permit assessment of the effectiveness of the action.

Consider whether pilot testing of a planned improvement should be conducted.

Improvements to reduce risk should ultimately be implemented in all areas where applicable, not just where the event occurred. Identify where the improvements will be implemented.

Action Item #1:	
Action Item #2:	
Action Item #3:	
Action Item #4:	
Action Item #5:	
Action Item #6:	
Action Item #7:	
Action Item #8:	

Source: © Joint Commission on Accreditation of Healthcare Organizations, 2005. Reprinted with permission.

Exhibit 1-31   A Framework for a Root Cause Analysis and Action Plan In Response to a Sentinel Event *(continued)*

Cite any books or journal articles that were considered in developing this analysis and action plan:

More information on JCAHO, sentinel events, and root cause analyses can be found in the Accreditation section that follows.

There are seven tools that those striving for quality improvement can use to accomplish the *Plan-Do-Check-Act* of total quality management. These tools are listed in Exhibit 1-32. These tools are useful, especially for visually adept people, to see a graphic depiction of a process. Visualizing an issue or process sometimes makes it easier to ascertain and pinpoint where the exact problem lies.[2]

Accreditation

Who looks after all the hospitals in the United States to ensure the quality of the services provided? There is a voluntary accreditation process in which hospitals that choose to participate may be surveyed to determine if the accreditation quality criteria have been met. Different types of hospitals have different accrediting organizations. Anyone who has worked as a nurse in a hospital for any period of time has heard of the Joint Commission on the Accreditation of Healthcare Organizations (JCAHO).

This accrediting body has continually grown since the first manual of hospital standards was published in 1926. Dr. Ernest Codman first described the concept known today as outcomes measurement, or measuring the success of the care provided based partially on the outcomes achieved. In 1951 the *Joint*

Exhibit 1-32   The Seven Tools for Continuous Improvement

1. Cause and Effect Diagram (fishbone chart or Ishikawa chart)—lists the causes of organizational problems.

2. Run Chart—used to determine a pattern or trend. Usually utilized at the completion of an improvement project to determine if there was actually improvement.

3. Flowchart—depicts processes pictorially, both the actual and ideal, in order to determine improvements that could be made.

4. Pareto Chart—compares multiple problems and shows which problems offer the greatest potential for improvement.

5. Histogram—a bar chart that shows the most likely cause of a problem within a process.

6. Scatter Diagram—shows how strongly two things are related.

7. Control Chart—monitors process improvements over time.

Source: Brassard, M., Ritter, D. (1994). *The Memory Jogger™ II, A Pocket Guide of Tools for Continuous Improvement & Effective Planning.* GOAL/QPC, Salem, NH.

---

[2]Please refer to the *Memory Jogger II,* by Brassard, Ritter, Rilter, and Oddo (1994). *Handbook for Improvement: A Reference Guide of Tools for Continuous Improvement & Effective Planning,* from Executive Learning and other such resources, for more detailed information.

Commission on the Accreditation of Hospitals was formed, governed by the American Hospital Association, the American College of Physicians, the American College of Surgeons, the Canadian Medical Association, and the American Medical Association (http://www.JCAHO.org). It is interesting to note that it is only recently that JCAHO added a nurse to their board. The Joint Commission accredits each area of healthcare as listed in Exhibit 1-33. According to the Joint Commission website, almost 17,000 organizations are accredited worldwide. To be accredited, the institution must achieve the standards by which health care quality is measured in America (www.JCAHO.org).

Earning accreditation is not just a nice plaque to have on the wall of the facility. The accreditation indicates that the facility has the ability to pursue continuous quality improvement and performance measures to obtain higher quality health care. Hence, it is a coveted plaque on the wall that can mean more customers, better reimbursement, higher quality physicians, nurses, and management staff, and an overall more successful and stable organization. Being accredited by the Joint Commission effects all five of the players in the health care system: consumers, providers, payers, suppliers, and regulators.[3]

For the years 2003 and 2004, the Joint Commission's major strategic initiative has focused upon patient safety. The specific goals for 2003 and 2004 are listed in Exhibit 1-34. Beginning January 2004, these goals were incorporated into expectations when organizations are surveyed (www.JCAHO.org).

Sentinel events, defined earlier in this chapter, are events that pose significant risks to the organization and quite possibly to patients and/or employees.

Exhibit 1-33   Beginning of JCAHO Facility Accreditation

1951 — Hospitals

1966 — Long-Term Care

1969 — Behavioral Health

1975 — Ambulatory Care

1979 — Laboratory

1988 — Home Care

1994 — Networks

2000 — Assisted Living

2001 — Office-Based Surgery

2002 — Critical Access Hospitals

2002 — Disease-Specific Care

Source: © Joint Commission on Accreditation of Healthcare Organizations, 2005. Reprinted with permission.

---

[3]Consumers, providers, payers, suppliers, and regulators are explained in detail in Dunham-Taylor and Pinczuk (2006) *Health Care Financial Management for Nurse Managers: Merging the Heart with the Dollar.*

Exhibit 1-34   National Patient Safety Goals for the Joint Commission Accredited Organizations

---

2003

---

1. Improve the accuracy of patient identification.

2. Improve the effectiveness of communication among caregivers.

3. Improve the safety of using high-alert medications (such as potassium-based drugs).

4. Eliminate wrong-site, wrong-patient, wrong-procedure surgery.

5. Improve the safety of using infusion pumps.

6. Improve the effectiveness of clinical alarm systems.

2004

All of the previous six plus an additional goal:

7. Reduce the risk of health care-acquired infections.

Beginning January 2004 surveyors can score a facility on the successful implementation of ways in which to achieve these goals.

Source: © Joint Commission on Accreditation of Healthcare Organizations, 2005. Reprinted with permission.

The Joint Commission has established a Sentinel Event Policy that enumerates exactly those procedures that are expected in each facility after a sentinel event occurs. According to Medical Risk Management Associates, LLC, if a sentinel event process is not already in place should a sentinel event occur, risks increase dramatically because the facility started out already behind (http://www.root-causeanalyst.com/costeffective.htm). In other words, after such an event occurs, without proper processes in place, inappropriate behaviors such as panic and/or crisis mode can follow (2001, p. 1).

The Sentinel Event Policy from the Joint Commission specifically states that hospital leaders are to have the processes established for the "identification, reporting, analysis, and prevention of sentinel events and for ensuring the consistent and effective implementation of a mechanism to accomplish these activities" (http://www.JCAHO.org/sentinel). Some sentinel events that have recently been highlighted as current problematic areas in 2002 and 2003 include:

- Preventing surgical fires,

- Infection control related sentinel events,

- Bed rail-related entrapment deaths,

- Delays in treatment, and

- Preventing ventilator-related deaths and injuries (http://www.JCAHO.org).

The occurrences that will be reviewed by the Joint Commission are listed in Exhibit 1-35.

When exploring sentinel events, a *root cause analysis* must be determined. This is a process, as defined by the Joint Commission, "that identifies the basic or causal (hence the name **root cause**) factors that underlie variation in performance, including the occurrence or possible occurrence of a sentinel event" (http://www.JCAHO.org). Most often, the root cause is not one particular person who makes a mistake or has an accident, but also involves improving other organizational processes to decrease the likelihood of similar events recurring. An example of an approach to assist in identifying and eliminating the true root of problems is called Six Sigma. This is a problem-solving methodology that focuses on quality, service delivery and revenue growth.

As stated previously, while the Joint Commission is one of the largest accrediting bodies within health care, there are others that accredit different types of agencies. For instance, rehabilitation facilities such as Albert Einstein Medical Center Moss Rehabilitation Hospital in Pennsylvania are surveyed by an organization known as the Commission on Accreditation of Rehabilitation Facilities (CARF). Much like Joint Commission, this voluntary accreditation certifies that the rehabilitation facility meets or exceeds the quality standards set by the Commission. This accreditation type applies to adult day rehabilitation services, assisted living rehabilitation services, some behavioral health services, and/or medical inpatient rehabilitation services. According to the Commission, 38,000 services have earned their accreditation (http://www.carf.org).

Osteopathic facilities also experience a different accreditation body. The accrediting agency for these health care facilities is the American Osteopathic Association (http://www.healthsciences.okstate.edu/center/student/campus.htm). For example, Oklahoma State University Health Sciences Center near Tulsa, Oklahoma, practices osteopathy. Both a teaching facility and a community health resource, this facility sees an influx of patients numbering about 20,000 annually.

Exhibit 1-35 JCAHO Reviewable Sentinel Events

---

1. Unanticipated death or major permanent loss of function OR
2. The event is one of the following:
   - Suicide while inpatient
   - Unanticipated death of a full-term infant
   - Infant abduction or discharge to wrong family
   - Rape occurring within the facility
   - Transfusion reaction with major blood incompatibilities
   - Surgery on the wrong body part

Source: © Joint Commission on Accreditation of Healthcare Organizations, 2005. Reprinted with permission.

Six Sigma is "a disciplined, data-driven approach for eliminating defects" which strives for perfection (http://www.isixsigma.com/sixsigma/six_sigma.asp). The number of defects can be no more than six standard deviations from the mean. How does this apply to a service industry such as healthcare? Well, "to achieve Six Sigma, a process must not produce more than 3.4 defects per million opportunities. A Six Sigma defect is defined as anything outside of customer specifications. A Six Sigma opportunity is then the total quantity of chances for a defect." Therefore, in healthcare a Six Sigma would involve no more than 3.4 disappointments per million customer expectations. WOW! That would be near perfection!!! Remembering of course, that customers for a hospital are not just the patients, but also include people such as family members, physicians, and vendors.

According to the Six Sigma LLC, the "fundamental objective of the Six Sigma methodology is the implementation of a measurement-based strategy that focuses on process improvement and variation reduction through the application of Six Sigma projects." (http://www.isixsigma.com/sixsigma/six_sigma.asp) Examples of Six Sigma Methodologies are DMADV (define-measure-analyze-design-verify) for new products or services and DMAIC (define-measure-analyze-improve-control) for existing products or services.

DMADV	Define	• Define the project goals and customer (internal and external deliverables).
	Measure	• Measure and determine customer needs and specifications.
	Analyze	• Analyze the process options to meet the customer needs.
	Design	• Design (detailed) the process the meet the customer needs.
	Verify	• Verify the design performance and ability to meet customer needs.
DMAIC	Define	• Define the project goals and customer (internal and external) deliverables.
	Measure	• Measure the process to determine current performance.
	Analyze	• Analyze and determine the root cause(s) of the defects.
	Improve	• Improve the process by eliminating defects.
	Control	• Control future process performance.

Source: http://www.isixsigma.com/library/content/c001211a.asp.

HIP What?

With so much emphasis on ensuring that hospitals are "leaner and meaner" and providing more quality in services rendered, it is no surprise that the United States government had to get in on the action. In the mid 1990s Congress took

Osteopathic treatment assesses and treats from the perspective of the whole body and seeks to restore the proper mobility of its component parts and re-establish synchronous and harmonious relationships among its systems (musculoskeletal, circulatory, digestive, pulmonary and neural). The patient is assessed and treated as a *whole person*.

Source: Definition of Osteopathy (2003). Retrieved November 12, 2003 from http://www.osteopathy-canada.com.

up the issue of health care reform, specifically in the areas of health information portability and patient information confidentiality. This was a necessity not only because of skyrocketing health care costs but also because an estimated 16 percent of Americans were uninsured, with still more being denied insurance based on pre-existing conditions (Mathis and Jackson, 2003). Simultaneously, due to economic declines, Americans were forced to change jobs more frequently.

Employees were being covered under new and different health care plans, which often required them to change to new providers and to transfer their confidential patient records to a new facility. In addition, technological advancements, such as emails, facsimiles, and scanners were making it easier for hospitals to obtain and disseminate private medical information. As technology improved, there was an increased need to protect a person's health information. To ensure a patient's privacy and insurance coverage, the Health Insurance Portability and Accountability Act (HIPAA) was enacted.

The Health Insurance Portability and Accountability Act protects the rights of employees while allowing them to change their health insurance plan from company to company without being penalized for pre-existing medical conditions (Root, Kabbe, Hubbard, and Hartley, 2002). Additionally, the law makes it illegal for a company to deny coverage to a sick employee and mandates that coverage be made available to those leaving a group plan (Mathis and Jackson, 2003). On August 21, 1996, President Clinton signed HIPAA, Public Law 104-191, into effect (Root et al., 2002).

The rules embodied within HIPAA are voluminous. HIPAA is one of the most complex and far-reaching set of federal regulations and has had the largest impact on health care since Medicare (Root et al., 2002). The primary objectives of HIPAA are to improve the efficiency of health care delivery, to protect the privacy of health care information by enforcing standards for privacy and security, and to empower individual clients with new rights related to their protected health information (Katten et al., 2001). HIPAA is also intended to provide a foundation for insurance reform. The goal of this insurance reform is to provide and improve portability and continuity of health insurance for individuals.

HIPAA is composed of three sections: the Transactions and Code Set, Security Regulations, and Privacy Regulations. The Transactions and Code Set Standards are designed to improve the efficiency of health plans and payment

Health Insurance Portability and Accountability Act (HIPAA)

- Improve the efficiency of health care delivery.
- Protect the privacy of health care information by enforcing standards for privacy and security.
- Empower individual clients with new rights related to their protected health information (Katten et al., 2001).

systems. This is accomplished through the establishment of common languages for data transmissions. The Security Regulations are designed to protect patient information from accidental or unauthorized disclosure, destruction, modification, or loss (Katten et al., 2001). These Security Regulations will certainly have an enormous impact as our technology continues to expand and to allow more individuals access to protected health information.

The Privacy Regulations were designed to govern the use and disclosure of patient information, and to grant individuals certain rights with respect to their protected health information (Katten et al., 2001). *Protected health information* (PHI) is defined as "information that is individually identifiable by virtue of its containing one or more patient identifiers, such as name, social security number, phone number, medical record number, or zip code" (Root et al., 2002). The rule names 18 such patient identifiers. Although first published in December 2001, the privacy standards were not fully implemented until April 14, 2003.

HIPAA guarantees certain rights and rules:

- The right to view one's own medical records.
- The right to confidential medical records.
- The right to control others' access to medical records.
- The law specifies all patient identifying information must be treated as protected health information (Katten et al., 2001).

These rules, under the Health Information Portability and Accountability Act (1996), create national standards that protect individual medical records and other health information. These privacy regulations assure patients that they have the right to control who can access their protected, identifiable health information. The privacy rules apply to all identifiable health information, whether electronic, paper, or oral (Katten et al., 2001). HIPAA helps to set boundaries and safeguards, outlining who can access privileged health care information, and holds accountable those releasing this information. For all health care arenas, communications with or about patients involving protected health information (PHI) must be private and limited to those who need this information to provide treatment, payment, or health care operations.

HIPAA Compliance

Implementing HIPAA privacy standards are requiring health care organizations to develop many new policies and procedures, create new documents, and decide how to integrate them into practice. Administrators have also been faced with deciding which employees will have access to protected health information (PHI), as well as to what extent and to whom reports may be shared. These concerns have imposed a heavy burden on smaller organizations that do not have the resources to dedicate to implementing these changes.

HIPAA changes cannot be a one-time change. Constant vigilance is necessary to ensure that compliance is maintained. In accordance with the privacy rules, HIPAA standards state that every covered entity must have a *privacy officer* on site (Root et al., 2002). The privacy officer must be knowledgeable about the clinical and administrative functions of the organization and know the laws surrounding the privacy of health information (Root et al., 2002).

The privacy officer is responsible for maintaining compliance with the privacy rules. The organizational lawyer assists with this task. Additionally, the privacy officer must establish compliance activities, and implement methods to effectively deal with complaints, develop policies and procedures, and coordinate with human resources the implementation and training component for all employees (Katten et al., 2001).

Before implementation can begin, the privacy officer should choose a privacy team. The members should represent each department. Essential training should begin with these members. HIPAA implementation should be divided into four phases (Root et al., 2002). The first phase involves learning HIPAA basics, defining job responsibilities, developing a documentation system that is HIPAA compliant, executing a budget, and setting a time line to meet objectives (Root et al., 2002). The second phase involves the translation of the privacy rules into documents for the entire health care organization. This phase involves understanding the flow of protected health information, developing a Notice of Privacy Practices, and drafting HIPAA policies and procedures (Root et al., 2002).

The third phase is referred to as the training phase. Here, a training program for all employees is developed, and employees are tested for understanding (Root et al., 2002). This phase is most important and therefore must receive appropriate attention. Employees need to be properly trained to know how to avoid HIPAA compliance violations. This way, costly sanctions that can be imposed on the violators and the organization as a whole can be avoided.

Phase four is the actual implementation of HIPAA. This involves developing authorization forms, obtaining signed acknowledgements, identifying your business associates, developing a business contract, and assessing the status of compliance (Root et al., 2002).

HIPAA violations can be very costly. Fines can be civil, criminal, or private, and can be imposed on the individual and/or the organization. Civil fines for a breach of privacy can be $100 per violation per subject and per person (Katten et al., 2001). Criminal penalties can be imposed if a person knowingly accessed, used, or disclosed protected health information improperly. These fines are much larger. For example, if a person inappropriately accessed protected health information, the fine could be as much as $50,000 and/or imprisonment for up to one year. If protected health information is accessed under false pretenses, the fine is $100,000 and imprisonment can be up to five years. If the protected health information was accessed for commercial reasons, the fine increases to $250,000 and the imprisonment may be for up to ten years (Katten et al., 2001). From the drastic punishment for infractions it is obvious that it is imperative to ensure that all staff members are properly trained. The training provided must be carefully documented and available for inspection by approved entities, monitors or agencies.

Conclusion

It is not difficult to understand how this chapter could have been much longer given the complex nature of health care. However, the overall goal of this chapter has been to provide a general idea of some basics concepts experienced by hospitals as care is delivered. I hope that there are topics covered within this chapter that have raised enough interest in your mind that you will read not only other chapters in more depth in this book, but pursue other avenues of learning as well. Health care is an ever-changing, evolving entity that requires constant literature reviews to remain current.

References

Aetna, Inc. (2003). Utilization review policies. Retrieved October 1, 2003 from http://www.aetna.com.

Aiken, L. H., Clarke, S. P., Sloane, D. M., Sochalski, J., & Silber, J. H. (2002). Hospital nurse staffing and patient mortality, nurse burnout, and job dissatisfaction. *Journal of the American Medical Association,* 288(16).

American Association of Colleges of Nursing (2003). Nursing shortage fact sheet. Retrieved December 12, 2003 from http://www.aacn.nche.edu/Media/Backgrounders/shortagefacts.htm.

American Hospital Association (2002, June). Challenges facing rural hospitals. *Trendwatch,* 4(1).

American Hospital Association (1994, 1998, and 2000). Annual survey. As cited in Kralovec, P. and Reczynski, S. (2000). Profile of U.S. Hospitals. *Hospital and Health Networks.* Retrieved May 18, 2003 from http://www.hospitalconnect.com.

American Organization of Nurse Executives (2003). Healthy work environments: Striving for excellence, volume II, Manassas, VA: McManis & Monsalve Associates.

American Organization of Nurse Executives (2002, November). CMS recognizes commission accreditation for critical access hospitals. *News update,* 8(15), 1.

American Productivity & Quality Center. (2001, January). *Impact of the new economy on benchmarking.* Retrieved August 15, 2003 from http://www.apqc.org/free/articles/dispArticle.cfm?ProductID=1285.

Anderson-Miles, E. (1994, September). Benchmarking in healthcare organizations. *Healthcare Financial Management*. 9, 1.

Bailey, K. D. (1994). Typologies and taxonomies: An introduction to classification techniques. Thousand Oaks, CA: Sage Publications.

Baker, G., Brooks, N., Anderson, G., Brown, A., Mckilltop, I., Murray, M., & Pink, G. (1998). Healthcare performance measurement in Canada: Who's doing what. *Hospital Quarterly*. Retrieved September 10, 2003 from http://www.longwoods.com/hq/winter98/feature2.html.

Baker, J. and Baker, R. (2000). Health care finance: Basic tools for non-financial managers. Gaithersburg: MD: Aspen Publishers, Inc.

Balanced Score Card in Healthcare (2000). Retrieved August 15, 2003 from http://www.fonendo.com.

Balicki, B., Kelly, W., and Miller, H. (1995, September). Establishing benchmarks for ambulatory surgery centers. *Healthcare Financial Management*. Retrieved March 5, 2002 from http://80- galenet.galegroup.com.ezproxy.etsu.edu.

Billows, L. A. (1997). Case management. As cited in Harris, M. (1997). *Handbook of home health care administration*. Gaithersburg, MD: Aspen Publishers.

Blumenthal, D. (2002). As cited in American Hospital Association (2002, May). Teaching hospitals—social missions at risk. *Trendwatch*, 4(2), 1.

Boles, K. E. and Neumann, B. R. (1999). Introduction to finance and managed care. *Managed care finance and managed care*. Retrieved September 4, 2003 from http://hmi.missouri.edu/Course_Materials/Residential_HSM/semesters/f99materials/hsm472/Chapter 1_Draft.doc.

Brassard, M., Ritter, D., Rilter, D., and Oddo, F. (1994). *The memory jogger™ II, A pocket guide of tools for continuous improvement & effective planning*. Salem, NH: Goal/QPC.

Brimson, J. (2002). *Why your Balanced Scorecard will not be successful-unless . . . Part 1*. Retrieved August 15, 2003 from http://www.systemcorp.com/framesite/downloads/frames/brimson_frame.html.

Brooks, C. A. (1999). Healthcare organizations. In Yoder-Wise, P. S. (1999). *Leading and managing in Nursing*. 2nd ed. St. Louis: Mosby, Inc.

Bullivant, J. (1994). *Benchmarking for continuous improvement in the public sector*. Essex United Kingdom: Longman Information and Reference.

Burns, L. P., Bazzoli, G. J., Dynan, L., and Wholey, D. R. (2000). Impact of HMO market structure on physician-hospital strategic alliances. *Health Services Research*. Retrieved December 8, 2003 from http://www.findarticles.com/cf_dls/m4149/l_35/62162629/print.jhtml

Busby, A. and Busby, A. (2001, June). Critical access hospitals: Rural nursing issues. *Journal of Nursing Administration*, 31(6), 301–310.

Camp, R. (1995). *Business process benchmarking*. Milwaukee: ASQC, Quality Press.

Cappozzalo, G., Hlywak, J., Kenny, B., and Krivenko, C. (1994, September). Experts discuss how benchmarking improves the healthcare industry. *Healthcare Financial Management*. Retrieved September 5, 2003 from http://80-galenet.galegroup.com.ezproxy.etsu.edu.

Cardinal, D. (2003, October). Benchmarks key in medical director pay-setting methods. *Physician Compensation Report*. Retrieved December 19, 2003 from http://www.findarticles.com.

Cartin, T. (1999). Principles and practices of organizational performance excellence. Milwaukee, WI: ASQ, Quality Press.

CASEMIX Quarterly (2003, June). *The 2003 CASEMIX Summer school.* Retrieved May 23, 2003 from http://www.casemix.org/act.asp?InizID=15.

Centers for Medicare and Medicaid Services (2002). Program information. Retrieved May 24, 2003 from http://www.CMS.hhs.gov/charts/default.asp.

Centers for Medicare and Medicaid Services (2003). Related change request. Retrieved May 6, 2005 from http://www.CMS.hhs.gov/medlearn/matters/mmarticles/2003/mm3036.pdf.

Christiansen, D. (2003, April). CAH designation earns deemed status. *Nursing Management, 34*(4), 18

Cohen, E. and Cesta, T. (2001). *Nursing case management: From essentials to advanced practice applications.* 3rd ed. St. Louis: Mosby, Inc.

Coile, R. C. (2003, September–October). 10 factors affecting the physician shortage of the future. *The physician executive,* 62–65.

Cooke, M. K. and Brodrick, T. M. (1997). Critical pathways. As cited in Harris, M. (1997). *Handbook of home health care administration.* Gaithersburg, MD: Aspen Publishers.

Cordes, S. (1996). Health care services and the rural economy. Chicago: Federal Reserve Bank of Chicago, as cited in American Hospital Association (2002, June). Challenges facing rural Hospitals. *Trendwatch, 4*(1), 2.

Czarnecki, M. (1994, September). Benchmarking can add up for healthcare accounting. *Healthcare Financial Management.* Retrieved September 5, 2003 from http://80-galenet.galegroup.com.ezproxy.etsu.edu.

Darves, B. (2003, November). Here come the hospitalists. Retrieved January 28, 2004 from http://www.nejmjobs.org/resource_center/Here_Come_the_Hospitalists.asp.

Duke University Health Systems Medical Center Information Systems (2002). Welcome to Duke University Health Systems Medical Center. Retrieved July 16, 2003 from http://www.mc.duke.edu.

Duke University Medical Center (2001). *Observation status Medicare rules.* Retrieved May 25, 2003 from http://www.jcaho.mc.duke.edu/obs.pdf.

Dunham-Taylor, J., & Pinczuk, J. (2006). *Financial management for nurse managers: Merging the heart with the dollar.* Sudbury, MA: Jones and Bartlett.

Ebener, M. (November–December, 1985). Reliability and validity basics for evaluating classification systems. *Nursing Economic$, 3,* 324–327.

Erwin, J. (1999, June). A simple plan: Discharge planning improves the odds. *Nurse-Week.* Retrieved August 29, 2003 from http://www.nurseweek.com/features/99-6/discharg.html.

Fischer, W. (1995). PCS and casemix types. Retrieved May 30, 2003 from http://www.fischer-zim.ch/notes-en/counts-of-PCS-Groups-9911.htm.

Fitzpatrick, M. (2002, March). Let's bring balance to healthcare. *Nursing Management, 33*(3), 35–37.

Gift, T., Stoddart, T., and Wilson, K. (1994, September). Collaborative benchmarking in a healthcare system. *Healthcare Financial Management.* Retrieved September 5, 2003 from http://80-galenet.galegroup.com.ezproxy.etsu.edu.

Gilbert, B. (1997, October). Study shows for-profit hospital conversions help communities by injecting capital. *Modern Healthcare.* Retrieved May 26, 2003 from http://www.uhsinc.com.

Ginter, P. M., Swayne, L. E., and Duncan, W. J. (2002). *Strategic management of health care organizations.* 4th ed. Malden, MA: Blackwell Publishers.

Giovannetti, P., and Mayer, G. (August 1984). Building confidence in patient classification systems. *Nursing Management,* 15(8), 31–34.

Gosfield, A. G. (2003, November). The stark truth about the Stark Law: Part 1. *Family Practice Magazine,* 10(10), 27–33.

Green, L. E. (1999). A simplified TQM model. Retrieved September 25, 2003 from http://www.skyenet.net/leg/legindex.htm.

Gulati, R. (1998). Alliances and networks. *Strategic Management Journal,* 19(2), 29–33.

Halasa, M. (n.d.). Door opens slightly to profit-sharing models. Retrieved December 16, 2003 from http://www.hcfinance.com/nov/5side1/html.

Hardin, S. and Langford, D. (2001). Telehealth's impact on nursing and the development of the interstate compact. *Journal of Professional Nursing,* 17(5), 243–247.

Hawthorne, D. (2003, July). *The business of healthcare report: Health care labor costs soar.* Retrieved November 20, 2003 from http://www2.texashealth.org/krld/2003/03-28_July2003.htm.

Health Care Financing Administration (now CMS). (2001, May). Medicare Hospital Manual. Retrieved June 4, 2003 from http://www.cms.hhs.gov/manuals/pm_trans/R772HO.pdf.

Hoffman, F. and Wakefield, D. S. (1986, April). Ambulatory care patient classification. *Journal of Nursing Administration,* 16(4), 23–30.

Hollreiser, E. (1997, January 3). Managed health care helps new drug development. *Philadelphia Business Journal.* Retrieved September 5, 2003 from http://80-galenet.galegroup.com.ezproxy.etsu.edu.

Hoppszallern, S. (2003). Health care benchmarking. *Hospitals & Health Networks.*

Hyatt, L. (2001, October). A venture in benchmarking. *Nursing Homes.* Retrieved September 5, 2003 from http://80-galenet.galegroup.com.ezproxy.etsu.edu.

Introduction to Benchmarking. (2002). Retrieved August 15, 2003 from http://www.benchmarking-in-europe.com.

Kaplan, R. and Norton, D. (2001). *The strategy focused organization: How Balanced Scorecard companies thrive in the new business environment.* Boston: Harvard Business School Publishing Corporation.

Katten Muchen Zavis (2001, October). How to begin the process of becoming HIPAA compliant. North Carolina Hospital Association. http://www.hospitalconnect.com/aha/key-issues.

Kippenbrock, T., Stacy, A., Tester, K., and Richey, R. (2002). Nurse practitioners providing health care to rural and underserved areas in four Mississippi Delta states. *Journal of Professional Nursing,* 18(4), 230–237.

Kirk, J. K., Michael, K. A., Markowsky, S. J., Restino, M. R., and Zarowitz, B. J. (1996). Critical pathways: The time is here for pharmacist involvement. *Pharmacotherapy,* 16(4), 723–733.

Kowal, N. S. and Delaney, M. (1996, May–June). The economics of a nurse-developed pathway. *Nursing Economic$*, 14(3), 156.

Larkin, H. (2003). The case for nurse practitioners. *Hospitals and Health Networks*. Retrieved August 20, 2003 from http://www.hospitalconnect.com.

Lee, D. T. F., Mackenzie, A. E., Dudley-Brown, S., and Chin, T. M. (1998). Case management: A review of the definitions and practices. *Journal of Advanced Nursing*, 27, 933–939.

Managed Care Concepts (2002). Precertification, utilization review, discharge planning. Retrieved September 22, 2003 from http://www.managedcareconcepts.com/utilization_management.html#pre-Certification.

Marks, T. (n.d.). Medicare hospital reimbursement. Retrieved June 4, 2003 from http://sitemaker.umich.edu/jbilli/files/medicare_part_a_briefing.ppt.

Massachusetts College of Emergency Physicians (2003). Ambulatory payment classifications. Retrieved June 3, 2003 from http://www.macep.org/practice_information/APCs.htm.

Mathis, R. L. and Jackson, J. H. (2003). Managing employee benefits. *Human Resource Management*. 10th ed. Mason, OH: South-Western.

Mazur, G. H. (2003). Total quality management. Retrieved September 25, 2003 from http://www.mazur.net/tqm/default.htm.

McCullough, A. C. (n.d.). *The Stark Law: Significant considerations for hospitals.* Retrieved December 19, 2003 from http://www.faegre.com/downloads/seminars/stark_law/mccullough.ppt.

Minge, D. (2001). Medicare payment disparities that adversely affect rural areas. As cited in Medicare Justice Coalition (2002, May). The impact of low payment rates on communities. Retrieved May 30, 2003 from http://www.mnseniors.net/_ftp/impactofadequatemedicarereimbursement020518.pdf.

Monarch, K. (2003). Magnet hospitals: Powerful force for excellence. *Reflections on Nursing Leadership*, Honor Society of Nursing, Sigma Theta Tau International.

Morrissey, J. (2002). Hospitals offer remote control. *Modern Healthcare*, 32(51), 32–36.

National Conference of State Legislatures (2002). Critical access hospitals. Retrieved May 30, 2003 from http://www.ncsl.org/programs/health/cawgreen.htm.

Nickols, F. (2000). *The accountability scorecard: A stakeholder approach to "keeping score."* Retrieved August 15, 2003 from http://www.systemcorp.com/framesite/downloads/frames/nickols_frame.html.

Oregon Health and Science University (2003). Office of rural health: The Medicare rural hospital flexibility program in Oregon. Retrieved May 23, 2003 from http://www.ohsu.edu/oregonruralhealth.cahinfog.html.

Peters, D. A. (1997). Classification: A tool from managed care. As cited in Harris, M. (1997). Handbook of home health care administration. Gaithersburg, MD: Aspen Publishers.

Powell, S. K. (2000). *Case management: A practical guide to success in managed care.* 2nd ed. Baltimore, MD: Lippincott, Williams, and Wilkins.

Prescott, P. A. and Soeken, K. L. (1996). Approaches to and uses of patient classification systems (Measuring nursing intensity in ambulatory care, part 1). *Nursing Economic$*, 14(1), 14–23.

Ramsey, C., Ormsby, T., and Marsh, T. (2000, December). Performance-Improvement strategies can reduce costs. *Healthcare Financial Management*. Retrieved August 15, 2003 from http://80-galenet.galegroup.com.ezproxy.etsu.edu.

Renholm, M., Leino-Kilpi, H., and Suominem, T. (2002, April). Critical pathways: A systematic review. *Journal of Nursing Administration,* 32(4), 196–202.

Report on Medicare Compliance (2003, September 18). Medical-director compliance flaws persist as scrutiny grows: Curtail iffy compensation. Retrieved December 12, 2003 from http://www.aishealth.com/Bnow/092303d.html.

Robinson, R. (2000, January 24). Balanced Scorecard. *Computerworld*. Retrieved August 15, 2003 from http://www.systemcorp.com/framesite/downloads/frames/robinson_frame.html.

Rohrbach, J. I. (1999). Critical pathways as an essential part of a disease management program. *Journal of Nursing Care Quality,* 14(1), 11–15.

Root, J., Kabbe, D., Hubbard, M., and Hartley, C. (2002). *Field guide to HIPAA implementation*. New York: AMA Press.

Sackman, K. (n.d.). *The rise of for-profit organizations*. Retrieved August 28, 2003 from http://www.afscme.org/una/nurse05.htm.

Senn, G. (1998, May). Clinical buy-in is key to benchmarking success. *Healthcare Financial Management*. Retrieved September 5, 2003 from http://80-galenet.galegroup.com/exproxy.etsu.edu

Simmons, C. W. (1998). Risk management (Managing standards). Retrieved October 1, 2003 from http://sparc.airtime.co.uk/users/wysywig/risk_1htm#INTRO.

Terry, K. (2002, August). The changing face. *Medical Economics,* 72–79.

United States Department of Health and Human Services (2001). Medicare hospital manual: Section 415.18 - Criteria and payment for sole community hospitals and for Medicare dependent hospitals. Retrieved June 4, 2003 from http://www.hhs.gov.

United States Department of Health and Human Services (2001). Behavioral health care system strives to handle increased demand. *Health Care Financing Review*. Retrieved September 5, 2003 from http://80-galenet.galegroup.com.ezproxy.etsu.edu.

United States Department of Health and Human Services (2002, April). What kind of doctor is a hospitalist? CMS publication: Baltimore, MD.

United States Department of Health and Human Services (2003). Bureau of health professions: American hospital workforce survey (2001). Retrieved August 28, 2003 from http://www.bhpr.hrsa.gov/healthworkforce/reports/default.htm.

Van Slyck, A. (2000). Patient classification systems: Not a proxy for nurse 'busyness.' *Nursing Administration Quarterly,* 24(4), 60–68.

Wachter, R. M. and Goldman, L. (2002, January). The hospitalist movement 5 years later. *Journal of the American Medical Association,* 287(4), 487–494.

Weber, D. (2003, January–February). Health care trends: What's hot, what's not, and what does the future hold? *The Physician Executive,* 6–14.

Young, D. (1998). Score it a hit. *CIO Enterprise Magazine*. Retrieved August 15, 2003 from http://www.systemcorp.com/framesite/downloads/frames/young_frame.html.

2

Using Inpatient Tools to Predict Cost and Measure Performance

Louise Gifford, MSN, RN

Introduction

This chapter focuses on key elements of the budget process and provides examples of budgeting tools for inpatient care. Each tool supports the budgeting process through various stages. Through standardization of these processes, departmental performance and planning occur in an organized, consistent manner from the unit level, department level, and divisional level.

The current climate in health care focuses on quality care, efficiency, and cost effectiveness. Managed care continues to squeeze costs (and arguably quality care) from health care organizations. Newspapers, journals, the media, and nearly every other form of communication contain articles and editorials proposing change, warning harm to growing elderly and other fragile populations, and focusing blame in every arena. While the debate ensues, health care organizations struggle to deliver quality care and survive financially.

The role of the nurse manager as a manager of both cost *and* quality continues to be an extremely important one. The nurse manager, in addition to strong clinical skills, must have a knowledge base in financial management specific to budget preparation and control procedures. Basic understanding of reimbursement, and of accounting and finance terminology, helps the nurse manager to build relationships with fiscal managers in the organization. Finally, the ultimate goal of an effective management team is to integrate actual financial performance with quality care indicators.

Learning about costing nursing services impacts several important areas of the nurse manager's realm of authority. Nursing hours, their supporting costs, and quality care, all link directly to the nurse manager. Any patient experience results in a consumer review, formal or informal, of the nursing and medical care received.

The nurse manager's role in patient satisfaction and in managing patient and family complaints offers balance to costs and care. While the consumer of health services does not often see a "line item" for nursing services on their bill, *patient satisfaction derives predominantly from direct nursing care.* Items such as drugs, time in the operating room and post-anesthesia unit, time with a therapist, laboratory tests, radiology tests and their interpretation, and many other line items only *imply* the presence of the expensive nursing resource. Imagine a nursing services' bill for emotional support, patient education, and nursing measures that directly prevent complications and longer lengths of stay! These essential elements of nursing care represent the expected level of service in health care.

The nurse manager's direct involvement in the budget process represents a more recent change in nursing roles and expectations. Moving the budget process to the same level as patient care pushes decision making to the point of care. The point of care then influences spending priorities and budget decisions. Managers contribute their abilities to integrate the financial, quantitative picture with the clinical picture. This integration advances the decision-making process to include important patient care issues such as safety, timely pharmacy and nutrition services, appropriate therapy services, patient satisfaction, and physician satisfaction. All of these areas represent important elements of cost and quality. The nurse executive and the nurse manager, through their planning and communication processes, create a holistic representation of the important elements of care through their knowledge and interpretation of patient care outcome data. *The nurse manager can relate changes in patient satisfaction to an inability to recruit adequate staff to maintain the budgeted nursing hours. This ties the process for selection and recruitment of qualified staff with how satisfied patients are with their care.*

Financial Responsibilities in Nursing

With ever-increasing responsibilities, the role of the nurse manager has expanded to both managing costs and dealing with the ways in which costs affect nursing quality. Some nursing administration departments have chosen to add a financial manager position. This individual may or may not be a nurse. Depending on the nurse executive, this role provides expertise and resources to the nurse manager in an effort to support both positive financial and patient care decisions.

As the nurse manager and nurse executive assume more financial responsibilities, they interact with finance department personnel. As both nursing and financial personnel grapple with difficult financial issues, sometimes the financial personnel think that "[nurse] managers do not always understand 'no'"(Zachry and Gilbert, 1992, p. 51). The concern for patient care quality, despite the need for financial success, suggests that there are situations in which "no" is unacceptable. The best solutions occur when the nurse manager and nurse executive possess a basic understanding of financial management and are involved in the discussion and planning to find more acceptable alternatives. Without the ability to suggest and quantify alternatives, safe patient outcomes can be at risk.

In recent literature, nurse educators and administrators have recognized the need for nurse executives to understand basic financial management concepts. Lemire (2000) discusses the importance of financial management education for graduate students in nursing administration. Jones (1994) states, "The nurse managers are increasingly being held responsible for meeting cost-containment objectives with their unit budgets" (p. 4). Although most authorities agree that neither the nurse manager nor the nurse executive needs a business degree, there is wide agreement that basic financial knowledge is required.

The potential impact nurse managers exert on their departmental counterparts suggests that even basic knowledge combined with collaboration skills can impact change. Caroselli (1993) suggests that economic awareness among nurse managers can have a positive impact on direct care staff. While the impact on direct care staff certainly seems achievable, the whole picture of influence is wider and potentially touches every department that provides services in the patient care arena. The opportunity for meaningful planning and effective strategies for change among first-line managers requires an executive team who is interested in real quality. The nurse manager and the individuals responsible for linens, solutions, medical supplies, office supplies, and respiratory supplies, create the potential for decision making based on both quality and efficiency.

Often, clinical nursing expertise is the sole reason for a person's promotion to a first-line managerial position. However, the knowledge of excellent patient care, combined with basic knowledge in financial management, achieves more balance in setting priorities for spending scarce resources. Another important nurse manager role is the development of collaborative relationships with financial managers. Then the nurse manager can learn and build on basic knowledge, while influencing the attitudes and priorities of the financial staff. Ray et al. (1995) suggest that nurse managers "through their ethical choices, can position an efficient health care delivery system grounded in caring and economic responsibility" (p. 50). They suggest strategies that "include reflection-in-action, mental models . . . covenantal relationship, and shared vision" (p. 50). The nurse manager fosters innovative communication and information processing systems that balance a bottom-line philosophy with patient care quality and employee satisfaction.

Building the Labor Budget

Most organizations use several key statistics to build the nursing patient care unit budget. These key statistics generally include:

- The nursing hour per patient day (NHPPD),
- The average patient census per day, and
- The percentage of registered nurse hours in direct care.

Other variables consistently reported include:

- Length of stay,
- Diagnosis-related group (DRG) reimbursements,
- Age,
- Race, and
- Sex.

Nursing departments identify their costs most frequently using some acuity system method (Eckhart, 1993). Unfortunately, definitions for key statistics are not uniformly used. An important request on the part of the nurse manager or nurse executive includes a list of definitions associated with key statistics and standard calculations used by the organization.

Direct Care Labor Costs

Direct care costs refer to labor costs associated with direct patient care. Direct costs can be aligned with the cost objective; that is, providing direct care to the patients on the unit or providing a particular service. Often the direct caregivers are the registered nurses, licensed practical nurses, and nursing assistants. *Indirect* caregivers are those individuals who *support the patient care delivery system*: the manager and the unit secretary.

There are basic principles that guide staffing, *but these principles will vary* from one organization to another. The American Nurses Association (ANA) suggests that critical factors associated with appropriate staffing include:

- The number of patients,

- Levels of intensity of the patients for whom care is being provided,

- Architecture and geography of the environment,

- Suitable technology, and

- The level of preparation of providers (Gallagher, Kany, Rowell, and Peterson, 1999, p. 50).

The ANA also suggests that organizational policies should recognize the various needs of patients and nursing staff. These principles and guidelines offer the nurse manager guidance in developing, implementing, planning, and evaluating budget performance.

Exhibit 2-1 shows the costing of the labor budget using a standard set of statistics and calculations for 6 South, a *fictional* surgical acute care nursing unit.

Exhibit 2-1, designed by the Nursing Department, provides vital statistics for the Nurse Manager. This data provides the base to build the total staff hours needed for direct patient care. The elements of Exhibit 2-1 are explained as follows:

Part I: Basic Statistical Data

Section A: **Total Open Beds**

This number represents the actual number of beds available on the cost center. Since 100% occupancy does not always occur, the average census per day is also calculated. In this illustration, 6 South has 22 beds but the usual census is lower.

Section B: **Average Census per Day**

The Nursing Department determines this statistic in a variety of ways. The acute care system generally tracks patient days by collecting the census each day.[1] The census statistic is created by simply adding all the daily census numbers for a given

---

[1]Observation patients (patients not admitted as inpatients) usually spend 23 hours or less in the hospital for observation of a specific diagnosis or group of symptoms, to determine if an admission to the hospital is necessary. Observation patients are usually *not* part of the census statistics because these patients are considered outpatients.

cost center and dividing by the number of days in the year (or the number of days in the month). In this example, 6 South has an average daily census of 20.

Section C: Percent Occupancy

Of the available beds on the floor, this number reflects the average number of beds actually filled each day ($20 \div 22$). 6 South averages 90.91% occupied beds.

Section D: Nursing Hours per Patient Day

The nursing hours per patient day (NHPPD) is a theoretical benchmark statistic provided by the organization's acuity system. This provides the number of nursing hours of *direct* patient care needed for one day per patient. This number is often determined by the patient classification system. Both for-profit and not-for-profit NHPPD benchmark statistics are available based on specific patient populations, i.e., rehabilitation, mother and baby, labor and delivery, medical, surgical, or behavioral health closed unit.

Exhibit 2-1   Budget Worksheet—Basic Statistical Data for 6 South

Part I—Basic Statistical Data

Cost Center#: 60101
Unit Name: 6 South

A	Total Open Beds	22
B	Average Census per Day	20
C	Percent Occupancy ($B \div A$)	90.91
D	Nursing Hours per Patient Day (NHPPD)	6.2
E	Percentage of Registered Nurses	59%
F	Daily Hours ($B \times D$)	124
G	Unit Staff per Day ($F \div$ hours/shift)	10.33
H	Productive Hours per Pay Period ($F \times$ days/pay period)	1,736

Part II—Direct Staffing per Pay Period

Section

I   Direct Care Staff—Productive Hours

Staff Category	Percent Allocation	Total Productive Hours (H)	Productive Hours per Category
RN	59%	1,736	1,030
LPN	33	1,736	570
Nursing Assistants	8	1,736	136
Total	*100%*		*1,736*

Exhibit 2-1   Budget Worksheet—Basic Statistical Data for 6 South *(continued)*

J   Direct Care Staff—Total Paid Time

Staff Category	Productive Hours per Category (I)	Times the Non-Productive Factor	Total Paid Hours per Category
RN	1,030	1.14	1,174.2
LPN	570	1.14	649.8
Nursing Assistants	136	1.14	155.04
Total	*1,736*		*1,979.04*

K   Full Time Equivalents (FTEs)

Staff Category	Total Paid Hours per Category (J)	Divided by the Number of Hours per Pay Period	FTEs
RN	1,174.2	80	14.68
LPN	649.8	80	9.12
Nursing Assistants	155.04	80	1.94
Total	*1,979.04*		*24.74*

Part III—Indirect Care Staff Hours

Section

L

Staff Category	Productive Hours	Times the Non-Productive Factor	Paid Hours	Divided by Hours per Pay Period	FTEs
Associate Manager	70.2	1.14	80	80	1
Support Associate	70.2	1.14	80	80	1
Administrative Associate	197.1	1.14	224.9	80	2.8
Case Manager	70.2	1.14	80	80	1
Total	*407.8*		*464.9*		*5.8*

Part IV—All Hours Summary

Section

M

Staff Category	Productive Hours	Times the Non-Productive Factor	Paid Hours	Divided by Hours per Pay Period	FTEs
Direct Staff	1,736	1.14	1,979.04	80	24.74
Indirect Staff	407.8	1.14	464.90	80	5.84
Total	*2,143.8*		*2,43.94*		*30.54*

Exhibit 2-1   Budget Worksheet—Basic Statistical Data for 6 South *(continued)*

N   Hours per Patient Day (HPPD)

	Paid Hours (J)	Divided by Days per Pay Period	Paid Hours per Day	Divided by the Average Census (B)	HPPD – Hours per Patient Day
Direct Staff	1,979.04	14	141.36	20	7.068

Wide variances in the NHPPD occur from as low as four or five NHPPD on a rehabilitation or post-partum unit to 15 or 16 NHPPD in a surgical intensive care unit. The NHPPD variations demonstrate the differences in patient acuity—the number of hours of nursing care the patient requires in a twenty-four hour period.

Additionally, significant differences exist depending on which database for NHPPD or hours per patient day (HPPD) is used to provide the comparative statistic (Cockerill, O'Brien Pallas, Bolley, and Pink, 1993, p. 348). For example, NHPPD might contain only direct care nursing hours while HPPD might include other indirect support staff such as division clerks. Alternatively, some NHPPD figures may include the nurse manager while others do not.

On 6 South NHPPD refers to staff giving *direct* nursing care—registered nurses, licensed practical nurses, and nursing assistants. The average NHPPD on 6 South is 6.2, a number determined from patient classification historical data.

Section E: Percentage of Registered Nurses

The percentage of registered nurses represents the ratio of registered nurses compared to all direct caregivers, a group which includes not only registered nurses, but also licensed practical nurses, nursing assistants, and other patient care support staff. In recent years, research has shown that RN ratios can affect patient outcomes.[2] This has prompted legislative efforts to mandate staffing ratios in certain states.[3] Although the author does not advocate mandating staffing ratios due to differing patient acuities and other factors, it is clear that staffing does affect patient outcomes. To date, however, such issues as NHPPD and the percentage of RN staff are neither consistently mandated nor standardized in their measurement. For 6 South, our percentages are 59% RNs, 33% LPNs, and 8% Nursing Assistants on nights.

---

[1]This is discussed in Chapter 20, Staff—Our Most Valuable Resource, in the book: Dunham-Taylor, J., and Pinczuk, J. (2006). *Health Care Financial Management for Nurse Managers: Merging the Heart with the Dollar.* Sudbury, MA: Jones and Bartlett.

[2]This is discussed in Chapter 19, Patient Classification Systems, in the book: Dunham-Taylor, J., and Pinczuk, J. (2006). *Health Care Financial Management for Nurse Managers: Merging the Heart with the Dollar.* Sudbury, MA: Jones and Bartlett.

It can be helpful to compare this type of data with other organizations. This comparative activity is called benchmarking. Choosing a benchmark involves a thorough investigation of the characteristics of the data elements in the benchmark data set. Be cautious and compare your organization to another entity which is not only similar in its characteristics, but also successful both financially and in terms of quality care. Organizational characteristics such as organizational size, teaching versus non-teaching status, delivery system of care, tertiary versus community hospital designation, and differences in role expectations for direct care staff are among the variables to consider. These variables help to ensure accurate benchmarking.

Section F: Daily Hours

Daily Hours is also a theoretical number. This calculation is made by multiplying the average daily census by NHPPD. The resulting number represents the hours of nursing care needed over a twenty-four hour period *for the currently identified patients* on the cost center. On 6 South, with an average of 20 occupied beds and an NHPPD of 6.2, 124 hours of nursing care are required per 24-hour period. (20 patients × 6.2 NHPPD = 124 nursing staff hours/day). *The daily hours provide the basis for the number of direct care nursing staff needed for each twenty-four hour period.*

Section G: Unit Staff per Day

The number of staff per day is calculated by dividing the daily hours by the number of hours the staff work per shift—take the daily hours and divide by 8 for eight-hour shifts or by 12 for twelve-hour shifts. On 6 South, all staff members work twelve-hour shifts. Therefore, dividing the daily hours by 12 indicates how many twelve-hour shifts staff will be needed to provide 6.2 hours of care to each patient. (124 nursing staff hours/day ÷ 12 hour shift = 10.33 nursing staff needed per day).

Next, unit staff hours are allocated to day and night shifts. For example, most units allocate approximately 60% of the daily hours to day shift and 40% of the daily hours to night shift. Critical care units, on the other hand, may find that 55% (days) and 45% (nights) are more appropriate ratios.

Assume that in this organization, medical and surgical nursing units allocate approximately 60% of the staff to days and 40% of the staff to nights. (Remember that this percentage will differ from one organization to another, or even from one patient care unit to another, depending on how patient care is planned throughout the twenty-four-hour period) (Keeling, 1999). Using 60% of the staff working the day shift, the staffing pattern for this patient care unit will require 6.2 staff on day shift. (10.33 nursing staff/day × 0.60 = 6.2 nursing staff on the day shift), and 4.13 nursing staff (0.4 × 10.33) on the night shift. The unit staff includes, then, six on days and four on nights.[4]

---

[4] 0.60 represents 60% of the nursing staff who will work the day shift.

Section H: **Productive Hours per Pay Period**

The productive hours in the pay period are the hours necessary to staff the unit for the pay period. In the worksheet example, the pay period is 14 days. To calculate productive hours in the pay period, multiply the daily hours (124) times the number of days in the pay period (14). On 6 South, there are 1,736 productive hours in this pay period. (124 nursing staff hours/day × 14 days = 1,736 productive hours in the pay period).

Part II—Direct Staffing per Pay Period

Section I: **Direct Care Staff–Productive Hours**

The data in Part I is based on staffing requirements per pay period. In Part II, direct care staff calculations are further divided into registered nurses, licensed practical nurses, and nursing assistants. To determine the number of hours of registered nurses needed for a census of 20 patients for one pay period, multiply the total productive hours (1,736) in the pay period by the percentage of hours (59%) needed for registered nurse coverage. (1,736 productive hours in a pay period × 0.59 = 1,030 RN direct care productive hours.[5])

The remaining non-RN direct nursing care hours (1,736 − 1,030 = 706) must be distributed as specified for the cost center. On 6 South, other direct staff are specified at 33% LPN and 8% nursing assistants. Thus, the remaining 706 productive hours for non-RN direct care staff are allocated as 570 hours of LPN direct nursing care (0.33 × 1,736), and 136 hours for nursing assistant hours (0.08 × 1,736 = 136 productive hours).[6]

Section J: **Direct Care Staff—Total Paid Time**

Since staff productive hours do not take into account paid, but non-productive time (such as sick and vacation time), we make one more calculation. Most organizations use a standard factor for non-productive time; this factor is usually available through the human resource department. On 6 South, the standard factor for paid, non-productive hours is approximately 14%.[7] By multiplying the productive hours on 6 South by 1.14 we add non-productive staff time such as holidays, vacations, and sick time (14%) to our productive time (100%), arriving at the *total paid hours* for direct nursing care. It is this figure, 1,979 total paid hours (1,736 × 1.14), that will be used to calculate salaries.

---

[5]Note that there is some rounding error. If you divide 1,030 by 1,736 you will get 59% (rounded). But when you multiply .59 × 1,736 you get 1,024. There is leeway on the floor as well in constructing your staffing plan.

[6]The 14% non-productive time figure is an estimate. Each year an actual calculation is made for 6 South that includes an extra leap year day, percent of overtime, on call time, etc., appropriate for that fiscal year.

[7]Note that when multiplying by a percentage it is expressed in hundredths, i.e., 33% = 0.33 and 8% = 0.08.

Section K: Full-Time Equivalents (FTEs)

Total full-time equivalents (FTEs) are given for each staff category. One FTE equals 2,080 hours of work each year (40 hours/week × 52 weeks/year = 2,080 hours). Generally, the FTE number includes both full-time and part-time personnel, so the actual number of people working on 6 South is larger than the number given in the FTE column.

The calculation of the full-time equivalents (FTE) involves dividing the total hours *paid* by 80 (the number of hours in a two-week pay period). For 6 South, 1,979 total paid direct care staff hours ÷ 80 hours = 24.74 FTEs.

Because the staff on 6 South work three 12-hour shifts per week, each staff member is 0.9 FTE. (36 paid hours per week × 52 weeks per year = 1,872 hours per year. 1,872 hours divided by 2,080 (one FTE) = 0.9 FTE.)

Part III—Indirect Care

Section L: Indirect Care Staff Hours

Indirect care staff support the nursing function, but do not actually give direct care. Indirect hours include clerical support, the unit manager, the clinical nurse specialist, and others. For 6 South, there is no nurse manager, but there is an associate manager, a support associate, an administrative associate, and a case manager. Other indirect support staff might include social workers, clerical staff, or clinical nurse specialists. *Note that indirect care hours are not represented in the NHPPD.* In fact, indirect hours are generally calculated in a different manner from direct hours. With direct patient care, the hours when staff must be on the floor to care for patients (productive time) are added to the non-productive time which will be paid but not worked. When direct care staff are off, whether for vacation, holidays, or sick time, they must be replaced. With indirect care staff, we generally start with a 40-hour week and *subtract* the non-productive time. Often, when indirect staff are gone for a day or even a week, we do not replace them. Indirect care hours will be added to the unit direct care nurse staffing.

Part IV—Summary

Section M: All Hours Summary

To complete the total labor budget for this patient care unit, move down to the "All Hours" summary. In the first column both direct and indirect care hours are added together. (For 6 South, 1,736 direct productive hours + 407.8 indirect care staff productive hours = 2,143.8 hours.) In the third column, hours include the 100% productive time plus the 14% non-productive time. In the fifth column, the total FTEs represent direct and indirect care total paid hours ÷ 80 hours in the pay period. (For 6 South, there are 24.74 direct staff and 5.81 indirect FTEs for a total of 30.54 FTEs.)

Section N: **Hours per Patient Day (HPPD)**

The final budget statistic is the HPPD—the numbers of hours provided by *direct* care staff per day to support the patient care unit's needs. Calculate the HPPD by dividing the direct care staff total paid hours by 14 (the number of days in the pay period) by the census per day for the unit. (For 6 South, 1,979 direct care staff total paid hours ÷ 14 days ÷ 20 patients = 7.07 HPPD.) Remember that HPPD may be defined differently in different institutions.

Labor Budget Implementation Plan

A number of very important factors drive a successful budget implementation plan—patient acuity, the nursing practice model, the skill mix of staff, and non-productive hours (Brown, 1999, p. 34). Developing a nursing delivery plan to assign staff clarifies the method of delivery for both the manager and the unit staff. Exhibit 2-2 shows how to plan the number of staff and track open and filled positions *to the budget*. This method allows the nurse manager to evaluate open positions continuously.

The ability to staff the unit effectively is directly related to having all staff positions filled. Each time a position is filled, the manager evaluates where the unit stands in relationship to the budget. The manager considers the unit's census activity and other factors to determine if the position is needed. If staff cannot be hired at one level (for example, LPNs) the nurse manager must consider whether adequate staffing requires that the positions be reclassified and filled with RNs.

Decisions such as altering the percentage of registered nurses to hire more licensed practical nurses or nursing assistants can also be made with this tool. For example, consider increasing the hours in practical nurses and decreasing the hours in registered nurses. Because of the difference in salary, the labor budget is reduced. However, this change also places more responsibility on the existing registered nurse staff. This decision may be effective if recruitment of registered nurses is problematic. With the difference in salary, the manager could hire more licensed practical nurses to keep up the number of staff members available to patients. These decisions need to be made with the nurse executive, because changing the registered nurse mix may, in fact, affect quality.

In Exhibit 2-2 the nurse manager has information readily available by type of staff. A *position, or job number,* is assigned to each job by the human resources department. In budgeting terminology, each of these position numbers is a *salary line.* This number does not change when the employee filling that position changes. The *filled* column indicates the total number of hours in a pay period for that salary line. The *shift* column indicates which 12-hour shift the employee typically works. The *date/hire* column is the date the employee was hired.

Exhibit 2-2   Current Position Control
Patient Care Unit: 6 South

Direct Care RNs	Employee	Job #	Position Control (PC) Hours	Filled Hours	Shift	Date Hired
	Jack Susani	3326	72	72	7 a	12/02/1999
	Sally Mason	3326	72	72	7 a	11/06/1988
	Olivia Fredericks	3326	72	72	7 a	
	Halley Johns	3326	72	72	7 a	
	Millie Quinn	3326	72	72	7 a	
		3326	72	72	7 a	
		3326	48	48	7 a	
		3326	72	72	7 a	
		3326	72	72	7 a	
		3326	72	72	7 p	
		3326	72	72	7 p	
			72	72	7 p	
			72	72	7 p	
			72	72	7 p	
			72	72	7 p	
			72	72	7 p	
			48	48	7 p	

RNs ➜ 2,000 Hours Filled = 1,176   2,000 Hours Budgeted = 1,174   Variance [1,174 – 1,176] = -2

Direct Care LPNs	Employee	Job #	Position Control (PC) Hours	Filled Hours	Shift	Date Hired
	Georgia O'Keeffe	3500	72	72	7 a	03/05/1995
	Richard Mondrian	3500	72	72	7 a	
		3500	32	32	7 a	
		3500	72	72	7 a	
		3500	72	72	7 a	
		3500	72	72	7 a	
		3500	72	72	7 p	
		3500	48	48	7 p	
		3500	72	72	7 p	
		3500	72	72	7 p	

LPNs ➜ 2,000 Hours Filled = 656   2,000 Hours Budgeted = 650   Variance [650 – 656] = -6

(Names are fictitious)

Exhibit 2-2   Current Position Control
                Patient Care Unit: 6 South *(continued)*

Direct Care Nursing Assistants	Employee	Job #	Position Control (PC) Hours	Filled Hours	Shift	Date Hired
	Mary Allen	684	80	80	7 a	06/12/1989
	Steve Marks	684	32	32	7 a	05/04/1982
	John Long	684	32	32	3 p	

NAs ➜ *2,000 Hours Filled = 144   2,000 Hours Budgeted = 155   Variance [155 – 144] = + 11*

(Names are fictitious)

At the end of each employee classification, the *total filled positions* indicates hours actually filled by hired employees. This number can be easily compared with the *budget allocation,* which contains the number of hours allocated (or allowed) for that employee classification. The *variance to budget* reflects the difference between the *actual hours filled* and the budgeted *hours allocated.*

Exhibit 2-3 provides a layout of 6 South along with the average daily census and the total beds. Assignments are made *by module* as specified in the unit layout. The *licensed caregiver ratio* is planned for each day using Exhibit 2-3. When this specified staffing assignment is not followed, the percentage of staff allocated to the shifts may be altered and may change the percentage of registered nurse staff needed for care assessment and planning.

The assignment plan specified in Exhibit 2-3 also provides a tool to help the nurse manager and staff anticipate how registered nurses, other licensed staff, and unlicensed staff, work together. Responsibilities for each role need to be *in writing* to clearly define each person's responsibilities. Registered nurses need to be skilled in delegation and communication. This approach also invites discussion about assignment planning and problem-solving for unusual situations. A plan for peak- or low-census periods may be beneficial as well.

The nurse manager and nurse executive must also plan for census fluctuation periods. In *written* departmental policies and procedures, use of *per diem* staff or agency staff needs to be defined as does the priority through which overtime is selected *in lieu* of *per diem* or agency staff.

Exhibit 2-4 describes the process through which the unit manager determines the plan to meet budget targets by unit census and percentage of registered nurses, licensed practical nurses, and nursing assistants.

When the census is 20, the direct care hours for patient care is 124 daily hours. This number is the result of the NHPPD (6.2) multiplied by the average census of 20. The unit manager knows that with a census of 20, six staff members will be needed for days and four staff members will be needed for nights.

Exhibit 2-3   Physical Layout of 6 South and Its Relation to the Staffing Plan

627 Private		620 Private
628 Private	ELEVATORS	621 Private
629 Semi-private		622 Semi-private
630 Semi-private	NURSE'S STATION	623 Semi-private
631 Semi-private		624 Semi-private
632 Semi-private		625 Semi-private
6323 Private		626 Private

Total Beds = 22
Average Daily Census = 20

	Days	Nights
Licensed Caregiver to Patients	5 : 22	3 : 22
RNs	4	1
LPNs	1	1
Nursing Assistants	1	1

Modular Staffing Plan	Days	Nights
Number of Sections and Room Numbers	2	2
	627–633 & 620–626	627–633 & 620–626
RNs	2/Section	1/Section
LPNs	1/Section	1/Section
Nursing Assistants	1/Section	1/Section

Exhibit 2-4   **Staffing to the Census**

Unit: 6 South
Beds: 22
HPPD: 6.
12 Hour Shifts

	Day Shift				Night Shift				
Census	Total Staff	RN	LPN	NA	Total Staff	RN	LPN	NA	Daily Hours
1–12	2	2	0	0	2	2	0	0	48
13–17	4	2	1	1	3	2	1	0	84
18–22	6	4	1	1	4	2	1	1	120

Census = 20 patients
NHPPD = 6.2
20 patients × 6.2 NHPPD = 124 daily hours
Since staff work 12-hour shifts,
124 daily hours ÷ 12-hour shifts = 10 staff needed/124 hours
Since 60% of staff are on days,
10 staff needed per 24 hours ÷ 0.6 = 6 staff needed for days
The remaining 4 staff (10 − 6 = 4) would be on nights

Using the percentage of RNs for this unit, multiply the total staff of six times the percentage planned for RNs. That equals 4.2. This means that 4 of the 6 staff members on days must be RNs. The remaining numbers for skill levels include 1 LPN and 1 NA (nursing assistant). On nights, using the same calculations, the night staff must include at least 2 RNs (4 times 0.59 = 2.4). Night shift will include 2 RNs, 1 LPN, and 1 NA.

The last step is to add all the hours together for 24 hours of care at a census of 20. The total of 10 staff members times the 12 hours each person will provide direct care to the patients equals 120 hours.

10 staff × 12-hour shifts = 120 hours of care.

Note that the budget allows 124 hours of direct care at the census of 20. The unit manager expects to be slightly under budget at 120 hours of direct care.

The census table is set in increments of the census with the at-budget-point near the middle of the census number range. Looking at Exhibit 2-4, note that the range of 18–22 patients provides the same number of staff for the census at 18, 19, 20 (budget), 21, or 22. The at-budget point (a census of 20) is at the center of the range.

What happens to the four hours that were allowed by the budget at a census of 20, but which were not used? Those hours come from the fraction of time that occurs when the number of staff per shift is calculated. Remember the calculation was 124 hours of direct care divided by 12 per/shift hours. These calculations resulted in uneven numbers. There were 10.33 staff members per 24-hour period, or 6.2 staff on days and 4.13 staff on nights. The budget target cannot be met exactly unless the unit manager decides to have someone come in for four hours sometime during the 24-hour period. *The census table is a guide. The manager uses these flexible hours to alter the staffing based on acuity.*

Acuity

The NHPPD reflects acuity, particularly if the organization conducts an assessment of acuity periodically, such as every three months. Some organizations conduct this assessment daily using a patient classification system. The rationale for conducting such assessments includes documenting changes in patient populations, changes in treatment modalities, proposing changes in nursing budgets, and changes in delivery system models. For example, this surgical unit may change over time as changes occur in the community. The NHPPD may differ when the predominant patient population is fragile elderly versus a more diverse population of younger and older patients. Obviously, the surgical NHPPD for a surgical unit within a community hospital may be quite different from the NHPPD at a teaching hospital.

The NHPPD is multiplied by the census to determine the allowed daily hours for direct patient care. The daily hours are then allocated, first by multiplying them by 60% for day shift and 40% for night shift, and then by distributing them between RNs, LPNs, and NAs.

There is a direct link between the information in Exhibit 2-4 and patient acuity. Exhibit 2-4 delineates staffing patterns and shows one way to estimate the points at which the staffing changes. This exercise assists the manager in anticipating staffing needs *before* any census deviation occurs. This staffing pattern tool, communicated with staff and supervisors around the clock, allocates staff for the unit according to the census for each shift; it provides a guide. Nevertheless, critical thinking and analytic skills are still necessary to meet patient needs. There are times when "going over budget" makes sense if a given group of patients needs more than 6.2 hours of patient care per day. The manager's rounds to assess patient care needs and appropriate staffing comprise the assessment necessary to make these decisions.

Exhibit 2-4 also gives the percentage of staff that must be registered nurses. Remember that the budget worksheet in Exhibit 2-1 used 59% registered nurses as the target for this patient care unit. Once the total number of staff is determined for the census number, approximately 59% must be registered nurses.

Learning how to decide when to use additional staff, or less staff, in comparison to a budget table, requires experience and nursing care quality information. Decision making around these issues includes assessment, planning, implementation, and evaluation on several levels. "Seeking only 'bottom line' solutions would seriously affect the well-being of nurses and clients" (Ray et al., 1995, p. 48). Among the factors the manager needs to consider are:

- Number of new staff in orientation that are supported by a preceptor;

- Quality information such as wound care and patient satisfaction;

- Number of open positions for all skills;

- Admission/Discharge/Transfer activity—time of day and numbers;

- Care of outpatients or observation patients not accounted for in daily census statistics;

- Level of intensity of the care;

- Architecture and geography of the unit;

- Available technology, such as fax, tube systems, errand services, pharmacy turnaround time, transportation services, and method of documentation;

- Tasks and procedures done by unit staff that are not calculated in patient classification;

- Discharge planning responsibilities; and

- Patient teaching responsibilities.

Monitoring and Analyzing the Labor Budget

Monitoring and analyzing budget performance requires that the organization provide its managers with data for the month or pay period. The nurse executive may require managers to submit a report on budget performance periodically (or immediately if budgeted levels fall too low or too high based on a predetermined standard).

The worksheet shown in Exhibit 2-1 can be used to demonstrate methods of budget monitoring and analysis. The manager needs certain statistics to determine budget performance:

- The actual number of patient days for the period;
- The number of productive hours used;
- The number of non-productive hours used;
- The ability to separate direct and indirect care hours; and
- The percentage of care provided by registered nurses in direct care.

Using the budget worksheet in Exhibit 2-5, a comparison of budgeted figures to actual figures in these areas can be established. Exhibit 2-5 provides such a comparison for 6 South.

The budget worksheet indicates that the NHPPD is 6.2, the average daily census is 20, and the expected use of productive hours is 1,736 for a 14-day pay period. The actual experience, however, was an average census of 22. The total productive hours and RN hours are shown in the third column. To compare the budget with the actual experience, budget numbers for a census of 22 patients are necessary. These figures are presented in column 4. Column 5 shows the difference between the budget for a 22-patient census and the actual

Exhibit 2-5   Budget Worksheet—Budget Versus Actual Performance

Unit: 6 South   *NHPPD: 6.2*

Item	Target Budget	Actual	Budget at Actual Census	Variance [Positive or (negative) difference]
Census	20	22	22	2
Productive Hours	1,736[1]	1,745[2]	1,910[1]	165
RN Productive Hours	1,024[3]	1,025[2]	1,127[3]	102
Percent RN Staff	59%[4]	58.7%[4]	59%[4]	0.3%
NHPPD[5]	6.2[5]	5.67[5]	6.2[5]	(0.53)

[1]NHPPD × Census = Daily Hours × Days in the pay period = Productive Hours.
[2]Based on actual hours worked.
[3]59% × total productive hours.
[4]Registered Nursing Hours ÷ Productive Hours.
[5]Productive Hours ÷ Days in the pay period ÷ Census.

experience. 6 South coped with its elevated census numbers with 165 fewer total hours, and 102 fewer RN hours when compared to budget. While finance will initially like this outcome, the negative impact can be seen in the NHPPD, which dropped from our standard of 6.2 down to 5.67. It is the nurse manager's job to determine whether this is an acceptable outcome (perhaps the patients on the unit were less acute than the typical census patients, or illness among staff prevented bringing staffing to the appropriate nursing hours) or whether these financial savings have come at a cost in terms of the quality and safety of the patient care.

Now let's use an example of actual monthly data on 6 South, illustrated in Exhibit 2-6. The manager assesses that the NHPPD for the pay period was 6.02, and 58.7% of productive hours were registered nurse hours. The unit was not staffed to the budgeted nursing hours of 6.2, and the registered nurse productive hours were somewhat below the 59% budget. The manager knows that the difference between the target hours of 3,348 and the actual hours of 3,250 represent a shortage of nursing hours—hours that the nursing unit needed to provide the expected level of care. The unit was understaffed for the pay period.

The manager needs to determine what caused this to occur. A review of the pay period may indicate things like two staff members on vacation, without replacement staff. Efforts to hire *per diem* staff or increase part-time staff to full-time do not always work. The manager may have open positions. Efforts to recruit for this particular position and shift may need additional analysis. As mentioned earlier, if LPNs cannot be hired, the position may need to be reclassified as an RN to meet needed levels of licensed caregivers.

If the manager were *over* budget, as seen on 6 North, several things might have occurred. There might be staff in orientation, supported by preceptors, where the manager is actually paying two salaries for the productivity of one person; the staff may not be following the census table; or perhaps the actual acuity on the unit exceeded 5.7 and the nurse manager was forced to use more hours and a higher percentage of highly trained nurses to meet the needs of quality patient care.

The use of overtime as an indicator demonstrates how well a manager is able to increase staffing when a sudden change occurs, such as someone calling in sick. Generally, the manager is likely to recruit staff for overtime hours. However, if the understaffing continues, unit staff may become tired and eventually refuse overtime. This also creates patient safety issues.

Monitors for all the key elements of the budget are necessary. The pay period census, the percentage of registered nurse staff, and the actual nursing hours should be reported regularly. Situations in which nurse managers are consistently unable to staff within the budget due to increasing census, inability to recruit staff to new positions, or inability to get staff to work overtime, signal serious problems. Johnson (1998) discusses ways to cope with census fluctuations. Most importantly, the recognition that several units have similar problems allows for more complete planning for the department as a whole.

Some payroll and scheduling software systems provide reports helpful to nurse manager analysis. For example, a system may provide managers with a monthly report on hours assigned to orientation, overtime, education, long-term illness versus short-term illness, paid time for holidays, and unit projects. Such a report would allow the manager to analyze the previous month or pay period to assess how paid hours were expended.

Additionally, the nurse manager needs to assess the position control report (Exhibit 2-2) to assess the number of open positions on the staff. This may reflect hours below or above budgeted positions. The manager may also need to reassess the census table and assignment planning tools. Are these tools accurate? Is the staff following the guidelines? If not, what are the reasons? Often staff devise their own ways of coping unless regular discussion of these issues occurs in staff meetings and during manager rounds.

Reporting Justification

Exhibit 2-7 represents one way to report variances from the budget. This tool requires the manager to determine if nursing hours per patient day and other vital statistics are at or near budget. Finding the patient care unit significantly under budget places an unnecessary burden on the organization, the staff, and the patients and their families. Exhibit 2-7 suggests a framework for developing a justification report that explains the various causes for failing to meet budget target figures.

It is important that the nurse manager keep regular key budget statistics for the unit. Each pay period per month one should track the actual census per day and per month, the actual nursing hours, and the actual percentage of registered nurse staff. The labor justification report needs to indicate how the unit compared to the budget plan. If pay period per monthly data reflect no problems, then nothing further needs to be done. However, when wide fluctuations occur, or when the data indicates that problems have occurred, further action is necessary. For example, if there are wide census fluctuations, patterns may evolve suggesting that the plan be changed. Or it is possible that units could be consolidated. All of this needs to be evaluated by the nurse manager and the nurse executive. It is important to establish a plan for over- and under-budget situations, and it is helpful to have open lines of communication with the staff and nurse executive about the plan. Continued performance in either direction, over-budget or under-budget, requires a plan that the staff understands. Solicit ideas from staff and the nurse executive as to possible alternatives to better deal with the problem. Sometimes a simple change in procedures (for example, a temporary errand service that replaces errands that the unit's staff currently perform) offers a savings in labor. Once plans are formed, communicate them to the staff. Plans may include such things as short-term contracts

Exhibit 2-6 Productivity Report

Unit	Average Census		Productive Hours[1] For a 30-Day Month			Nursing Productive Hours[2] Per Patient Day (NHPPD)			RN Hours[3]		
	Target Census	Actual Census	Target Budget	Budget at Actual	Actual	Target Budget	Budget at Actual	Actual	Target Budget	Budget at Actual	Actual
6 South	20	18	3,720	3,348	3,250	6.2	6.2	6.02	2,195	1,975	1,852
6 North	28	33.2	4,788	5,472	5,610	5.7	5.7	5.84	2,633	3,010	3,050

[1] Census (Budget and Target) × NHPPD × Days in the Month = Productive Hours (Budget and Target)

[2] Productive Hours (Budget, Target, and Actual) ÷ Days in the Month ÷ Census (Budget, Target, and Actual) = NHPPD (Budget, Target, and Actual)

[3] 59% (the predetermined RN rate for 6 South) × Monthly Hours for 6 South and 55% (the predetermined RN rate for 6 North) of Monthly Hours for 6 North

Exhibit 2-7 Nonproductive Time Report

Unit: 6 South

Sick	Unpaid Sick	Long-term Sick	Paid Holiday	Jury Duty	Funeral Leave	Workshop Hours	Orientation Hours	Scheduled Overtime	Total		
									Budget	Actual	Difference
287	234	111	156	0	24	16	204	12	603	1,044	-441

for extra hours, taking time off, or other efforts to improve the support services for the unit. Simultaneous communication over a department or division reassures staff that consistency and standardization occur throughout the nursing department.

Connect the performance for all nursing indicators together—budget and quality. The whole picture reinforces that the organization's leadership believes in efficiency *and* quality. Recognition for participation in these plans and activities, and for performance improvement, encourages staff to commit to efficient, quality care.

Materials and Supplies

Assessment of Needs

The material and supplies budget details those items charged to the patient care unit, i.e., paper, forms, leased equipment, IV supplies, linen, fax machine toner, patient education materials, equipment repairs, postage, equipment maintenance, drugs in stock supplies, medical supplies, instruments, office supplies, and purchased services. The actual items charged, the categories in which the items are based, and the associated numbers and systems vary from one organization to another. Generally, this year's budget is based on last year's usage. The nurse manager's challenge is to understand how and what is billed to the unit and to understand how to control and manage these expenses.

Planning a budget for materials and supplies creates a process through which ongoing comparisons occur between budget and actual expenditures. This process involves cost management, decreased waste, and adjustments in how work is accomplished. Strasen (1987) describes the major budget functions as: planning, management of activities, and control of spending. The nurse manager's role engages these functions into the development of key processes at the patient care level. The nurse manager plans and assesses costs, manages activities and programs at the unit level, and controls spending. An effective nurse manager has a set communication and education plan that has included unit staff in the process.

It is helpful for the nurse manager to assess the patient care unit's needs and usage patterns months *before* the actual budget process starts. The purpose of the assessment is to support the unique needs of the patient population on the unit; establish a pattern of usage; ensure that safe, working equipment and supplies are available; and establish accurate charging systems.

The rationale for conducting a detailed assessment to develop materials and supply cost plans are numerous. Staff members who have supplies easily available to them do not find it necessary to hoard their own supply inventory deep in cupboards, closets, and drawers—a practice that leads to problems like the use of outdated inventory and a higher supply expenditure than is actually needed. Finding the supply item *in the same place each time it is needed* saves staff time, decreases staff frustration, prevents delays in care to patients, and decreases physician wait time. A manager who possesses intimate knowledge of supply item needs saves personnel valuable time by focusing on specific problems with a specific plan for each problem. Finally, managing this budget provides the manager with an opportunity to uncover systems that are not working well and that waste the time and energy of a busy staff.

Conduct the assessment using several avenues. First, interview the staff about patient needs and ask questions about what is appropriately or inappropriately stocked. Search the unit's storage areas for worn or broken equipment, outdated inventory, and overstocked supplies. Interview the distribution manager to review usage patterns and par levels. Physician complaints can offer a key to supply problems. If your unit is a surgical unit, talk to a number of surgeons about their assessment of supplies. If your unit is a telemetry unit, talk to the physician users about their observations of the inventory. Rounds in patients' rooms can also provide a clue to what is needed for bedside equipment and furniture. Include the patients and their families in the assessment of supply needs. Look in the conference room and consider the reference books on the shelves and the furniture used by staff, physicians, patients, and families. Try to see the unit through the eyes of a visitor or patient. The unit manager is likely to develop a list of needs, including such things as repairs to wallpaper, and plans to replace carpeting or furniture over a number of years.

The most tedious job involves the review of several months of information system reports that the organization offers its managers. Develop an understanding of the patterns of usage and the costs for particular accounts. Compare the activity over several months or per quarter.

Contact financial staff in the organization to define what categories of supplies and materials are used and request the category definitions. Compare your unit with another, similar unit. Looking at the differences and similarities may be helpful to develop ideas and discover things that need the manager's attention. This initial assessment may uncover things like errors in coding by finance staff, lost charges due to complicated procedures followed by staff, failure to rotate stock by date, poor communication on discontinued items and forms, failure to allocate the work to the most appropriate person, and many others.

Developing the Budget Worksheet

In the budget process, each patient care unit submits an estimated budget for the upcoming year based both on last year's budget and on the anticipation of specific changes in the organization or physician practice patterns. Exhibit 2-8 shows a list of items and the estimated cost for the year. The manager increases or decreases each category by reviewing the performance last year, anticipating upcoming changes, and submitting the budget for approval. As the nursing department sets goals for the new budget year, the nurse manager also makes changes to accommodate departmental goals.

Exhibit 2-9 lists some questions the manager can use to anticipate changes in the new materials and supplies budget. The answers to these questions, a list of goals for the nursing department, and the results of the manager's assessment of the unit's needs, provide a basis for budget decisions. Remember, these are estimates. The nurse manager needs to provide justification for the anticipated expense.

Some organizations review budgeted costs to unused budget monies at the end of the year and use "surplus" funds to replace furniture or purchase stock items in bulk. The manager gets the needed furniture or carpeting now, instead of adding it to the budget for next year, and the whole organization benefits by improving the environment and saving money by purchasing in bulk supply.[8]

Finally, the nurse manager should anticipate a request to further reduce the budget. The finance department adds up everything submitted by managers and often faces a huge request list. There is temptation to overestimate in anticipation. Some managers even develop two budget submissions at the same time. The nurse executive, as the leader of the nursing department, sets the tone for the approach to budget preparation. The nurse manager, through participation in the budget process, communicates integrity. This author's recommendation is to *honestly estimate the budget* at each step of the process. A well-documented approach to budgeting and thorough communication with the nurse executive are in the best interests of all concerned. The notes saved from the assessment of need, the goals of the organization, and the answers to questions like those in Exhibit 2-9, offer a systematic method for prioritizing need and reducing expense.

Monthly Monitoring of the Budget

The organization generally provides a number of reports, including a monthly summary, with totals spent in each account and a comparison of actual expenses to budget. Another report, probably received weekly, gives details on what has been charged to the patient care unit. Take the time to scan this report. Big mistakes are easily picked up when it is obvious to the manager that a particular item is never used, or the account number is not one that the unit uses. For example,

---

[8]Organizations have different rules when it comes to allowing monies to be shifted from one "line-item" (for example, telephone and postage) to another line-item (for example, supplies). Your ability to use "surplus" funds at year-end will depend in part on the amount of freedom you have to move budgeted monies from one category to another.

Exhibit 2-8 Supplies List

Item: Initial Materials and Supplies Submission
Unit: 6 South
Manager: Nancy Nurse
Cost Center #: 56229

Account Number	Account Description	Estimated New Budget	Estimated Monthly Cost
001	Billable Supplies	$ 23,193	$ 1,933
002	Medical Supplies	62,000	5,167
003	Instruments	30	3
004	Sutures	300	25
005	IV Sets	18,915	1,576
006	General Operating Supplies	9,540	795
007	Office Supplies	4,500	375
008	Forms	12,000	1,000
009	Paper and Plastic Supplies	4,000	333
010	Copier Supplies	300	25
011	Linen Products	11,000	917
012	Dietary Supplies	4,300	358
013	Drugs: Stock	3,000	250
014	Solutions	6,800	567
015	Purchased Services	30,000	2,500
016	Leased Equipment	1,500	125
017	Books	100	8
018	Equipment Repairs	150	13
019	Equipment Maintenance	600	50
020	Postage	12	1
021	Other Expenses	50	4
	Total	**$192,290**	**$16,025**

Exhibit 2-9   A Few Questions to Ponder

- Are new pathways coming out next year?
- Is your patient population going to change?
- Will physicians be using new techniques or therapies?
- Does the copy machine have a contract?
- Are you responsible for the fax machine supplies—toner and paper?
- Are your nursing references over 5 years old?
- Do you have a pharmacy reference on the unit?
- Will some of your patients become outpatients in the near future?
- Are you responsible for information systems—personal computers and software licenses?
- Has a new level of care opened in the organization that affects your patient population?
- Will you be responsible for consultant visits?
- Are leased services part of the unit's budget?
- Is your linen charged the unit?

cardiac stents charged to a medical unit must be a mistake. Follow up; this is a very expensive mistake.

Generally, the nurse executive requests written justification for variances in the range of 5–10% over or under budget. If percentages are not given on the financial reports, create your own:

1. Divide each budget total by 12 (the months in the year) to arrive at a monthly estimate.

2. Calculate the *difference* between the monthly budget and the actual.

3. Divide the *difference* by the monthly budget number to get a *percentage* variance.

   Note: As a *cost* center, all amounts *over* budget are *negative* variances. All amounts *under* budget are *positive* variances.

Now, evaluate the results:

- Concentrate on the specific sub-accounts that are potentially incorrect. Errors in charging to the unit may occur and need to be corrected. Sudden usage changes often signal an error of this kind. Sometimes a coding error occurs. These are recognized as decimal point errors (called "slides" by accountants). For example, the cost is exactly 100 or 1,000 or even 10,000 higher or lower than usual. Another easy finding is dollars associated with a sub-account number never seen on this report in the past.

- Other significant differences can signal a change in the patient population. For example, overflow from the medical units or surgeons at a national conference may be the justification for changes in patterns in the budget.

- Assure that the distribution department charged the unit for supplies that are appropriate to the unit. If necessary, develop your own statistics to help you know when your budget is off.

The example in Exhibit 2-10 demonstrates one way to organize an analysis of costs by sub-account. The manager, using this self-devised system, monitors only those areas that are over budget or that seem unusual. Of the five items listed, the manager investigates three. One item represents an error. The $7,349 was posted to the monthly summary of expenses by mistake. One item is justified due to an increase in patient census. The forms account seems wrong since the census was over budget. And, finally, the linen overage requires attention from the manager. This unit's average number of patients per day was 33 this month, instead of 28. Through the initial assessment, the manager's familiarity with what each material or supply item means, and how the patient care unit uses the item, helps to quickly identify changes in normal usage patterns.

Plan feedback at staff meetings to recognize accurate charging and use of supplies. A short discussion on this topic keeps staff aware of their own importance in the processes that keep costs accurate. Some organizations reward these behaviors by offering a small gift to the unit with quantifiable improvement or sustained accuracy. Lunch or dinner from the hospital administration for a great job recognizes the staff on how well they are doing. Communication that is clear and direct enhances the feeling of respect and genuine appreciation. "Good communications do more than enhance the feeling of respect—they also boost motivation and productivity" (Rosen, p. 41).

Summary

The role of the nurse manager in the budget process is pivotal to the financial health of the organization. Clinical and administrative skills are essential for the developing unit manager. The workplace relationships that the unit manager develops include the clinical staff and staff related to the units human and supply resources. Knowing the distribution staff, finance staff, purchasing staff, and contract staff demonstrates the evolving role of the unit manager. In addition to payroll and overtime sheets, the nurse manager also reviews reports on labor costs for direct and indirect care staff, and material and supply costs. Involvement in the whole picture of the patient care unit pulls the manager into decision making that prioritizes how to decrease unnecessary costs and propose necessary costs with clinical rationale. The experienced nurse manager helps the organization realize *why* and *how* nursing input to financial decisions, within the framework of clinical care, results in successful cost management.

Exhibit 2-10 Cost Analysis of Supplies by Account—Adjusted and Unadjusted for Census Variations

Unit:	6 South		Month:	June, 2000
Manager:	Nancy Nurse		Budgeted Census:	28
Cost Center #:	56229		Actual Census:	33

| | | | Unadjusted for the Census | | | Adjusted for the Census (e) | | | |
Account Number	Account Description	Actual Monthly Cost	Budget (a)	Dollar Variance (b)	% Variance (c)	Adjusted Budget (+18%)	Dollar Variance (b)	% Variance (c)	Rationale
008	Forms	$ 729	$1,000	($271)	(27 %)	$ 1,180	($451)	(38%)	Needs checking. Does not match the census.
009	Paper and Plastic Supplies	390	333	57	17 %	393	3	1%	Explained by the increase in the patient census.
011	Linen Products	2,351	917	752	82 %	1,082	1,269	138%	Needs checking. Increase is too large to be explained by the census increase.
013	Drugs: Stock	298	250	48	19 %	295	3	1%	Explained by the increase in the patient census.
031	Special Order Supplies	7,349	0	7,349	(d)	0	7,349	(d)	Special order supplies are *never* used on this unit. This is a billing error.

(a) From Exhibit 2-8 on a per-month basis

(b) Budget (estimated monthly cost) minus actual

(c) Dollar Variance ÷ budget (estimated monthly cost)

(d) You cannot divide by zero. Mathematically, this variance is *infinitely* large!

(e) Budget − Actual ÷ Budget = 28 − 33 = 5 ÷ 28 = +18%

References

Brown, B. (1999). How to develop a unit personnel budget. *Nursing Management*, 30(4), 34–35.

Caroselli, C. (1993). Economic awareness of nurses: Relationship to budgetary control. *Nursing Economic$*, 14(5), 292–298.

Cockerill, R., O'Brien Pallas, L., Bolley, H., & Pink, G. (November–December 1993). Measuring nursing workload for case costing. *Nursing Economic$*, 11(6), 243–249.

Dunham-Taylor, J., & Pinczuk, J. (2006). *Health care financial management for nurse managers: Merging the heart with the dollar*. Sudbury, MA: Jones and Bartlett.

Eckhart, J.G. (1993). Costing out nursing services: Examining the research. *Nursing Economic$*, 11 (2), 91–98.

Gallagher, R., Kany, K.A., Rowell, P., & Peterson, C. (1999). ANA's nurse staffing principles. *American Journal of Nursing*, 99(4), 50, 52–53.

Johnson, S.H. (1998). Coping with census fluctuations. *Nursing Management*, 29(10), 48L.

Jones, K.R. (March 1994). Direct and indirect costs. *Seminars for Nurse Managers*, 2(1), 4–5.

Keeling, B. (1999). How to allocate the right staff mix across shifts. *Nursing Management*, 30(9), 16–17.

Lemire, J. (2000). Redesigning financial management education for the nursing administration graduate student. *Journal of Nursing Administration*, 30(4),199–205.

Ray, M.A., Didominic, V.A., Dittman, P.W., Hurst, P.A., Seaver, J.B., Sorbello, B.C., & Stankes Ross, M.A. (1995). The edge of chaos: caring and the bottom line. *Nursing Management*, 26(9), 48–50.

Rosen, R.H. (1992). *The Healthy Company*. New York: Putnam Publishing Group.

Strasen, L. (1987). *Key Business Skills for Nurse Managers*. Philadelphia: J.B. Lippincott.

Zachry, B.R., & Gilbert, R.I. (1992). Director of nursing planning and finance: A new role. *Nursing Management*, 12(23), 50–52.

3

Ignoring the Patient Classification System— Another Way to Staff

Kathryn W. Wilhoit, MSN, RN, CNAA, FACHE
Jane M. Mustain, MSN, RN
With Special Recognition to
Deborah McInturff, Financial Analyst

Introduction to Nursing Hours per Patient Day-Based Staffing

Today's nurse manager is asked to make a variety of difficult staffing-related decisions, knowing that those decisions will be well scrutinized by other organizational leaders. The wise nurse manager makes use of many tools and systems to improve decision making by providing timely, precise, and accurate information.

A number of nurse managers and their organizations use some form of patient classification system to calculate staffing needs based on patient acuity.

Phillips, Castorr, Prescott, and Soeken (1992) noted in the *Journal of Nursing Administration* that two factors must be considered when measuring nursing resource use: the volume of services, and the skill level at which those services are provided. They further noted that most patient classification systems "address only the volume of care needed and do not consider the complexity of care and the associated skill level of providers required" (p. 47). This can lead to underestimation of the cost of patient care being provided.

This is one reason that a growing number of nurse managers and their organizations are deserting patient classification systems, believing them to be an inaccurate, resource-wasting exercise in futility. This chapter examines a staffing process based on nursing hours per patient day (NHPPD), seeking to answer the question, *can the NHPPD-based staffing process provide timely and accurate information?* If so, the facility can have quality patient care and satisfied patients, and provide a standard measure that can be compared and studied to yield information on best nursing practice.

Personal Reflections: Why Choose This Method

Until the year 2001, our facility had used some form of patient classification to identify acuity in making staffing decisions for over two decades. This process began with a manual version of the GRASP® patient acuity identification system in the late 1970s. "GRASP® is a well documented, research-based methodology with a 20-plus year history of accurately capturing work requirements" (www.graspinc.com). The process was automated somewhat by moving to scanning sheets used with the ANSOS (Automated Nurse Scheduling and Operating System) in the mid-1980s. The addition of GRASP® software in 1997, combined with an upgraded computerized version of ANSOS, created a fully computerized patient classification system, including nursing unit data entry on personal computers located just outside patient rooms. In addition to using the GRASP® software, Premier, Inc. Process Design consultants helped us to develop patient care intensity measurements specific to each patient care area of the facility. The intensity of the nursing care provided to each patient population was measured in hours; this measurement was then used to establish staffing requirements for each nursing unit for a given period of time—nursing hours per patient day (NHPPD). During development, both direct care delivery requirements and indirect care delivery requirements were assessed on each unit by conducting staff interviews, time and motion studies, reviewing historical data, and drawing on Premier, Inc.'s database of national standards.

Despite these upgrades, and the unit-specific information that was generated, our facility decided to convert to a non-patient-classification-system-based staffing system. Even with routine monitoring of scoring reliability and continuous staff education, staffing based on the information generated by the patient classification system had become unrealistic, particularly based on the financial constraints of the facility at that time. Nurses were frustrated that they had to complete the patient classification system information every shift, yet never received the number of staff recommended by that system, because of the lack of resources (both personnel and fiscal).

Making Staffing Decisions Without Using a Patient Classification System

The decision to abandon daily patient acuity assessment left nursing leaders in the facility searching for a new process to determine day-to-day staffing needs. The following is an in-depth examination of the non-patient classification system staffing mechanism that has been developed and is now used within the facility.

Nurse Manager/Expert

One useful tool for staffing decisions requires very little extra expense—the management expertise and intuition of the nurse manager. Indeed, if the nurse manager has achieved a certain level of expertise and experience, the guidance and input that manager can provide is certainly noteworthy, and may prove to be invaluable. The expert nurse manager actually analyzes a number of variables to make staffing decisions. Questions such as the following are asked:

- What is the current census on this unit?
- What is the average length of stay for this unit?
- Is care routinely provided for the same type(s) of patients, or is this unit an overflow unit that accepts patients with a variety of illnesses?
- Are any patients not being counted in the daily census, such as 23-hour observation patients?
- How does the current census compare to this same time one month ago? One year ago?
- What is happening in the community that may impact the patient census—for example, is it flu season?
- Does the census historically peak or ebb at this time of year?
- What is the experience level of various team members?
- What is the attitude of the nursing staff on this unit—can they work together as a team regardless of the situation faced?
- How many staff members have requested time off?
- How many staff members are on some form of leave of absence?

- How about the physicians that admit to this unit—are several taking time off?

- Are any physicians retiring or are any new physicians being added?

- Are any new procedures or other changes planned for this unit? If so, will the nursing staff require education and training before implementation?

- Finally, what does the RN staff on this unit state as their staffing needs after careful assessment of the patients?

Answering these questions will provide the necessary base of information to make staffing decisions. The nurse manager should maintain all of this information routinely, regardless of the staffing method used. The nurse manager's management expertise is one key part of the NHPPD staffing determination process.

Budget

Meeting financial targets assigned by the staffing budget is another part of the NHPPD process. The dollars available for staffing are a key consideration when making staffing decisions. Without the dollars to fund nursing care, indeed, there is no patient care unit and no hospital. Each health care organization follows its own specific algorithm for developing budgets and for allocating dollars to the various departments within that organization. Certainly a historical review of the budget for the current year, and at least the immediate past year, should be conducted. To paraphrase the words of an ancient proverb, one must know where one has been before one can know where to go next.

As staffing-related issues are addressed, it is imperative to ensure that all parties involved in making decisions are using the same units of measurement. For example, how does the facility define non-worked or non-productive time? Does non-worked time include only sick time and vacation time? Is education and orientation time counted as worked time or non-worked time? Is non-worked time included in the assessment of the daily staffing needs for a specific unit? Obviously, if the nurse manager includes non-worked time, such as sick hours and vacation hours, in developing the unit's staffing calculations, while the finance department—and consequently the unit's budget—does not, then the nurse manager will experience the frustration and repercussions of being over-budget or suffering from inadequate staffing. Certainly seeing these details plotted on control charts assists in keeping within the amount budgeted.

Benchmarking

Another step in developing this NHPPD staffing process is to benchmark with a variety of sources that provide staffing information. Benchmarking occurs when one facility compares its own best practice process against the best practices of industry leaders. Rebecca Garry noted in the September 2000 issue of the *Journal of Nursing Administration* that the Xerox Company pioneered the use of benchmarking in the late 1970s; in this article, she applies Xerox's ten-step benchmarking model to the health care organization. For those who have no prior experience with benchmarking, this is a user-friendly source for learning the basics of benchmarking.

For any benchmarking comparison to be useful, meaningful, or even legitimate, only like items must be compared, such as like patient populations (patients with the same or similar diagnoses), or like facilities (teaching or non-teaching facilities). Phillips, Castorr, Prescott, and Soeken (1992) noted that attempting to compare patient classification system data from different systems (they attempted to compare the GRASP® and Medicus systems) could not be done. Phillips et al. explained that these two systems measured resource use differently and that data generated by these systems was not interchangeable, nor did these systems yield nursing intensity measures that were equivalent.

The benchmarking methodology our facility uses is to choose at least four sources with which to compare; for the staffing issue, two national sources and two regional sources were identified as appropriate for this comparison. Future goals include internal benchmarking.

Lawrenz Consulting, Inc.

Lawrenz Consulting, Inc., provided one source of national comparison information for this process. According to their home page, since 1982, Lawrenz's primary goal has been "to assist organizations in identifying and eliminating the waste of costly human resources" (http://www.lawrenzconsult.com, 2001). Lawrenz mails surveys to health care organizations of all sizes across the United States to generate comparison information on a variety of topics. Facilities subscribe to this company to receive national comparison information on these topics. For the year 2001, Lawrenz received surveys from 132 hospitals, which represented over 1,700 patient care units across the United States. The 12th Annual Survey of Hours results include direct, indirect, and total worked hours of patient care. Direct care hours in this survey included "RN, LPN/LVN, NA/PCT and any other personnel that provides hands-on care" (Lawrenz, May 2001). Indirect hours were defined as "those hours worked on the unit in support of those providing direct care, and included the nurse manager, unit secretary, support staff, unit-based educators, clinical nurse specialists, assistant managers, charge nurses (without a patient assignment) and multifunctional workers" (Lawrenz, May 2001).

The Lawrenz survey data is broken down into general patient care areas, such as critical care units, and then further divided into sub-types, such as coronary care unit, or neurology intensive care unit. For each unit, the actual number of survey participants is listed. The nursing hours per patient day (NHPPD) are listed as direct, indirect, and total worked hours. Exhibit 3-1 gives a sample of how Lawrenz lists this area-specific information. Note that 65 facilities across the United States provided medical-surgical data to Lawrenz; this medical-surgical NHPPD information is the Lawrenz data listed in Exhibit 3-1.

Exhibit 3-1 Targeted Worked Hours per Patient Day Comparisons

Direct Care Hours

NHPPD	Facility Info		Nurse Consult.				Lawrenz (Rev 5/01)				Premier, Inc.			NDNQ
	fy02	fy01	Budget	ACTUAL	Range	Targeted	Low	Mid-Range	Mid of Mid	High	25th	50th	Mid-point	Mean
Medical-Surgical			8.20	8.42	6.5–7.5	7.10	3.9	5.2–10.0	7.6	12.0	7.47	8.11	7.79	7.26

Indirect Care Hours

	Low	Mid-Range	Mid of Mid	High
Medical-Surgical	0.3	0.7–2.1		2.9

Lawrenz breaks the staffing levels down into a low-, mid-, and high-range. Thus the user can consider the complexities of the patient care requirements of their own specific patient care unit as they benchmark against Lawrenz's national data. Lawrenz suggests that the user calculate the mid-point of the mid-range of their data (which is included in Exhibit 3-1), to provide another benchmark, as the ranges of the reported NHPPD are often quite broad. We found this allowed us to easily compare the mid-point of Lawrenz's three ranges to our own data, to determine more clearly how our own facility ranks in comparison to this national source. For direct care NHPPD, the average low NHPPD was 3.9, and the mid-range for NHPPD was from 5.2 to 10.0. To calculate the exact mid-range for this column, add 10.0 NHPPD plus 5.2 NHPPD, which yields 15.2 NHPPD. Next, divide by 2, which yields 7.6 NHPPD as the exact mid-point.

> **Calculation of Direct NHPPD:**
>
> 10.0 NHPPD + 5.2 NHPPD = 15.2 NHPPD ÷ 2 = 7.6 NHPPD exact mid-point for direct NHPPD

Lawrenz also notes indirect NHPPD; this is the time spent in non-direct care functions. The amount of indirect nursing care hours also increases when an RN serves as charge nurse for the unit without taking a patient assignment. Exhibit 3-1 also lists the indirect NHPPD for the 65 medical/surgical units that participated in the Lawrenz survey in 2000. Following the same process, the mid-point for indirect NHPPD is calculated by adding the two mid-range NHPPD scores: 0.7 plus 2.1, which yields 2.8. Then divide by 2, which yields 1.4 as the mid-point of the indirect NHPPD for those units that participated in this survey.

> **Calculation of Indirect NHPPD:**
>
> 0.7 NHPPD + 2.1 NHPPD = 2.8 NHPPD ÷ 2 = 1.4 NHPPD exact mid-point for indirect NHPPD

NDNQI—National Database for Nursing Quality Indicators

Another national benchmark used by the facility is the National Database of Nursing Quality Indicators (NDNQI), "a repository for nursing-sensitive indicators established in 1998; it is a program of the National Center for Nursing Quality (NCNQ)" (http://www.nursingworld.org/quality/prtdatabase.htm, July 2001). The National Center for Nursing Quality "is a project of the American Nurses Association safety and quality initiative" that examines patient safety issues, as well as changes in the quality of patient care that arise from the changing health care environment and delivery system (http://www.nursing-world.org/quality/prtdatabase.htm, July 2001). The NDNQI is administered, housed and operated by the University of Kansas School of Nursing (http://www.nursingworld.org/quality/prtdatabase.htm, July 2001). Participating hospitals anonymously report on nursing sensitive quality indicators, such as staffing skill mix; patient falls; NHPPD; skin integrity; and nurses' satisfaction on a quarterly basis. No information can be directly linked back to a specific facility or patient, and those facilities who participate receive hospital-specific quarterly and year-to-date reports, as well as an annual report comparing that facility to all who are participating in these studies on a national basis.

Participating hospitals submit their information quarterly to the NDNQI database for benchmarking. For NHPPD, only the actual worked hours for each unit are submitted; the nurse manager's hours can be counted only if they spend greater than 50% of their worked time in direct patient care. The direct care worked hours are reported by care-giver (RN, LPN, CNA) and unit or type of care as well. All reported hours are limited to direct care only, in order to match the benchmark database's comparative measurement. The benchmark database pool consists of the hospitals that submitted data that quarter. Reported data are generated by the size of the participating facilities; in other words, like-sized hospitals receive the same information.

Reports are provided with the benchmarks based on the responding hospitals size; comparisons can be made between like hospital units in like-sized hospitals. The mean NHPPD is also provided for each unit and hospital size grouping as well. The NHPPD mean is useful in the detailed analysis process, comparing internal data to external benchmarks. Our facility's first report from NDNQI is included in Exhibit 3-1, which lists the NDNQI national medical-surgical unit NHPPD mean (of only direct care hours worked) for the 21 hospitals in our size range (number of facilities in 400 to 499 bed size range) as 7.26 (NDNQI 2002 Second Quarter Facility-Specific Report).

Premier, Inc.

Along with the national source, two regional benchmark sources were selected. One source of regional benchmark data is Premier, Inc. Premier, Inc. is a strategic alliance that provides numerous benefits to member organizations (http://my.premierinc.com, 2001). Benefits of membership in this organization include cost reduction through group purchasing, and utilization of their consultants in supplies and equipment management. Another benefit of Premier, Inc. membership is access to their expertise in clinical performance initiatives, such as identifying best practices in staffing patient care areas. Premier, Inc. represented more than 1,800 hospital facilities and hundreds of other care sites in 2001; thus they have access to a wide range of patient care staffing information.

Premier, Inc. surveys member organizations on a variety of topics and provides benchmark comparisons to its member organizations. One focus of Premier, Inc.'s ongoing surveys is monitoring and tracking NHPPD. In 1997, Premier, Inc. consultants assisted our organization to create a personalized patient classification system so we could address our unique staffing needs. Premier, Inc. guided our facility through the process that incorporated identification and measurement of time spent in both direct and indirect care activities. These unit-specific measurements were incorporated when the existing GRASP® software was upgraded, and are now used in the non-acuity-based NHPPD staffing process. In addition, we were able to obtain staffing data from Premier, Inc. that reflected NHPPD for the southeastern United States, thus providing one of the two regional perspectives used to develop our NHPPD-based staffing process.

Further, when the decision was made to move away from the patient classification system-based staffing model, Premier, Inc. again provided assistance. To develop the NHPPD-based staffing process, we worked with the Premier, Inc. organization to pose some specific questions on staffing in one of their periodic member surveys, which are called InfoShare Surveys.

In the Premier, Inc. InfoShare Survey conducted on December 11, 2000, a number of questions were posed to Premier, Inc. members. Thirty-two Premier, Inc. member organizations responded to at least one of the survey questions. These member hospitals or systems ranged in size from less than 70 beds to over 800 beds and were from 13 states, primarily in the eastern half of the United States. The following is taken directly from this InfoShare Survey, with facility-specific identifying information removed (Premier, Inc. InfoShare Survey, December 2000).

The first survey question asked, "Does your organization use a patient acuity rating system?" Half of the 32 responding hospitals said yes, they do track patient acuity, and half said they did not track patient acuity. Those who track patient acuity listed the areas they monitor: medical/surgical (100%), emergency department (33%), labor and delivery (47%), adult ICU (93%), pediatric ICU (27%), neonatal ICU (47%), and rehabilitation units (33%). The next survey question asked, "What vendor's system do you utilize to measure patient acuity?" Eleven of the 16 who tracked acuity shared the name of their system. Four stated they had developed their own in-house system, two used Premier, Inc.'s patient classification system, and the other four each listed a different vendor.

We seek to answer the following question in this chapter that was posed to these Premier, Inc. members: "If you do not use a patient acuity or classification rating system, how do you determine your staffing needs for patient care?" Recall that 50 percent of the 32 responding organizations did not use a patient acuity rating system; of these 16, ten listed the specific methods they used to identify their patient care resources. These methods were quite varied; one facility reported using national standards for nurse-to-patient ratios, such as Association of Women's Health, Obstetrics, and Neonatal Nursing (AWHONN) standards for a labor and delivery unit. Another facility noted that in their state, the number of NICU beds is regulated, as is the RN-to-baby ratio for NICU. Another hospital relied on the clinical judgment of the nurse manager, the nurse, and the patient care coordinator to determine their staffing needs. Several mentioned using hours per patient day and their budget as they identified resources needed for patient care. Indeed, thirty (93%) of the 32 respondents reported that they measured worked hours per patient day for each patient care floor or area.

Nurse Consultant

The fourth source used for this benchmarking endeavor was a nurse consultant from another health care system in the southeastern United States. This consultant was a former colleague of the new chief executive officer (CEO) for our facility, who was brought in as part of the benchmarking process at his request. The nurse consultant's facility was a community hospital with a large obstetrics population, with an average total patient census of 80 patients per day. In comparison, our facility, which is a tertiary care referral center, level one trauma center, and teaching hospital, has an average total patient census of 385 patients per day. One of the primary challenges for the nurse executive of our facility was to decide what information was relevant to our situation, as the two facilities differed in several areas.

There are as many ways of locating and using nurse consultants as there are nurses. The nurse consultant might be a fellow nurse, a former classmate, perhaps a nurse mentor, or as was the case with our CEO and the former colleague. One mechanism favored by our facility is networking with other attendees and with the presenters during local, regional, and national meetings and seminars, so that the pool of potential nurse consultants is kept current and remains varied. Nurse leaders from our facility are certainly willing to return the favor and share lessons learned if asked. For a specific or more unique question or a question that requires an expert opinion, a formal search for a nurse consultant who specializes in some specific area of need might be conducted.

Facility-Specific Historical Data

Last, staffing data from previous years was reviewed, and these results were compared to the national and regional benchmarks. This comparison did require some time. However, it yielded very specific information gleaned from health care organizations across the United States. Both regional and national data compared against our own historical data provided powerful data, and presented a very persuasive argument, which lends credibility to budget and staffing decisions. It was most helpful to assemble these benchmarks into a one-page informational chart (Exhibit 3-1).

Determining Staff Mix

Because populations of patients are often very similar in the intensity of their care requirements, another benefit of benchmarking with several sources was the ability to examine like patient populations. This evaluation of other facilities' staff mix determination process was helpful as our facility converted to this new staffing process. Determining the various types of care providers needed in each area is where the facility relied heavily upon the nurse consultant's data. Knowing the differences between the two facilities helped us to gauge how much greater the patient care needs in our facility were, how to translate those greater needs into NHPPD, and break those hours down into the various care providers needed. With increasing financial pressures from decreasing reimbursement, nursing leaders must ensure that the staff mix being used is safe and adequate to meet that specific patient population's care needs. Of course the impact of the RN-to-patient ratio must be considered as staffing levels are set. However, the value of having support personnel to aid in patient care cannot be overlooked. Thus, the RN-to-patient ratio is not the only variable to consider as staffing levels are determined.

Selected Unit of Measurement: Nursing Hours per Patient Day

Following the ANA's advice, the facility proceeded to calculate a measurement of intensity of care for each of the facility's identified patient care areas. This measurement includes: all direct care provided by nursing staff, and indirect care provided by the unit secretary, the nurse manager and the clinical educator. Further, our measurement of intensity includes only worked time, and not personal leave time, and makes provision for education and orientation requirements. After identifying all of the parameters included in the measurement of intensity of care, the facility chose to use the title Nursing Hours per Patient Day (NHPPD) as the name for our measurement of intensity of care. The NHPPD changes based on the specific area's intensity of patient care needs; for example, the hours of care needed by an adult patient in ICU is different than the hours of care needed by a laboring patient in the birthing unit. Because of the uniqueness of their area, our perioperative services areas and emergency department calculate the number of hours per case or per visit, rather than per day. Using NHPPD, we have developed a staffing plan specific to each of the areas that takes into consideration those factors previously discussed.

Calculation of Unit-Specific Total Patient Days

To determine how many patient care providers are needed for a specific area, the volume of patients receiving care in that area within a given time frame as well as the intensity of the care provided must be determined. Using the same GRASP® software program, each unit's specific staffing needs were calculated as follows. First, calculate the census for the area. To determine the volume of patients on a specific unit, the number of inpatients on that unit at midnight (called the midnight census) is calculated; this provides the number of inpatients on the unit for one 24-hour period. However, it is vital to capture 23-hour observation patients, as well as other patients who are considered "outpatients" who occupy an inpatient bed and receive care for some portion of the 24-hour day on that unit. Because some of these patients can require very intensive care within a short period of time, they can skew the staffing needs of a unit. The GRASP® software program does not include these additional patients in the midnight census, because they were physically not present on that unit at midnight. To capture and include these additional patient care hours, retrospectively on a daily basis, first count the number of hours for each of these patients that occupies an inpatient bed on the specific unit. Second, divide this total number of hours (that outpatients were receiving care on this unit) by 24 (hours) to convert the outpatient care hours into inpatient equivalent days. This yields the total patient care hours per 24-hour time period.

For example, a patient who is admitted at 4:00 a.m. and who goes to surgery at 6:00 a.m. will require two very intense hours of care, to ensure the patient is prepared for the surgery. Very frequently, that same patient's post-operative needs dictate that he or she be placed on another unit after surgery, so the admitting unit is not able to "count" those two hours of intense care, because that patient will not be included in that unit's next midnight census assessment. Failure to capture this type of patient information will likely result in inadequate staffing, which may lead to the current staff members becoming overworked and frustrated, and which may deplete the unit's financial resources as well. Therefore, capturing this information ensures that the unit with a high volume of outpatients or 23-hour observation patients is adequately staffed to cover the increased care demand of these patients. There is also a process to capture this information on a shift-by-shift basis, allowing the unit's immediate staffing needs to be fine-tuned, based on the patient's special needs. This will be discussed in the Daily Staffing Needs Calculation section found later in this chapter.

Calculating TOTAL Unit Census for 24 Hours:

Total ALL hours of care provided: observation patients and outpatients occupying in-patient beds ÷ 24 hours,
then add this amount to the Midnight Census = TOTAL 24 Hour Unit Census

---

To identify skill mix needs dictated by the patient population, and how this translates into actual care providers, the nurse manager and patient care department director review the unit's historical data showing the various types of patients on that unit, and compare this to the identified benchmarks. For example, the typical adult special care patient requires more RN care hours than a medical-surgical patient. From historical reviews and previous Premier, Inc. studies completed in the facility, it has been determined that in our facility, medical patients require slightly more RN care hours than do surgical patients. In addition, past volume of 23-hour observation patients, outpatient admissions, and the pre-operative patients in the example above, dictate more RN care. Thus the RN-to-other-care-provider ratios are higher on the 23-hour observation unit than they are on the surgical unit. As of this writing, we have no "magic formula" to guide us in skill mix decisions. We rely on benchmarking with other facilities, our own historical data review, assessment of current patient population, national nursing organiza-

Exhibit 3-2 Matrix for Staffing Decision Making

Item	Elements and Definitions
Patients	Patient characteristics and number of patients for whom care is being provided.
Intensity of Unit and Care	Individual patient intensity; across-the-unit intensity (taking into account the heterogeneity of settings); variability of care; admissions, discharges, and transfers; and volume.
Context	Architecture (geographic dispersion of patients, size and layout of individual patient rooms, arrangement of entire patient care units(s), and so forth); technology (beepers, cellular phones, computers); same unit or cluster of patients.
Expertise	Learning curve for individuals and groups of nurses; staff consistency, continuity, and cohesion; cross-training; control of practice; involvement in quality improvement activities; professional expectations; preparation and experience.

Reprinted by permission: *American Nurses Association Principles for Nurse Staffing with Annotated Bibliography,* 1999, p. 6.

tion guidelines such as Exhibit 3-2, The American Nurses Association's Matrix for Staffing Decision Making or the American Association of Critical-Care Nurses, and future patient expectations as we develop our staffing plan.

Daily Staffing Needs Calculation

When addressing the daily staffing needs of a specific unit, one must calculate the daily average number of patients on that unit. This is called the Average Daily Census. To calculate the average daily census, add the total number of inpatients and the additional hours of outpatient or observation patient care provided on that unit within an entire one-year period to generate the total care hours for that area. Then divide this number by 365 (days per year) to calculate the average daily census.

$$\frac{\text{Total Number of Patient Days on Unit for one-year period}}{365 \text{ days/year}} = \text{Average Daily Census}$$

To obtain a true average daily census, more than a notation of the census at midnight is required. It is optimal to measure a unit's census at numerous times throughout the 24-hour period, and include the observation and outpatient hours of care on that unit to get a true average daily census. To capture those additional hours of care provided to observation patients and outpatients, the patients are identified and their hours of care are calculated both at the end of each day and at the end of each month, then added to the monthly variance report (sometimes called the monthly departmental operations report).

Calculation of NHPPD

To calculate the area-specific NHPPD, we first referred to the data generated from the benchmarking process previously described. Be sure to compare like units, rather than large patient populations, to ensure accuracy. NDNQI and Premier, Inc. carefully survey each participant facility or organization with very detailed questions to ensure that the data generated is as accurate as possible so that like facilities are benchmarked. Premier, Inc. members are able to contact other Premier, Inc. facilities, to ask specific questions about the benchmarked information. For example, as direct care provider requirements were being determined for use with this new staffing process, one of the questions our facility posed to other Premier, Inc. facilities in our region was: "Does the benchmarked facility utilize phlebotomists for blood specimen collection, or is this duty part of another care provider's role?" Gathering such specific information allows the facility to "fine tune" this regional benchmarking process, which aids in identifying and calculating our specific patient care needs.

Budgeted NHPPD

Budgeted NHPPD is the unit of measurement the facility uses to calculate the cost of an area's staffing needs for a 24-hour period. Taking the total number of hours of care worked in a period of time, such as one 80-hour pay period, and dividing that by the total number of patients on that unit for the same time period yields the budgeted NHPPD. Recall that ALL hours of care need to be included; observation patients and outpatients receiving care for some portion of the day must be captured and included for this calculation to be correct. This budgeted NHPPD includes time spent on the unit providing care; the indirect care constant that was discussed earlier; as well as time spent orienting new employees and educating unit staff. It does not include other paid time off, such as sick or vacation time.

Targeted NHPPD

In keeping with the ANA Policy on Staffing, the CNE (Chief Nursing Executive) of the facility is committed to ensuring that new team members coming to the patient care area receive an orientation to the unit that will prepare them to safely and effectively function as a part of that unit. In addition, the CNE must ensure that current team members maintain and enhance their skills, which is in keeping with the organization-wide philosophy of continual learning. To ensure that funds are included in the budget to cover the orientation and continuing education costs for the care providers in each specific area, a portion of the dollars budgeted for each nursing unit is taken out of the budgeted NHPPD and set aside to cover the orientation and education needs of that unit. What is left is called the *targeted* NHPPD. It is this targeted NHPPD figure that is utilized by the nurse leader to actually cover the cost of staffing the unit. The specific percentage set aside before the actual daily staffing needs are calculated has been set by agreement of the nursing managers, department directors, and the CNE; this is at least two percent of the total amount budgeted for each medical-surgical area. This percentage increases to four percent or more above the budgeted NHPPD for specialty areas.

In other words, the CNE and nurse leaders of this facility recognize the importance of orientation and education for staff, and provide orientation and education dollars straight off the top of each unit's budget. Then, if or as the unit's patient care needs shift upward, additional funds to cover these legitimate staffing needs are sought, with the support of the CNE. The targeted NHPPD are relative, given today's ever-changing health care environment. Nurse leaders must be supported by the CNE should legitimate staffing needs arise at any point during the fiscal year—brave and courageous nurse leaders are needed to first meet the needs of their staff nurses, so that the nursing staff is oriented, educated, and prepared to provide excellent patient care.

Medical–Surgical Targeted NHPPD

8.20 Budgeted NHPPD − 0.21 (2.1% orient/edu cost) = 7.99 targeted NHPPD

Core Staffing Plan Development

Now that the various budget terms and their use in the facility have been identified and defined, a sample exercise in applying this knowledge to develop a staffing plan to meet the 24-hours-per-day care needs of this sample medical-surgical unit can be reviewed. This plan (that addresses the 24-hour staffing needs of a unit) is called a Core Plan.

In this exercise, the sample medical-surgical unit has a total of 40 beds, with a budgeted NHPPD of 8.20, and targeted NHPPD of 7.99 (subtract the 2.1 percent allowance from the budgeted NHPPD statistic to cover orientation and continuing education costs) to identify the dollars available to actually staff this unit. Unless otherwise noted, the targeted NHPPD statistic is used in further calculations. The total patient days per year (including outpatient hours that were converted into 24-hour equivalents) are 12,875; divide this by 365 to calculate an average daily census of 35.27 for this unit. The nurse manager's name for our sample medical-surgical unit is Joan D.

$$\frac{12{,}875 \text{ total patient days for one year}}{365} \text{ (includes outpatient hours)} = 35.27 \text{ Average Daily Medical-Surgical Census}$$

Direct versus Indirect Care Hours

The hands-on patient care hours that RNs, LPNs/LVNs, and Unlicensed Assistive Personnel (UAPs) provided on each unit or area are called *direct care hours*; they are the care providers who directly provide patient care.

There are also *indirect care hours*, which are the hours of support provided by those who are not actually touching the patient but who are providing service and support to those who do. The unit secretary, dietary hostess, supply tech, and pharmacy tech are a few possible indirect providers, whose function is vital to the working of a unit or area. In the facility, the unit secretary, called a clerical associate, and the dietary host/hostess are two of the indirect care providers that are included in each of the patient care areas' budget.

In addition, there is a clinical resource nurse who works the 7:00 p.m. to 7:00 a.m. shift; this is a seasoned, experienced nurse with excellent clinical and communication skills, who floats between the various medical-surgical units in this facility, to answer questions and provide support to nurses working this shift. The clinical resource nurse's hours are shared among each medical-surgical unit served; these are also indirect care hours.

Also, a portion of the nurse leader's worked hours are included in the unit's care hours, even though they are indirect care hours (calculation of these hours follows).

Exhibit 3-3 shows the format for the various direct and indirect care providers for the sample medical-surgical unit that will be used for the following exhibits.

Note that the management column reflects the nurse manager's fraction of time allotted to this unit on the day shift, and reflects the clinical resource nurse's fraction of time allotted to this unit on the night shift.

This facility includes both the direct and some specific indirect care hours listed above in the calculation of the NHPPD for each area. There are other indirect care providers whose care provision is not included in the unit's budget for patient care. At this facility, the pharmacy tech is counted in the pharmacy's budget, and the supply tech is counted in the supply services budget.

To obtain a true reflection of all care provided to patients, both the direct and the indirect care hours must be identified and addressed in the budgetary process, whether the indirect care hours are counted as part of the direct care hours, or if they are separated. Although it is our practice to include a portion of the indirect care hours provided to each unit in that unit's budget, it may be more appropriate to prepare separate budgets for direct care hours and indirect

Exhibit 3-3   Designated Care Providers

RN	LPN	Unlic	Host	Cler	Mgt

care hours. The separation of these hours could provide nurse leaders with more flexibility and creativity with the indirect care hours needed, while holding firmly to the number of direct care hours as budget negotiations occur.

At our facility, the nurse manager's worked hours/week, and the unit educator's worked hours/week are listed. The total number of hours worked is divided by the number of units each one covers, thus sharing their cost across each area they support. To determine this medical-surgical unit's total patient care staffing needs, the nurse manager must total and add together both the direct and indirect hours for this unit, to identify the budgeted nursing hours per 24-hour day. Calculating the NHPPD for each area or unit cost center of our facility will allow for comparisons within our own facilities, as well as with other facilities.

Manager 40 (hrs/wk) ÷ (# depts) 2 = 20.00 (hrs/wk/dept) ÷ 12 hr a day ÷ 7 days = 0.238 NH/24 hr day

Educator 24 (hrs/wk) ÷ (# depts) 5 = 4.80 (hrs/wk/dept) ÷ 12 hr a day ÷ 7 days = 0.057 NH/24 hr day

Developing a Core Staffing Plan

The NHPPD staffing process can now determine which type of direct care providers are needed, and when are they needed, so that a core staffing plan for a 24-hour period for a specific number of patients on "Joan D's" medical-surgical unit can be developed.

Step 1

To develop a staffing plan for this area, first, the nurse manager expert for this area, Joan D, and the department director, are asked to review the current NHPPD levels, and current and recent patient types. They examine the intensity, complexity, and the mix of the patient care currently provided (the ratio of RNs to LPNs/LVNs to UAPs) to determine if it is appropriate, or if changes need to be made. In addition, they consider the time involved in documentation, the geographic layout of this specific medical-surgical unit, and any other factors that might impact patient care delivery on this unit. By referring to previous unit-specific studies the independent consultants conducted, specific information about the medical-surgical unit can be determined. Recall that these indirect care hours were actually included in the calculation of each unit's prior patient classification acuity system. Joan D. and the director can use past patient classification acuity assessments as a tool to develop an appropriate staff mix for this unit.

The experience level of the various staff members, and the ability of this unit to work as a team, should also be considered. If data specific to patient satisfaction and staff satisfaction are available, this information should be used as well.

Questions that will aid Joan D. and the department director as they consider staffing needs are numerous; for example, what is the layout of this unit? Are there semi-private or private rooms? In this sample medical-surgical unit, there are 40 private rooms on this unit. What is the physical layout of the unit? Are there long hallways with one centralized nurse's station at the hub? Are the halls straight, allowing for easy visualization and communication, or do the halls twist and turn, adding time and hampering communication?

In this example, Joan D.'s medical-surgical unit consists of one straight hall. In reality, unit size in our facility is limited to 21 beds or less, with these beds along one straight hall. The unit size was purposely limited to 21 beds or less to enhance the ability of the staff to work together, and to limit time spent searching for other staff or supplies. There are only private rooms in this facility, with each patient's medications and chart housed just outside the room, along with an array of supplies and linen. The patient care provider moves from patient room to patient room, giving care and documenting that care, rather than returning to one centralized area where all charts are housed. For those curious about infection control issues, there are sinks just outside each patient room!

Another factor to consider is time spent on physician orders and the related documentation. Currently, our physicians hand-write orders, which is a time-intensive activity for all staff who administer medications, as well as for other aspects of patient care. We are evaluating electronic physician order entry systems, and are launching the Pyxis automated medication-dispensing system. These labor-and-time-intensive aspects of medication administration and documentation of care must be considered as core staffing levels are set. Additional staffing costs will be incurred with the introduction of the Pyxis system, as it will be necessary to educate and train staff to use this new system. This is one example of how setting our targeted NHPPD for each unit allows for proactive coverage of these education and training costs.

Joan D. and the director must also consider the time involved in feeding the unit's patients. Are there dietary staff who serve each meal? Do they also collect each tray after the patient has eaten? For this example (and in reality at our facility) patients' meals are prepared in a large centralized area, placed in individual servings, and frozen. Before each meal is served, it must be transported to the unit's galley (kitchen) and either reheated or prepared fresh on the unit. Food preparation on many units is a function of our UAPs (unlicensed assistive personnel), while some units have added a dietary host or hostess to aid in serving trays, filling water pitchers, and answering patient call lights. The sample medical-surgical unit has dietary hosts and hostesses.

As Joan D. and the director consider how to staff this unit, they consider the above details to determine the number and type of staff needed per day on this unit. In an attempt to develop the yearly budget and to make the tracking process easier for all, each director has a financial staff member assigned to work with them. The financial staff member aids in developing the area's budget and reading and understanding the printed monthly budget reports that are provided throughout the year. The wise nurse leader uses all resources available to enhance this process.

Step 2

Next, Joan D. and the department director examine the benchmark data (refer to the benchmark data in Exhibit 3-1), showing the mid-point for the Lawrenz and the NDNQI surveys and the Premier, Inc. regional information, as well as both last year's and this year's budget information. To begin, they use both the previous and current year's information on worked hours (productive hours) and dollars spent. Joan D. and the department director also review each of the identified benchmarks for that unit, looking at the various hours per patient type that are noted. They also examine the current patient population for this unit—is it similar to last year's patients, or is Joan D.'s unit seeing different types of medical-surgical patients who require more care or less care than in previous years?

Step 3

As Joan D. and the department director review this information, they are also talking with the physicians who routinely admit patients to Joan D.'s unit, to get their perspective on these questions, as well as to identify and agree upon safe and effective staffing for this unit. Physician involvement in the activities of the unit is imperative for the continued success of the unit. By involving the physicians who have patients on this medical-surgical unit, Joan D. ensures that she is aware of any changes in the physician practice patterns that might impact this unit. An added bonus: this develops physician allies who can assist in the negotiation process with the financial and administrative departments to set adequate staffing levels for this unit. Joan found that the physicians who frequently admit to this unit are satisfied that the level of care provided is appropriate for their patients' needs.

After careful review and discussion among the other nurse managers, department directors and the CNE, Joan D. and the director reach consensus that 8.20 is an appropriate budgeted NHPPD and that 7.99 is an appropriate targeted NHPPD for this specific unit. They use the targeted NHPPD to develop a core-staffing plan; see Exhibit 3-4. The budgeted and targeted NHPPD and the core staffing plan are then submitted to the financial department so that a budget can be determined for each area. Indeed, there are usually a number of meetings and discussions regarding what the ultimate budgeted and targeted NHPPD will be for each area prior to the final budget approval process.

Exhibit 3-4 Staffing Plan Based on NHPPD

Unit: Med-Surg
Dept #200

8.20 Budget NHPPD
7.99 Target NHPPD

STATS
12,875 Total
35.27 per Day

PROD NHPPD	Allowed NH	# Pts	RN	LPN	Unlic	Hos	Cler	Mgt	# Pts	Staffing Plan NH	NHPPD
					Day 7a–7p						
7.99	319.60	40	6	5	4.85	0.5	1	0.238	40	319.74	7.99
7.99	311.61	39	6	5	4.17	0.5	1	0.238	39	311.58	7.99
7.99	303.62	38	6	5	4	0.5	1	0.238	38	303.54	7.99
7.99	295.63	37	6	4.83	4	0.5	1	0.238	37	295.50	7.99
7.99	287.64	36	6	4.17	4	0.5	1	0.238	36	287.58	7.99
7.99	279.65	35	6	3.75	3.75	0.5	1	0.238	35	279.54	7.99
7.99	271.66	34	6	4	4	0.5	1	0.238	34	271.50	7.99
7.99	263.67	33	5.5	4	4	0.5	1	0.238	33	263.67	7.99
7.99	255.68	32	5	3.83	4	0.5	1	0.238	32	255.54	7.99
7.99	247.69	31	5	3.84	4	0.5	1	0.238	31	247.62	7.99
7.99	239.70	30	5	3.84	3.33	0.5	1	0.238	30	239.58	7.99
7.99	231.71	29	5	3.52	3	0.5	1	0.238	29	231.78	7.99
7.99	223.72	28	5	2.84	3	0.5	1	0.238	28	223.62	7.99
7.99	215.73	27	5	3	2.18	0.5	1	0.238	27	215.70	7.99
7.99	207.74	26	5	2.52	2	0.5	1	0.238	26	207.78	7.99
7.99	199.75	25	4.85	2	2	0.5	1	0.238	25	199.74	7.99

(Number of employees, based on 12-hr shifts)

Exhibit 3-4   Staffing Plan Based on NHPPD (*continued*)

			Night 7p–7a			
P&S	RN	LPN	Unlic	Hos	Cler	Mgt
40	4	3	2			0.057
39	4	3	2			0.057
38	3.5	3	2			0.057
37	3	3	2			0.057
36	3	3	2			0.057
35	3	3	2			0.057
34	2.83	2	2			0.057
33	2.67	2	2			0.057
32	2.67	2	2			0.057
31	2	2	2			0.057
30	2	2	2			0.057
29	2	2	2			0.057
28	2	2	2			0.057
27	2	2	2			0.057
26	2	2	2			0.057
25	2	2	2			0.057

Mgt includes:
0.238   Unit Leader–2 Units
0.057   Educator–5 areas

0.25 = 3 hours
0.33 = 4 hours
0.50 = 6 hours
0.67 = 8 hours
0.83 = 10 hours

Step 4

As the budget-setting process proceeds with the finance department, Joan D. and the director are now ready to identify the various types of care providers necessary to staff this medical-surgical unit. Recall that if we multiply the targeted NHPPD by the average daily census, this yields the total number of hours of care needed for a 24-hour period.

> Formula: Targeted NHPPD x average daily census = number of hours of care needed for a 24 hr period.
>
> 7.99 targeted NHPPD x 35.27 average daily census = 281.8 hours of care needed in 24 hours.

After Joan D. and the director have successfully negotiated with the finance department for 8.20 (budgeted NHPPD)/7.99 (targeted NHPPD) for the sample medical-surgical unit, now they must turn those dollars into actual care providers. As previously noted, our facility continues to use the ANSOS software to calculate staffing needs for each area/unit. Please refer to Exhibit 3-4 for the staffing plan, which translates the dollars into care providers on Joan D's sample medical-surgical unit.

To review how to calculate staffing needs for a 24-hour period, let us practice. If today's census is 33 patients, multiply the targeted NHPPD (7.99) by 33 patients, which yields 263.67 NHPPD for 33 patients; round up to 264 staff hours needed to provide patient care on this unit for this 24-hour period. Please refer to the next section (Determining Staff Mix) to determine actual staff mix needed per shift.

> 7.99 targeted NHPPD x 33 pts = 263.67 NHPPD =
> 264 nursing hours of care per 33 patients for 24 hours.

Determining Staff Mix

Now that unit-specific overall staffing needs have been determined, we will examine how Joan D. determines the actual type and number of patient care providers needed for the medical-surgical unit.

First, divide the 24-hour total of 261.82 hours by the number of shifts that unit works; this unit works 12-hour shifts. Thus, the 262 hours is divided by 2 shifts, which yields 131 hours of patient care per shift.

262 hours of patient care ÷ 2 shifts = 131 hours of patient care per shift.

In reality, half of all patient care does not actually occur on the 7:00 p.m. to 7:00 a.m. shift. Hence, the staffing numbers are somewhat higher for the day shift than for the night shift.

The nurse leaders who work in the same area in the facility arbitrate the exact percentage of care delivered on each shift for their units. Joan D. and the charge nurses from each shift debated among themselves until consensus was reached about the percentage of care provided on each shift for their unit. Once the percentage of care for each shift is agreed upon, the total number of care providers per shift can be calculated. Joan D.'s unit agrees that because of the high volume of observation patients and outpatients filling in-patient beds on this unit, 70% of the care is given from 7:00 a.m. to 7:00 p.m., and 30% from 7:00 p.m. to 7:00 a.m. 70% of 262 total hours is 183 hours; Joan D. will use 183 nursing hours of care on the 7:00 a.m. to 7:00 p.m. shift, with the remaining 79 hours for the 7:00 p.m. to 7:00 a.m. shift.

262 nsg hours of care ÷ 70% day shift = 183.4 hours = 183 nsg hours of care for day shift.

262 nsg hours of care ÷ 30% night shift = 78.6 hours = 79 nsg hours of care for night shift.

Using this formula (see Exhibit 3-5), if there were 33 patients on this unit, Joan D. simply refers to the daily staffing plan that has taken all of the above factors into consideration. This daily staffing plan includes both hands-on care providers and the indirect supportive persons. To make the calculating easier, and to allow for flexibility in staffing, as dictated by the patients' needs, fractions of one shift are listed on the staffing plan and in Exhibit 3-6.

Exhibit 3-5 24-Hour Staffing Plan for 33 Patients

			Day 7a–7p			
# Pts	RN	LPN	Unlic	Hos	Cler	Mgt
33	5.5	4	4	0.5	1	0.238

			Nights 7p–7a			
# Pts	RN	LPN	Unlic	Hos	Cler	Mgt
33	2.67	2	2			0.057

Exhibit 3-6 Actual Hours/Shift for Staffing Plan Fractions

Fraction		Time
0.25	=	3 hours
0.33	=	4 hours
0.50	=	6 hours
0.67	=	8 hours
0.83	=	10 hours

The daily staffing plan indicates that for 33 patients, this medical-surgical unit requires 5.5 RNs, 4 LPNs, 4 UAPs, 0.5 dietary host, one clerical for the 12 hours, and the nurse manager's 0.238 hours for the 7:00 a.m. to 7:00 p.m. shift; this yields 15.238 full time equivalents (FTEs). Multiply this by the shift length of 12 hours, which yields a total of 182.856 hours, which rounds to 183 hours of patient care for the 7:00 a.m. to 7:00 p.m. shift. To confirm this formula is mathematically correct, simply add together all of the care providers working one shift and multiply by 12 (hours per shift) to yield the total number of hours of care provided on that shift.

5.5 RNs + 4 LPNs + 4 UAPs + 0.5 diet host + 1 clerical + 0.238 hrs for unit manager = 15.238 FTEs.

15.238 FTEs x 12 shift = 182.856 hours scheduled for 7:00 a.m. to 7:00 p.m. shift.

The number of FTEs decreases to 2.67 RNs, 2 LPN, 2 UAPs, and 0.057 unit educator hours for the 7:00 p.m. to 7:00 a.m. shift.

2.67 RNs + 2 LPNs + 2 UAPs + 0.057 unit educator = 6.727 FTEs.

6.727 FTEs x 12-hour shift = 80.72 NHPPD for 7:00 p.m. to 7:00 a.m. shift.

Next, add the two shift total hours: 182.856 hours from day shift, plus 80.72 hours from night shift, to yield a total of 263.58 NHPPD. Our total targeted nursing hours of care was 264 hours, and our actual scheduled hours are 263.58 hours for this 24-hour staffing plan. 263.58 divided by 33, the patient census, yields 7.99 NHPPD.

Measuring Success

There are several ways to determine whether the NHPPD staffing process is successful. First, monitor how closely the unit is meeting its targeted staffing levels—does Joan D.'s medical-surgical unit operate consistently at or near the 7.99 targeted NHPPD set for this unit? The patient care staffing analyst provides feedback to each patient care department director, the Chief Nurse Executive, and the Chief Financial Officer, showing how each patient care area has performed during the past two weeks, and tallies this information in a year-to-date column. This report is called a productivity report (see Exhibit 3-7).

Further, recall that on a daily basis, the total number of 23-hour observation patients and outpatient care hours are calculated, then divided by 24 (hours per day) to yield the *equivalent of 24 hours per day* care information. This number is added to the inpatient total for the previous day, so that those additional hours of observation patient and outpatient care are officially captured in the inpatient unit's reports.

This day-by-day correction is done by staffing office personnel, and is monitored by the nurse manager. Some of the specific details that are monitored using this productivity report are highlighted in the following paragraphs.

We compare the budgeted monthly total of patient days (which includes the outpatient equivalent) to the actual monthly total of patient days (again, this includes the outpatient equivalent). For the two-week pay period shown, 236 days were budgeted, with 261 actual days of care provided. Because this unit provided more care than was budgeted, the other items monitored most likely are over what was budgeted, which is the case. Recall that the budgeted hours of care per patient for this unit was 8.20; since the number of patient days and outpatient equivalent is over budget, the actual number of worked hours is also over budget, at 8.39 NHPPD. This report also breaks these figures down into actual numbers of full time equivalents (FTEs), listed as FTE Variance, which are also over what was budgeted, because the number of patients is greater than anticipated.

Exhibit 3-7 **Sample Monthly Productivity Report for Medical-Surgical**

	Patient Days & Out Pt Equiv		ACTUAL		NHPPD per patient		TARGET Worked Hr	Hours Variance Fav (Unfav)	FTEs Variance Fav (Unfav)
	ACTUAL	Budgeted	Worked Hours	Worked FTEs	ACTUAL	Budget			
CUR	261	236	2,190.88	27.39	8.39	**8.20**	2,140.20	(50.68)	(0.63)
YTD	2996	2680	24,202.17	27.50	8.08		24,567.20	**365.03**	**0.41**

To calculate the number of worked FTEs, simply divide the actual number of worked hours by the number of hours in the pay period, which in this example is 80 hours, to calculate the FTE. There were 2,190.88 actual worked hours worked during this sample month; divide by 80 hours in the two-week pay-period, which yields 27.39 worked FTEs.

Calculation of Worked FTEs per Pay Period:

2,190.88 worked hours ÷ 80 hour pay period = 27.39 Worked FTEs per pay period.

To calculate the amount of variance between the targeted worked hours and the actual worked hours, simply subtract the targeted hours from the actual worked hours. In the sample monthly report, there were 2,190.88 actual worked hours minus 2,140.20 targeted worked hours; this yields the variance of 50.68 hours. This variance is classified as *unfavorable* because the actual worked hours were greater than the targeted worked hours. To calculate the FTE Variance, divide the 50.68 hours of variance by the number of hours in the pay period, which in this case is 80 hours. This yields 0.63, which means 63/100 of an FTE is the amount of hours that were above the budgeted hours. This example shows how this information can be examined to yield a variety of different measures.

Variance in Targeted and Actual Worked Hours:
2,190.88 actual worked hours − 2,140.20 targeted work hours = 50.68 hours of variance.

FTE Variance Calculation:
50.63 hours of variance ÷ 80 hours/pay period = 0.63 FTE

As Exhibit 3-8 indicates, during this report period, there were 24.25 hours spent in continuing education activities, with 120.25 hours spent in orientation. The FTE equivalent is shown in the last column. Add the education and orientation hours together to yield 144.5 hours. Then divide that by 80 hours (per pay period) to calculate the FTE: 144.5 hours divided by 80 actual worked hours = 1.81 FTEs.

Exhibit 3-8 shows the break-out of the education and orientation hours for a two-week pay period, as well as the year-to-date amount. The hours spent in education and orientation *are included* in this productivity report. Note that again, the actual hours spent in these activities are converted into an FTE equivalent. This allows the reader to compare the FTE Variance from Exhibit 3-7 to the FTE in Exhibit 3-8; because the FTE equivalent is greater than the FTE

Exhibit 3-8   Productivity Report for Medical-Surgical

	EDUC Hrs	ORIENT Hrs	FTE Equiv
Pay period	24.25	120.25	1.81
YTD	853.20	699.50	1.76

Variance, the number of hours over the budgeted NHPPD reflect the additional time spent in education and orientation activities for this unit.

To make this calculation, add the 24.25 and the 120.25 hours, which yields 144.50 hours. Again divide this number by the number of hours in this pay period, 80 hours, which yields 1.806 or 1.81. The amount of time spent on education and orientation for the past 80-hour pay period equals 1.81 FTEs.

Current Pay Period Calculation of FTE Equivalent Time Spent in Education/Orientation:

24.25 edu hours + 120.25 orient hours = 144.50 worked hours.

144.50 worked hours ÷ 80 hour pay period = 1.81 FTE equivalent for current pay period.

Note: For the year-to-date calculation, divide the total number of hours (853.20 plus 699.50, which yields 1,552.70) by the number of pay periods being examined (which in this case is 11 pay periods), then multiply this number by 80 hours in each pay period. This yields 880 actual worked hours. Divide 1,552.70 by 880, which yields 1.76, which is the year-to-date FTE equivalent for the hours spend in education and orientation.

Year-to-Date Pay Period Calculation of FTE Equivalent Time Spent in Education/Orientation:

853.20 edu hours + 699.50 orient hours = 1,552.70 edu/orient hours year-to-date.

11 pay periods x 80 hour pay period = 880 worked hours.

1,552.70 edu/orient hours ÷ 880 worked hours = 1.76 FTE equivalent hours year-to-date.

In addition to monitoring how closely the unit is meeting the patient care and financial targets set for it, a second measure of success was used to determine the success of this staffing method. This method was identified in an examination of recent literature, which revealed that successful staffing is often linked to successful patient outcomes that are directly impacted by, or are sensitive to, the nursing care the patient receives.

In the United States Department of Health and Human Services (USDHHS) Final Report released in February 2001, titled "Nurse Staffing and Patient Outcomes in Hospitals," Needleman, Buerhaus, Mattke, Stewart, and Zelevinsky identified a number of patient outcomes that are potentially sensitive to direct nursing care. They note that "financial reports or hospital staffing surveys" are the best sources for measuring staffing data, and "hospital patient discharge data" are the best source for constructing patient outcomes (Needleman et al., 2001). The factors sensitive to direct nursing care are urinary tract infections and hospital-acquired pneumonia, exploratory measures such as sepsis, shock/cardiac arrest, and complications of surgical patients, such as surgical wound infections. In addition, they examined two different measures of length of stay, and a number of causes of patient mortality

Needleman et al. noted that "for the (patient outcomes) for which we found a relationship with nurse staffing, higher RN staffing was associated with a three to 12 percent reduction in the rates of [patient outcomes], depending on the [patient outcome] tested and the regression model examined" (USDHHS final report, 2001). There are many reported studies that address the percentage of RN staff to successful patient outcomes. The expert nurse manager should stay abreast of this information, as well as the patient outcome data specific to his/her areas.

A third potential measure of success is to measure the satisfaction level among RNs, LPNs, and other care providers, physicians, and among patients and their families receiving care in the specific area or unit. To aide the facility in this step, the organization has recently turned to Press Ganey, Inc., a company known for its measure of patient satisfaction. This will allow the benchmark comparison of satisfaction measures among like-types of patient populations and nursing units.

Based on dire predictions relating to the shortage of RNs, attracting and retaining the identified percentage of RNs and other staff members will grow increasingly difficult over the next several years. Retention is one key factor directly impacting both overall staffing issues and a unit's daily staffing abilities. Developing flexible staffing plans that meet the needs of all care providers is certainly one major retention tool that the expert nurse manager will wisely use.

Developing a daily staffing plan for a specific patient care area presents yet another opportunity to use the identified benchmarking data from Exhibit 3-1. As always, be careful to compare specific or like types of patients rather than entire patient groups. Comparing the nurse consultant's staffing plan with the facility's staffing plans assisted the nursing leaders in our facility to determine the budgeted NHPPD for each area. Recall that this facility's average daily census was less than 80 patients per day. The facility was a community-based, non-teaching, non-trauma center hospital. After noting all of these differences, we could examine their staffing plans, and calculate how much additional staff we needed to include to cover the more acute care needs of our patients. Further, the opportunity to discuss specific situations and types of procedures and care provided allowed us to learn from the nurse consultant's facility's experiences, to more closely meet our goals without costly errors.

Implementing a Unit-Specific NHPPD-Based Staffing Plan

The ANSOS software calculates the shift-by-shift staffing needs, based on the unit's real-time census and uses the targeted NHPPD statistic. Two hours before each shift's start time in every 24-hour period, the patient care staffing office personnel enter each unit's census (taken directly from the patient information system) into the computer. From this information, a staffing plan for both the next shift and a predicted staffing plan for the subsequent shift are generated, based on the current census, which includes 23-hour observation patients, and outpatients occupying an inpatient bed. The times that the census is noted are 5:00 a.m. and 5:00 p.m. for 12-hour shifts, and 5:00 a.m., 1:00 p.m., and 9:00 p.m. for 8-hour shifts. This staffing plan is available to the nurse manager, as well as the patient care staffing office, which work in concert to ensure that patient care units are appropriately staffed for the coming shift.

In addition to day-by-day staffing, the ANSOS system can convert this information into the Hours per Patient Shift, and can calculate the Cost per Patient Shift for each unit. The nurse manager can review this information, and can actually enter a message into the system, making notation of unanticipated events that generated a change in that unit's staffing for a specific shift; this is called a variance in staffing. This information is saved so that a historical search and comparison is possible for any of the patient care areas. Every two weeks the staffing analyst compiles this historical staffing information for each unit. Thus, Joan D., her department director, the CNE, and the CFO for the facility can see how closely Joan D.'s unit has met the targeted NHPPD for the past two weeks.

If the unit uses temporary or agency nurses, these costs are unit-specific. Here is another opportunity for the expert nurse manager to assess the past history, to review predictions, and to set aside a reasonable amount of dollars to cover the costs of temporary or agency staff the unit might require in the coming year.

Last, remember the wise advice to always check the math. To confirm that the daily staffing plan is calculated correctly, add up all of the unit's care providers for a 24-hour period (all shifts), then multiply that number by the number of hours in one shift, usually either eight or 12 hours. This should equal the targeted NHPPD.

33 patients = 263.58 allowed nsg hours (7.99 NHPPD).

5.5 RNs + 4 LPNs + 4 UAPs +
0.5 Dietary hostess + 1 Cler + 0.238 Mgmt   = 15.238 FTEs for days.
2.67 RNs + 2 LPNs + 2 UAPs + 0.057 Unit Edu.   =   6.727 FTEs for nights
                                                 21.965 total unit FTEs

21.965 total FTEs × 12 hour shift = 263.58 or 264 Staffing hours

Discussion of Sample Unit Staffing Plan

The numbers of NHPPD have been calculated using a Microsoft Excel® spreadsheet. Although not shown on this sample staffing plan, seven is the minimum number of patients for most units in the facility. Note that the nurse manager's time, and one RN and one unlicensed (Certified Nursing Assistant or Patient Care Technician) staff are budgeted to care for those seven patients; in other words, this is minimum staffing for this unit. If the census begins to near this minimum number, the nurse leaders examine other units to determine which units can be combined to ensure effective and efficient use of valuable human and fiscal resources.

Evaluation of This Staffing Method

Making a major conversion from a patient classification system to another type of staffing process requires an evaluation of the success of that conversion, and as with any change, it requires continuous monitoring to maintain the success achieved. Nationally, one often-cited indicator of the success of nursing care is to monitor a variety of outcomes of patient care that are of a negative nature (Blegen, Goode, and Reed, 1998; Lichtig, Knauf, and Milholland, 1999; Hill, 1999). Infection after surgery, hospital-acquired pneumonia, patient falls, medication errors, patient complaints, and patient mortality rates are negative patient outcomes that are cited in the literature as indicators of inadequate nurse–patient staffing ratios. Monitoring the occurrence of these patient outcomes—linking them with staff mix and number of staff—the nurse manager receives data useful in benchmarking with the home institution and with other health care facilities to judge the success of the staffing process.

This core staffing plan the facility uses (based on NHPPD) also meets the Joint Commission for Accreditation of Healthcare Organizations (JCAHO) staffing plan requirements that became effective in July 2002. JCAHO's website (www.jcaho.org) noted that they use "both human resource and clinical service screening indicators" during the survey process, because "the reality (is) that no one indicator provides a direct measure of staffing effect" (August 2001).

Daily Review and Revision

The *key* to this NHPPD staffing plan is the twice-daily review and revision for twelve-hour shifts, and three times per day review and revision for eight-hour shift units. These reviews capture the individual patient's special or unanticipated needs, and allow the staff on each unit to increase or decrease based on the patient's needs. Nurse managers (or an identified representative from each unit), nursing department directors, the nursing house supervisor, and the executive leader taking administrative call for that day meet twice per day during the work week to examine staffing needs per unit per shift for that day.

This twice-daily meeting is called the "State of the House" meeting. During this meeting, each unit's actual staff is compared to the current and projected census. Patient diagnoses and patients' special needs are examined. The staffing office secretary attends these meetings and as staffing changes are made, a spreadsheet is generated that lists by unit the current staff and that unit's projected needs for the coming shifts. This ability to assess the current staffing plus the projected needs of patients unit by unit also allows last-minute fluctuations in staffing due to staff call-ins to be captured. Thus, units that are over-staffed can share staff with units who need to flex up their staff numbers because of patients' needs or unexpected absences. This twice per day review also allows for proper patient placement throughout the facility; this review facilitates the best possible placement of surgical cases, emergency admissions, and medical procedure cases that require admission after the procedure, and ensures that the receiving unit is staffed appropriately to care for these patients as they move into and throughout the patient care areas in the facility.

A second type of daily monitoring of the NHPPD staffing plan is also included on the spreadsheet generated during the "State of the House" twice-daily meeting. Each area's number of team members actually providing direct care, plus those participating in either educational events or orientation, is noted. Recall that orienting team members are not "counted" as part of that unit's actual staff while in their unit-specific orientation. Listing each unit's actual worked NHPPD compared to the targeted NHPPD allows for easy benchmarking against the unit's targeted NHPPD.

The ANSOS software program originally used in the patient classification system has been modified, and the facility now uses it to track and document staff that are working. This process is relatively easy and efficient. The ANSOS system is also interfaced with the time and attendance system, so that actual time-worked information is downloaded into ANSOS every morning for the previous 24-hour period. Thus, the nurse manager can use ANSOS to view actual worked hours; an ANSOS-like example is shown in Exhibit 3-9 below, listing each staff member's name and title on this report.

The nurse manager and/or nursing department director reviews this information on a routine basis (daily, if possible), to ensure the data is correct. If staff forgets to clock in or out of the unit, or fails to transfer their time worked between units, the ANSOS system captures this mistake and the unit-specific

Exhibit 3-9   Example of ANSOS Printout Listing Actual Worked Hours

Day Shift		Night Shift	
T = 4.8 A = 4.6		T = 3.4 A = 3.0	
CEN = 15		CEN = 17	
Doe, J	R	Gray, J	R
Smith, P	R	Moss, K	R
Jones, F	L	Turner, B	L
Hughes, D	A	Floyd, S	A
Mills, A	C		

Note: T = Target NHPPD calculated per shift, A = actual number of staff working that shift. CEN = Patient Census for that shift. R = RN, L = LPN, A = CNA, C = Clerical.

data generated is distorted. For example, if an RN works on the medical-surgical unit for the first eight hours of a shift, then is reassigned to the cardiovascular unit for the last four hours of a shift, and fails to transfer those last four hours to the cardiovascular unit, the staffing history for both units for this shift is incorrect.

By logging into the ANSOS system on a daily basis, the nurse manager or department director can view the past 24 hours of staffing for this unit, as well as identify any time-clock related issues that might distort the data for this unit's staffing. The nurse manager makes daily corrections to reflect the actual worked time, and any unusual patient care demands or events that occurred during the shift; perhaps a patient coded, or another situation occurred that required much staff time. Events resulting in increased or decreased need for staff are logged into the system to explain the variance from target staffing. The nurse manager makes the worked time corrections in the time and attendance system, which will be downloaded into ANSOS in the next day's report; frequently, the nurse manager also makes these corrections directly in the ANSOS system. In the facility, a variance of 15 hours above or below the budgeted NHPPD is acceptable; if the variance is greater than 15 hours, the nurse manager must document the reason or cause of the variance. This can be done quickly and easily by making notes directly in the ANSOS system.

Trending of Staffing Data

One mechanism to evaluate the success of this staffing method is to trend a variety of data over time, benchmarking against the target set for the specific unit, as well as against the previously identified benchmarks used by the facility.

For example, Joan D., nurse manager for the sample medical-surgical unit discussed previously, and other nursing leaders in the facility review this unit's staffing data (along with the other units in the facility) in a variety of ways.

Another way to evaluate the success of this staffing method is to monitor both weekly and quarterly the types of patients admitted to each unit; this data is trended and monitored for changes. As this first year of using this staffing method is ending, there were no major changes in patient populations that would have dictated a reassessment and/or adjustment of the sample medical-surgical area's budget. Examples of events that could dictate such a major change would be the decision to change the type of patients placed on the unit, or the loss of a major physician group, with the resultant change in the type(s) of patients coming to that unit. Another possible reason to restructure a unit's budget is if a major financial change occurs in the facility, that resulted in the decision to merge or actually close units.

Bi-Weekly Review

Joan D., the nurse manager, and the nursing department director should also review staffing data on a bi-weekly, per-pay-period basis. Following is a control chart showing a sample three-month block of time graphed by the two-week pay-periods. The first chart, Exhibit 3-10, compares the actual worked hours versus the targeted NHPPD as compared to the actual patient census for the medical-surgical unit. This first chart includes the time staff spent in educational or orientation activities in the actual worked NHPPD.

The next chart, Exhibit 3-11, shows the same sample data over the same time period, and deletes the number of hours spent in educational/orientation activities from the actual worked NHPPD. For the most part, the NHPPD closely follows the actual patient census for this area, as would be expected.

As shown in Exhibit 3-11, when the hours spent in educational/orientation activities are removed, the worked NHPPD and the actual census more closely reflect the targeted NHPPD for this unit, as they more closely mirror each other. The desired goal is to see the actual worked NHPPD line move in the same direction as the patient census line, perhaps as overlapping lines, depending on how closely the unit can match its staffing to the patient census and those individual patient's needs.

Monthly and Longer-Term Review

It is at least as important for the nurse manager to compare trends in the unit's staffing over a prolonged period of time as it is to review each day's staffing. Just as patients' temperatures are trended (often using some form of graphic sheet) during their hospital stay, so too will the wise nurse manager or director trend the

Exhibit 3-10 Unit 2A Medical-Surgical Nursing Hours per Patient Day
Includes Education & Orientation Hours

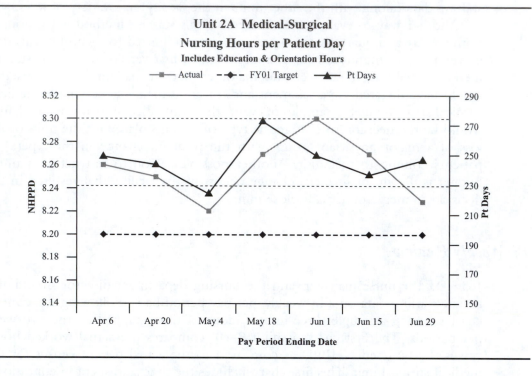

Exhibit 3-11 Unit 2A Medical-Surgical Nursing Hours per Patient Day
Does NOT INCLUDE Education & Orientation Hours

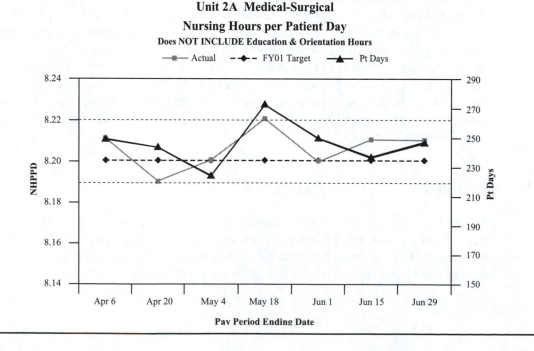

unit's staffing data over time. Using control charts to compare the unit's actual worked NHPPD to the targeted NHPPD for some period of time allows for trending of this data. Thus, variances outside the accepted range can be identified and investigated. Further, it will be helpful to compare the unit's actual worked and targeted NHPPD to the number of hours of time staff spent in educational/orientation activities. Certainly the weeks following graduation of RNs and LPNs will show increased time in orientation and education as these new graduates are being oriented to the unit.

Following is a sample staffing history report, Exhibit 3-12, that the nurse manager or director might generate to trend a unit's staffing information over time. In the following example, six sample months were chosen at random for review. Row one lists the census for the six months being reviewed. Row two lists the number of actual worked hours (productive hours), excluding time spent in orientation or educational activities. Row three divides the productive hours listed in row two by the census in row one, to determine the productive NHPPD. Row four provides six months of actual worked versus targeted NHPPD for the medical surgical unit, which includes time spent in education and orientation activities.

Another longer-term review of staffing data used in the facility is called a productivity report. Reviewing productivity reports may assist the nurse manager or director in obtaining a clear picture of the unit's staffing history. Exhibit 3-13 shows three months of productivity data for the sample medical-surgical unit.

In this sample productivity report, note that the column labeled patient days includes those outpatients who were occupying an in-patient bed on this unit for some portion of a 24-hour period. This unit's actual census exceeded the budgeted census two of the three months reviewed above; as the number of patient days was above budget, so too were the number of NHPPD and the actual worked hours. Recall that the education and orientation hours are **INCLUDED** in the budgeted worked hours column. Because this unit exceeded the budgeted NHPPD of 8.20, these variances are listed as unfavorable. Recall that when the educational/orientation hours, listed in the three columns at the far right, are subtracted from the actual worked hours for the month, the total is below the budgeted worked hours identified for each month.

Therefore, it is vital to track the time spent in these necessary activities, so that variances in productivity can be monitored and addressed. For example, in the Sample Productivity Report for April, the total number of education hours was 32.25, and orientation hours was 206.75; add the two columns together for a total of 239 hours spent in education/orientation. Then subtract these hours from the actual worked hours: 4,560 actual worked hours minus 239 education/orientation hours = 4,321 corrected worked hours. Divide 4,321 by the actual census of 552 to determine that the NHPPD for this month was in reality 7.83, which is under both the targeted NHPPD of 7.99 and the budgeted NHPPD of 8.20 for the sample medical-surgical unit.

Exhibit 3-12 Sample Medical-Surgical Staffing History Report

Sample Medical-Surgical Unit

Unit	Sept	Dec	Feb	Mar	May	June	TOTALS
Med-Surg Census	583	605	556	609	593	571	3,517
Productive Hours	4,900	4,854	4,215	4,726	4,845	4,781	28,321
Productive NHPPD	8.40	8.02	7.58	7.76	8.17	8.37	8.05
Productive NHPPD— Orient & edu included	6,480	6,612	5,462	5,277	5,853	4,622	

Exhibit 3-13 Sample Medical-Surgical Productivity Report

Sample Medical-Surgical Unit

	Patient Days & Outpatient Equivalents		Actual Worked Hours	NHPPD per patient		Budgeted Worked Hours	Hours Variance Fav (Un)	FTEs Vari. Fav (Un)	Edu Hrs	Orient Hrs	FTE Equiv
	Actual	Budget		Actual	Budget						
APRIL	552	554	4,560	8.26	8.20	4,526.40	(33.60)	(0.42)	32.25	206.75	2.99
MAY	593	547	4,891	8.25	8.20	4,862.60	(28.40)	(0.36)	45.25	160.00	2.57
JUNE	571	552	4,725	8.27	8.20	4,682.20	(42.80)	(0.54)	29.00	201.25	2.88

32.25 edu hours + 206.75 orient hours = 239 total edu/orient hours.

4,560 actual worked hours − 239 edu/orient hours = 4,321 corrected worked hours.

4,321 corrected worked hours ÷ 552 actual census = 7.83 corrected NHPPD for April.

Chief Nursing Executive Evaluation

Others within the acute care facility review staffing data from specific units, and across various departments. Perhaps the one person most critical to the successful delivery of quality patient care is the CNE for the facility. The CNE often serves as the nursing department's ambassador when dealing with others within the health care institution. For these dealings to be effective, the CNE must have current knowledge of a variety of topics, including staffing-related issues. One tool the CNE of our facility uses is a spreadsheet that lists the following monthly data for each patient care unit: volume, productive work hours, NHPPD, and NHPPD with education and orientation hours excluded. In addition, a control chart that combines all patient care areas actual worked NHPPD compared to the targeted NHPPD calculated for all combined patient care areas is prepared. Please refer to the following as examples of these charts. See Exhibit 3-14.

The first chart includes all educational/orientation hours worked, while the second chart excludes these hours. See Exhibit 3-15.

**Exhibit 3-14   Report for Chief Nursing Executive
All Patient Care Areas Combined**

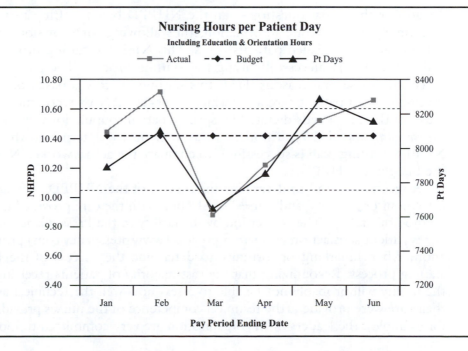

Exhibit 3-15 Report for Chief Nursing Executive
All Patient Care Areas Combined

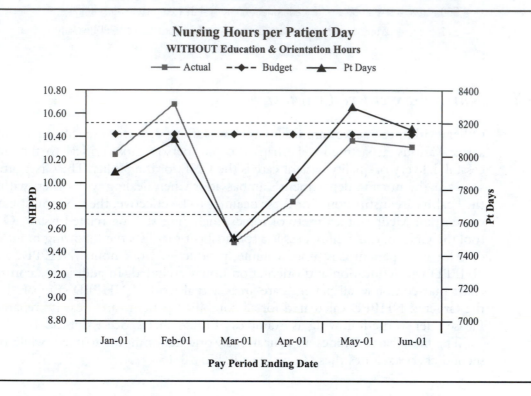

Nursing Hours per Patient Day
WITHOUT Education & Orientation Hours

Conclusions: Judging This Plan's Success

To answer the initial question—can the NHPPD-based staffing process provide timely and accurate information, thus allowing for provision of quality patient care and satisfied patients?—yes. This NHPPD staffing process works, and our facility is successfully using this staffing process. The plan is deemed successful for several reasons. First, this staffing process is based on NHPPD specific to each patient care area, which meets the ANA's recommendation to measure the care needs dictated by specific patient populations (*Principles for Nurse Staffing*, 1999). Another measurement to determine whether the NHPPD staffing plan is successful is to compare the actual worked NHPPD to the budgeted NHPPD.

A second method to determine the success of the NHPPD staffing process is to monitor patients' and nurses' satisfaction with the care provided under this method of staffing. The conversion by the facility to the Press, Ganey and Associates patient satisfaction evaluation process (www.pressganey.com) provides yet another benchmarking opportunity to determine the success of the NHPPD staffing process. Recognizing that the vast majority of patients receiving care in the facility will probably not be able to assess how well the technical aspects of their care were provided (the technical competence of the nurses providing care, for example), the leaders of the organization are very committed to monitoring *how* patient care is provided from the aspect of the caring experience provided by the nurses to their patients.

As of this writing, the first quarter report from Press, Ganey has been received; our benchmarking process begins with comparing our first quarter results with similar health care systems' first quarter results. We realize that at this point, one quarter of data is not much to benchmark against in terms of patient satisfaction. Although measuring patient satisfaction is somewhat nebulous, our theory is that if the NHPPD staffing process is successful, patients will be satisfied with the care provided, and our Press, Ganey scores will reflect this by increasing over time.

Third, the nursing division in the facility has also recently joined the National Database of Nursing Quality Indicators (NDNQI), housed at the National Center for Nursing Quality (NCNQ). Participating in another national database provides another national source for benchmarking for the facility, and is a part of this facility's quest for Magnet Hospital recognition, another initiative that is presently underway. This is a new venture for our facility; at this writing, our first benchmarking results are in-hand. We anticipate that this new benchmark will provide a valuable guide to our facility as we begin using this performance improvement tool to improve our patient outcomes and fine-tune this new NHPPD-based staffing process.

Fourth, along with this change in the staffing process, is the commitment of the CNE to ensure that education and training costs are included in each nursing unit's budgeted patient care hours. By reviewing benchmarks such as the NDNQI mean and the Premier, Inc., mid-of mid range for the various nursing areas, the CNE is then armed with specific information to use in negotiating NHPPD for the facility. Further, the facility is using the RN Case Manager assigned to each nursing area or department to assist in documenting the improvements made in the quality of patient care being provided. Data is reviewed and categorized so that specific details relating to the nationally identified patient outcomes measures can be captured and trended over time. Presently, this data collection occurs in a piece-meal fashion, with a number of areas focusing on area-specific details, and with no one area gathering enough information to yield a "big picture" of what patient outcomes are facility-wide; as the outcomes monitoring process improves, so will the ability to assess the success of the NHPPD staffing process.

The key to measuring the success of this NHPPD staffing process, or any staffing process, is to use a combination approach; by combining daily staffing needs review and adjusting up or down, shift to shift, as well as benchmarking staffing trends over various time periods, we are using the best of two methods rolled into one! Nurses providing hands-on care do not spend time completing acuity ratings each shift, yet have the ability to flex staffing up or down as the patients' needs dictate. To keep the NHPPD method successful, it is essential that the time spent in education and orientation be monitored separately from the actual worked NHPPD. The NHPPD staffing process has become more user-friendly than the patient classification system, because the individual nurse on a unit does not spend time "doing dot sheets" either manually or via computer, and because the nurse manager can monitor the real-time staffing needs of each unit's patients, and adjust that unit's staffing level based on the patients' needs.

References

American Nurses Association (1999). *Principles for nurse staffing.* Washington, DC.

About GRASP® systems. Retrieved August 2, 2001 from http://www.graspinc.com.

Blegen, M., Goode, C., & Reed, L. (1998). Nurse staffing and patient outcomes. *Nursing Research, 47*(1), 43–50.

Garry, R. (2000). Benchmarking: a prescription for healthcare. *Journal of Nursing Administration*, 30(9), 397–398.

Hill, M. (1999). Outcomes measurement requires nursing to shift to outcome-based practice. *Nursing Administration Quarterly*, 24(1), 1–16.

JCAHO Tests model for new staffing effectiveness standards. Retrieved August 7, 2001 from http://www.jcaho.org.

Lawrenz Consulting Healthcare Management Solutions. (2001). Lawrenz Consulting, Inc. Retrieved July 12, 2001 from http://www.lawrenzconsult.com.

Lawrenz 12th annual survey of hours. (May 2001). *Perspectives on Staffing and Scheduling*, 20(3), 1–6.

Lichtig, L., Knauf, R., & Milholland, K. (1999). Some impacts of nursing on acute care hospital outcomes. *Journal of Nursing Administration*, 29(2), 25–33.

National Database of Nursing Quality Indicators. (2001). Retrieved July 12, 2001 from http://www.nursingworld.org/quality/prtdatabase.htm.

Phillips, C., Castorr, A., Prescott, P., & Soeken, K. (1992). Nursing intensity going beyond patient classification. *Journal of Nursing Administration*, 22(4), 46–52.

Public Newsroom. Retrieved July 12, 2001 from http://mypremierinc.com.

US Department of Health and Human Services Health Resources and Services Administration Final Report (February 28, 2001). *Nurse staffing and patient outcomes in hospitals.* Needleman, J., Buerhaus, P., Mattke, S., Stewart, M., & Zelevinsky, K. Authors.

Acuity-Based Flexible Nursing Budgets

Coy L. Smith, ND, MSN, RN, CNAA, CHE

Introduction

This chapter assists managers to develop meaningful acuity-based variable budgets, focusing on labor budgets, but non-salary flexible line items are also covered. Additionally, fixed expenses are developed to create an annual financial plan or budget for the nursing unit. Patient classification acuity levels become the products "produced" on the nursing unit. Each acuity level is related to the other by the number of hours per patient day (HPPD) assigned to each level. Nursing hours become the statistics[1] by which the variable portion of the budget is flexed. The variable components of cost per product or statistic are explored, assisting the manager to explain variances in the costs

---

[1]A statistic is defined as the smallest unit of measure to describe resources required for each product produced. For example, a patient is classified as a Level 3 acuity on a given day of stay. In this example, 8 hours of care (direct and indirect care) are needed for a Level 3 patient. Eight Units or statistics were consumed to produce the level.

per statistic. Finally, relationships between cost accounting systems, nursing information systems, general ledger, patient classification systems, and their interfaces are explored.

The *flexible* (or *variable*) *nursing budget* is a type of budget that changes on a periodic interval based on the historical needs of patients. The budget "flexes" up or down based on the volume generated for the time period. One type of flexible budget adjusts the monthly budget up and down by the number of visits or patient days in acute care. When each patient day or visit is adjusted for the intensity of service required, or acuity, then the monthly budget more closely reflects the resources needed. When patient volume or acuity changes, there is a subsequent increase or decrease in the variable portion of the patient care unit budget.

Well designed acuity-based variable budgets provide for a more precise monthly budget than static budgets, which are based on previously set annual levels. The variable workload for nursing care is most often measured in nursing hours per patient day (NHPPD). The nursing hours of care is then the benchmark unit or relative value unit of measurement—1 RVU = 1 hour of staff time. A reliable and valid patient classification system must be used to capture the acuity level. The required hours of care associated with each level in the acuity system then provide the units or statistics for that day of care. As an illustration of the variable budget, Exhibit 4-1 gives a simplistic view of the result of a monthly flexible budget report.

In this example, during April, Med/Surg One generated a higher volume (6,240 required hours of care) than was budgeted (5,400 hours of care). Naturally, more dollars were spent than were budgeted to meet both the increase in acuity and volume of patients. When calculating the variable cost per statistic, the actual performance in April was $20.83, $2.31 better than was planned.

Exhibit 4-1   Summarized Variable Budget Report for Med/Surg One

Hometown Hospital

Apr-0X Med/Surg One	MTD Actual	MTD Budget	MTD Standard Variance	MTD Flexed Budget	MTD Flexed Variance
Variable Dollars	$ 130,000.00	$ 125,000.00	$ (5,000.00)	$ 144,456.00	$ 14,456.00
Volume	6,240	5,400	(840)	6,240	
Cost per Statistic	$ 20.83	$ 23.15	$ 2.31	$ 23.15	$ 2.32
Fixed Dollars	$ 15,000.00	$ 15,000.00	$	$ 15,000.00	$
Total	$ 145,000.00	$ 140,000.00	$ (5,000.00)	$ 159,456.00	$ 14,456.00
Average Daily Census	32	30			
Average Acuity	6.5	6			

MTD = Month to date

The flexed budget for variable dollars was calculated by multiplying the new volume by the budgeted cost per statistic (6,240 × $23.15 = $144,456).

Actual performance in April (cost per statistic) was $20.83, $2.31 better than was planned.
$23.15 (budgeted) − $20.83 (actual) = $2.31

To calculate Variable Dollars:

6,240 (volume) x $23.15 (cost per statistic) = $144,456

This cost center became more efficient with increasing acuity and volume. Instead of being $5,000 over budget, the way the static budget would reflect this information, the cost center was $14,456 under budget. Note that the planned fixed dollars ($15,000) were spent as planned regardless of the volume.

Variable, Fixed, and Overhead Expenses

Exhibit 4-2 describes the various components of cost. Both *fixed labor (FL)* and *variable labor (VL)* contain productive and non-productive components. It is useful to know both the productive and non-productive hours. Non-productive hours are paid hours when not caring for patients, i.e., holiday, sick, or vacation time. The productive hours are those on the schedule for work either as variable or fixed labor. Most often, direct care HPPD are associated with productive Variable Labor (VL) components. Typically a person's job description is either Variable or Fixed. For example, the unit clerks, clinical nurse specialists, and managers do not flex based on volume and are considered "fixed." Their *non-productive time*, made up of vacation, holiday, sick time (VHS), and

Exhibit 4-2   Components of Expense Associated with Cost Accounting

Variable Expenses

Variable Labor (VL)
Variable Supplies (VS)
Variable Overhead (VO)

Fixed Expenses

Fixed Labor (FL)
Fixed Supplies (FS)
Fixed Overhead (FO)

education time is also considered fixed. Those direct caregivers such as RNs, LPNs, CNAs, Technicians, Physical Therapists, Respiratory Therapists, Radiology Technologists, and so forth, are considered "variable," because the numbers of hours they work can change based on patient needs, and thus so does their non-productive time.

The view taken here assumes that all Variable Labor continues to increase or decrease based on the volume and acuity of patients, or acuity-adjusted patient days. In scenarios where the unit is very small, or on the off-shift, there is a minimal staffing pattern required to keep the unit open. Should the volume of care needed drop below this minimal staffing pattern, then these staff become fixed and they do not continue to "flex" down with the volume on the unit. One can design the budget so that this minimal staffing falls into Fixed Labor. However, the general trend is toward moderately-sized units to gain logical staffing efficiencies, even in times where volume and acuity drop.

Typically the nurse manager oversees the variable and fixed labor and supply budgets, but does not regularly receive reports on *the overhead expenses*, also known as indirect expenses. Overhead for a given patient care unit is based on some accepted costing method. Typical overhead expenses would be utilities, insurance, and the cost of support departments not producing patient chargeable expenses, such as administration, finance, information services, housekeeping, engineering, and security. Generally overhead is factored in when creating a profit and loss statement for a given unit or patient type. Sophisticated cost accounting systems, called decision support systems (DSS), factor in revenue and all components of cost to each patient discharge. If properly maintained, these systems can give the manager a true view of profitability for the unit, or specific patient types, at the close of each month.

There are many software packages called nursing information systems (NIS), which can code and archive hours paid, as well as give the required HPPD, the actual HPPD, and the variance between the two values. These systems are used to project needs for future shifts, or for future fiscal years. The variable portion of Nursing Information Systems "flex" is based on volume and acuity. Fixed hours such as manager hours, the clerical hours, consultant hours, or the constant hours for stocking and doing counts, do not flex, and are added into Total HPPD at a constant rate. Note that some budgeting methodologies assume that unit maintenance activities (reporting, maintaining records, setting up charts, stocking, counting, and so forth) are all 100% flexible based on the number of patients and their associated care needs or hours. The Nursing Information System may or may not track non-productive hours. Many of these systems are interfaced with the time-keeping or payroll system and serve as the report writer for all hours and payroll expense in total.

A large component of cost per day in acute care is nursing variable labor. Calculations can only be accurate if the daily acuity rating is entered into the Decision Support System and the Nursing Information System for every patient, every day. The appropriateness of the HPPD must therefore be considered (Mayo and

Van Slyck, 1999). Appropriate HPPD can be determined in a number of ways: using patient classification data, using nurse administrator/manager/staff experience, or using benchmark data or research data that ties staff mix with patient outcomes. Clearly one method to do this is to complete baseline and ongoing activity summaries at some necessary interval.

Variable Cost Centers and Products

All *variable or direct cost centers* in hospitals are either product producing and/or revenue producing. These cost centers provide direct care to patients. They are in contrast to the *fixed or indirect cost centers* such as Finance, Information Systems, Administration, and others because each of these revenue centers has a patient chargeable event. Workload varies based on the number of products produced. For the patient care unit, the product or statistic used to flex the budget is the acuity adjusted patient day. Recovery rooms or operating rooms often use operating room or recovery room minutes as products. Diagnostic areas use procedures as their product and units of measure. The term "cost center" is a generic term for all general ledger groupings. In many facilities, those centers that generate revenue are termed "revenue centers." Patient Care Units should indeed be termed revenue centers. The term "cost center" here is used in the generic sense.

Note that there are often mixed components of cost from other variable cost centers such as Pharmacy and Dietary. In these examples, a meal or medication is directly charged or associated with the patient. These revenues and expenses show up in the Pharmacy and Dietary cost centers, however, there are items of floor stock that are shared by all patients. These items are expensed on the nursing unit when they are sent to the floor. This expense is considered variable supplies (VS) on the patient care unit. Variable supplies, as actual expense, are spread evenly to all products generated on the patient care unit.

Usually they are related algebraically by the associated hours of labor each product consumes, and converted to relative value units. For the purposes of the nurse manager and the inpatient nursing unit, volume is handled directly in hours, and hours per patient day. Each acuity classification has different hours of care associated with it. Each hospital has a slightly different way of representing and relating products internally and the nurse manager has to become familiar with each hospital's methodology.

Establishing the Variable Budget

In establishing the variable nursing budget, the manager clarifies with administration, and often the Finance Department, the variable or fixed status of each position. The following list of questions can serve as a guide for establishing the parameters of your budget:

- How are educational and orientation hours dealt with?

- Is vacation, sick, holiday time (VHS), and education time a constant for all positions, or unit-specific historical hours? If a historical basis is to be used, were there unusual circumstances that made the historical values too high or too low?

- What historical time frame will serve as a basis for volume and acuity of patients?

- What new treatments or optimal treatment guidelines will be in effect for the new fiscal year that will drive the total HPPD up or down?

- Will changes in length of stay (LOS) be a factor?

- What line items in the non-salary budget are fixed and which are flexible? (Typically pharmaceuticals, laundry/linen, dietary, and medical/surgical supplies are all considered variable.)

- Is a new supply or medication anticipated for the treatment of patients? Has the cost of this item been adequately captured in the historical base?

- What volume assumptions did Finance use in establishing the Revenue Budget for the new time period?

Most managers can obtain, or already record, the number of vacation, holiday, continuing education, orientation, and sick hours from the previous fiscal year and can annualize a year-to-date number from the current fiscal year. If the payroll system keeps this information and generates reports for the manager, the manager has to spend less time keeping these records. A common problem that often forces nursing units to be over budget is that staff replacement (non-productive time) for all of the above reasons is not adequately represented in the staffing budget.

Staff Nurse Involvement in designing staffing patterns and mix of RN, LPN, and support staff, is very important so the assumptions used in designing the budget for a given patient care unit can be verified. The forces of excellence, or magnetism, show that the most successful hospitals incorporate practicing RN involvement in budget development (American Nurses Credentialing Center, 2003).

Projecting Budgeted Volumes

The first step in setting up the flexible budget is to determine the total number of statistics (hours of care) planned in the next fiscal year.

The following information now needs to be gathered for the patient care unit:

- Projected patient days (usually finance supplies this based on revenue assumptions);
- Historical mix of patient classification (from the current FY NIS); and
- Hours of care assigned to each classification for the unit.

In Exhibit 4-3, a 24-bed, general medical unit is expected to have 7,300 patient days next fiscal year.

The mix of classification (obtained from the patient classification system) on a 6-level acuity system for the most recent 6 months was:

Class 1 = 0%
Class 2 = 24%
Class 3 = 46%
Class 4 = 24%
Class 5 = 6%
Class 6 = 0%

in proportion to 100% of patient days. The second column shows standard hours of care assigned to each classification:

Class 1 = 3.25 hours
Class 2 = 4.75 hours
Class 3 = 5.75 hours
Class 4 = 8.25 hours
Class 5 = 12.50 hours
Class 6 = 21.00 hours

(47,559.50 hours of care ÷ 7,300 patient days = 6.515 average budgeted NHPPD)

The 7,300 patient days on this unit will require 47,559.50 hours of care. To determine the average HPPD, divide the total hours by the patient days.

The average budgeted nursing hours per patient day are 6.515. This number represents the direct and indirect care provided to a patient for each 24-hour day. It does not include those support or fixed roles, or non-productive time. Non-productive time is defined as vacation, holiday, sick, and education time.

Exhibit 4-3   Volume Budget Example

7,300 Total Days projected for new FY

	Patient Days		Hours of Care		Total Hours
Class 1	0	×	3.25	=	0.00
Class 2	1,752	×	4.75	=	8,322.00
Class 3	3,358	×	5.75	=	19,308.50
Class 4	1,752	×	8.25	=	14,454.00
Class 5	438	×	12.50	=	5,475.00
Class 6	0	×	21.00	=	0.00
Total	**7,300**				**47,559.50**

Developing the Variable and Fixed Salary Budget

To complete the variable salary budget, the manager needs to add vacation, sick, holiday time, and education/orientation non-productive time for the variable positions. The fixed hours for unit clerks, clinical nurse specialists, and nurse managers need to be calculated. If these positions are replaced when they are off-duty, such as unit clerks, then the non-productive rate has to be added to the HPPD. Note that the clinical nurse specialist/educators and nurse manager are usually not replaced when off duty.

Exhibit 4-4, Variable and Fixed Staffing Audit Spreadsheet with Non-productive Time, illustrates a spreadsheet model that separates out fixed and variable staff, and VHS, adds a factor of 16.07 percent to cover non-productive time (holiday, sick, or vacation time, or education/orientation expenses). Recording

Exhibit 4-4   Variable and Fixed Scheduling Audit Spreadsheet

SA200Y	Fiscal 200Y Nursing Budget Preparation based on Staffing Patterns		
1/1/200X	Nursing Unit: Tele1	Average Daily Census 20	
	Head Nurse: Jamie Doe		

Allowance for Paid Time Off

	Days/Yr	% Allowance		
Vacation	17	7.59%		
H/E	11	4.91%	**Direct**	**Direct**
			RN %	**CGHPPD**
Sick time	8	3.57%	524.00	6.54
		57.2%		
Total	36	16.07%		

Exhibit 4-4 Variable and Fixed Scheduling Audit Spreadsheet (*continued*)

Staffing Patterns—Day Shift

Positions	Sun.	Mon.	Tues.	Wed.	Thurs.	Fri.	Sat.	Man days/Wk	Average Staffing	FTEs/Wk.	Hours of Care/Pt Day	Total Hours Worked	Total Percent of Staff
Care Providers													
Coordinator		1	1	1	1	1		5.00	0.71	1.00	0.29	40.00	7.09%
RN	4	3.5	3.5	3.5	3.5	3.5	4	25.50	3.64	5.10	1.46	204.00	36.17%
LPN								0.00	0.00	0.00	0.00	0.00	0.00%
CNA								0.00	0.00	0.00	0.00	0.00	0.00%
Tech	3	3	3	3	3	3	3	21.00	3.00	4.20	1.20	168.00	29.79%
Psyc Tech								0.00	0.00	0.00	0.00	0.00	0.00%
Pt Care Spec.								0.00	0.00	0.00	0.00	0.00	0.00%
Care Givers	7.00	7.50	7.50	7.50	7.50	7.50	7.00	51.50	7.36	10.30	2.94	412.00	73.05%
Hours/Pt Day	2.80	3.00	3.00	3.00	3.00	3.00	2.80	2.94	2.94				
Total Hours Worked	56.00	60.00	60.00	60.00	60.00	60.00	56.00					412.00	
PSA	1	1	1	1	1	1	1	7.00	1.00	1.40	0.40	56.00	9.93%
HN		1	1	1	1	1		5.00	0.71	1.00	0.29	40.00	7.09%
UC	1	1	1	1	1	1	1	7.00	1.00	1.40	0.40	56.00	9.93%
Clinical Nur. Spec								0.00	0.00	0.00	0.00	0.00	0.00%
Support Staff	2.00	3.00	3.00	3.00	3.00	3.00	2.00	19.00	2.71	3.80	1.09	152.00	26.95%
Hours/Pt Day	0.80	1.20	1.20	1.20	1.20	1.20	0.80	1.09	1.09				
Total Hours Worked	16.00	24.00	24.00	24.00	24.00	24.00	16.00					152.00	
Total Staff	9.00	10.50	10.50	10.50	10.50	10.50	9.00	70.50	10.07	14.10	4.03	564.00	100.00%
Total Hours/Pt Day	3.60	4.20	4.20	4.20	4.20	4.20	3.60	4.03	4.03				
Total Hours Worked	72.00	84.00	84.00	84.00	84.00	84.00	72.00					564.00	

Exhibit 4-4 Variable and Fixed Scheduling Audit Spreadsheet *(continued)*

Staffing Patterns—Evening Shift

Positions	Sun.	Mon.	Tues.	Wed.	Thurs.	Fri.	Sat.	Man days/ Wk	Average Staffing	FTEs/ Wk.	Hours of Care/ Pt Day	Total Hours Worked	Percent of Staff
Care Providers													
Coordinator								0.00	0.00	0.00	0.00	0.00	0.00%
RN	3	3	3	3	3	3	3	21.00	3.00	4.20	1.20	168.00	53.50%
LPN								0.00	0.00	0.00	0.00	0.00	0.00%
CNA								0.00	0.00	0.00	0.00	0.00	0.00%
Tech	2	2	2	2	2	2	2	14.00	2.00	2.80	0.80	112.00	35.67%
Psyc Tech								0.00	0.00	0.00	0.00	0.00	0.00%
Pt Care Spec.								0.00	0.00	0.00	0.00	0.00	0.00%
Care Givers	5.00	5.00	5.00	5.00	5.00	5.00	5.00	35.00	5.00	7.00	2.00	280.00	89.17%
Hours/Pt Day	2.00	2.00	2.00	2.00	2.00	2.00	2.00	2.00	2.00				
Total Hours Worked	40.00	40.00	40.00	40.00	40.00	40.00	40.00					280.00	
PSA	0.25	0.25	0.25	0.25	0.25	0.25	0.25	1.75	0.25	0.35	0.10	14.00	4.46%
HN								0.00	0.00	0.00	0.00	0.00	0.00%
UC		0.5	0.5	0.5	0.5	0.5		2.50	0.36	0.50	0.14	20.00	6.37%
CNS								0.00	0.00	0.00	0.00	0.00	0.00%
Support Staff	0.25	0.75	0.75	0.75	0.75	0.75	0.25	4.25	0.61	0.85	0.24	34.00	10.83%
Hours/Pt Day	0.10	0.30	0.30	0.30	0.30	0.30	0.10	0.24	0.24				
Total Hours Worked	2.00	6.00	6.00	6.00	6.00	6.00	2.00					34.00	
Total Staff	5.25	5.75	5.75	5.75	5.75	5.75	5.25	39.25	5.61	7.85	2.24	314.00	100.00%
Total Hours/Pt Day	2.10	2.30	2.30	2.30	2.30	2.30	2.10	2.24	2.24				
Total Hours Worked	42.00	46.00	46.00	46.00	46.00	46.00	42.00					314.00	

Exhibit 4-4 Variable and Fixed Scheduling Audit Spreadsheet (*continued*)

Staffing Patterns—Night Shift

Positions Care Providers	Sun.	Mon.	Tues.	Wed.	Thurs.	Fri.	Sat.	Man days/ Wk	Average Staffing	FTEs/ Wk.	Hours of Care/ Pt Day	Total Hours Worked	Percent of Staff
Coordinator								0.00	0.00	0.00	0.00	0.00	0.00%
RN	2	2	2	2	2	2	2	14.00	2.00	2.80	0.80	112.00	50.00%
LPN								0.00	0.00	0.00	0.00	0.00	0.00%
CNA								0.00	0.00	0.00	0.00	0.00	0.00%
Tech	2	2	2	2	2	2	2	14.00	2.00	2.80	0.80	112.00	50.00%
Psyc Tech								0.00	0.00	0.00	0.00	0.00	0.00%
Pt Care Spec.								0.00	0.00	0.00	0.00	0.00	0.00%
Care Givers	**4.00**	**4.00**	**4.00**	**4.00**	**4.00**	**4.00**	**4.00**	**28.00**	**4.00**	**5.60**	**1.60**	**224.00**	**100.00%**
Hours/Pt Day	1.60	1.60	1.60	1.60	1.60	1.60	1.60	1.60	1.60		1.60		
Total Hours Worked	32.00	32.00	32.00	32.00	32.00	32.00	32.00					224.00	
PSA								0.00	0.00	0.00	0.00	0.00	0.00%
HN								0.00	0.00	0.00	0.00	0.00	0.00%
UC								0.00	0.00	0.00	0.00	0.00	0.00%
CNS								0.00	0.00	0.00	0.00	0.00	0.00%
Support Staff	**0.00**	**0.00**	**0.00**	**0.00**	**0.00**	**0.00**	**0.00**	**0.00**	**0.00**	**0.00**	**0.00**	**0.00**	**0.00%**
Hours/Pt Day	0.00	0.00	0.00	0.00	0.00	0.00	0.00	0.00	0.00				
Total Hours Worked	0.00	0.00	0.00	0.00	0.00	0.00	0.00					0.00	
Total Staff	**4.00**	**4.00**	**4.00**	**4.00**	**4.00**	**4.00**	**4.00**	**28.00**	**4.00**	**5.60**	**1.60**	**224.00**	**100.00%**
Total Hours/Pt Day	1.60	1.60	1.60	1.60	1.60	1.60	1.60	1.60	1.60		1.60	224.00	
Total Hours Worked	32.00	32.00	32.00	32.00	32.00	32.00	32.00					224.00	

Exhibit 4-4 Variable and Fixed Scheduling Audit Spreadsheet (continued)

Staffing Patterns—All Shifts

Positions Care Providers	Sun.	Mon.	Tues.	Wed.	Thurs.	Fri.	Sat.	Total Man days/Wk	Average Daily Staffing	Working Total FTEs/Wk.	Hours of Care/Pt Day	Total Hours Worked	Percent of Allowance Staff FTEs/Wk	NWR Allowance FTEs/Wk	Total Recommended FTEs/Wk	PTO Hrs. Only Per Pt. Day	Hours of Care Paid/Working & PTO
Coordinator	0	1	1	1	1	1	0	5.00	0.71	1.00	0.29	40.00	3.63%	0.16	1.16	0.05	0.33
RN	9	8.5	8.5	8.5	8.5	8.5	9	60.50	8.64	12.10	3.46	484.00	43.92%	1.94	14.04	0.56	4.01
LPN	0	0	0	0	0	0	0	0.00	0.00	0.00	0.00	0.00	0.00%	0.00	0.00	0.00	0.00
CNA	0	0	0	0	0	0	0	0.00	0.00	0.00	0.00	0.00	0.00%	0.00	0.00	0.00	0.00
Tech	7	7	7	7	7	7	7	49.00	7.00	9.80	2.80	392.00	35.57%	1.58	11.38	0.45	3.25
Psyc Tech	0	0	0	0	0	0	0	0.00	0.00	0.00	0.00	0.00	0.00%	0.00	0.00	0.00	0.00
Pt Care Spec.	0	0	0	0	0	0	0	0.00	0.00	0.00	0.00	0.00	0.00%	0.00	0.00	0.00	0.00
Care Givers	16.00	16.50	16.50	16.50	16.50	16.50	16.00	114.50	16.36	22.90	6.54	916.00	83.12%	3.68	26.58	1.05	7.59
Hours/Pt Day	6.40	6.60	6.60	6.60	6.60	6.60	6.40	6.54	6.54								
Total Hours Worked	128.00	132.00	132.00	132.00	132.00	132.00	128.00					916.00					
PSA	1.25	1.25	1.25	1.25	1.25	1.25	1.25	8.75	1.25	1.75	0.50	70.00	6.35%	0.28	2.03	0.08	0.58
HN	0	1	1	1	1	1	0	5.00	0.71	1.00	0.29	40.00	3.63%	0.00	1.00	0.00	0.29
UC	1	1.5	1.5	1.5	1.5	1.5	1	9.50	1.36	1.90	0.54	76.00	6.90%	0.31	2.21	0.09	0.63
CNS	0	0	0	0	0	0	0	0.00	0.00	0.00	0.00	0.00	0.00%	0.00	0.00	0.00	0.00
Support Staff	2.25	3.75	3.75	3.75	3.75	3.75	2.25	23.25	3.32	4.65	1.33	186.00	0.17	0.59	5.24	0.17	1.50
Hours/Pt Day	0.90	1.50	1.50	1.50	1.50	1.50	0.90	1.33	1.33								
Total Hours Worked	18.00	30.00	30.00	30.00	30.00	30.00	18.00					186.00					
Total Staff	18.25	20.25	20.25	20.25	20.25	20.25	18.25	137.75	19.68	27.55	7.87	1,102.00	100.00%	4.27	31.82	1.22	9.09
Total Hours/Pt Day	7.30	8.10	8.10	8.10	8.10	8.10	7.30	7.87	7.87								
Total Hours Worked	146.00	162.0	162.0	162.0	162.0	162.0	146.0					1,102.00					

Exhibit 4-4 Variable and Fixed Scheduling Audit Spreadsheet (*continued*)

Paid Time Off Analysis

Day Shift-Hour/Wk Evening Shift-Hours/Wk Night Shift Hours/Wk All Shifts/Hours/Wk All Shifts FTEs/Wk

Positions	Vacation	Holiday	Sick	Total Day Shift	Vacation	Holiday	Sick	Total Evening Shift	Vacation	Holiday	Sick	Total Night Shift	Vacation	Holiday	Sick	Total All Shifts	Vacation	Holiday	Sick	Total
Coordinator	3.04	1.96	1.43	6.43	0.00	0.00	0.00	0.00	0.00	0.00	0.00	0.00	3.04	1.96	1.43	6.43	0.08	0.05	0.04	0.16
RN	15.48	10.02	7.29	32.79	12.75	8.25	6.00	27.00	8.50	5.50	4.00	18.00	36.73	23.77	17.29	77.79	0.92	0.59	0.43	1.94
LPN	0.00	0.00	0.00	0.00	0.00	0.00	0.00	0.00	0.00	0.00	0.00	0.00	0.00	0.00	0.00	0.00	0.00	0.00	0.00	0.00
CNA	0.00	0.00	0.00	0.00	0.00	0.00	0.00	0.00	0.00	0.00	0.00	0.00	0.00	0.00	0.00	0.00	0.00	0.00	0.00	0.00
Tech	12.75	8.25	6.00	27.00	8.50	5.50	4.00	18.00	8.50	5.50	4.00	18.00	29.75	19.25	14.00	63.00	0.74	0.48	0.35	1.58
Psyc Tech	0.00	0.00	0.00	0.00	0.00	0.00	0.00	0.00	0.00	0.00	0.00	0.00	0.00	0.00	0.00	0.00	0.00	0.00	0.00	0.00
Pt Care Spec.	0.00	0.00	0.00	0.00	0.00	0.00	0.00	0.00	0.00	0.00	0.00	0.00	0.00	0.00	0.00	0.00	0.00	0.00	0.00	0.00
Care Givers	31.27	20.23	14.71	66.21	21.25	13.75	10.00	45.00	17.00	11.00	8.00	36.00	69.52	44.98	32.71	147.21	1.74	1.12	0.82	3.68
Support Staff	4.25	2.75	2.00	9.00	1.06	0.69	0.50	2.25	0.00	0.00	0.00	0.00	5.31	3.44	2.50	11.25	0.13	0.09	0.06	0.28
HN	0.00	0.00	0.00	0.00	0.00	0.00	0.00	0.00	0.00	0.00	0.00	0.00	0.00	0.00	0.00	0.00	0.00	0.00	0.00	0.00
UC	4.25	2.75	2.00	9.00	1.52	0.98	0.71	3.21	0.00	0.00	0.00	0.00	5.77	3.73	2.71	12.21	0.14	0.09	0.07	0.31
CNS	0.00	0.00	0.00	0.00	0.00	0.00	0.00	0.00	0.00	0.00	0.00	0.00	0.00	0.00	0.00	0.00	0.00	0.00	0.00	0.00
Support Staff	8.50	5.50	4.00	18.00	2.58	1.67	1.21	5.46	0.00	0.00	0.00	0.00	11.08	7.17	5.21	23.46	0.28	0.18	0.13	0.59
Total PTO Hours	39.77	25.73	18.71	84.21	23.83	15.42	11.21	50.46	17.00	11.00	8.00	36.00	80.60	52.15	37.93	170.68	2.01	1.30	0.95	4.27
Total PTO FTEs	0.99	0.64	0.47	2.11	0.60	0.39	0.28	1.26	0.43	0.28	0.20	0.90	2.01	1.30	0.95	4.27				

Exhibit 4-4   Fiscal 200Y Nursing Budget Preparation based on Staffing Pattern

Nursing Unit: Tele 1   Date: 11-15-0X
Head Nurse: Jamie Doe

Labor Dollar Calculator

Variable Positions	Rate	Productive	Non-Prod.	Total
NCC	$22.00	$45,760.00	$7,354.29	$53,114.29
RN	$20.00	$503,360.00	$80,897.14	$584,257.14
LPN	$15.00	0.00	0.00	0.00
CNA	$11.00	0.00	0.00	0.00
Tech	$12.00	$244,608.00	$39,312.00	$283,920.00
Psyc Tech	$11.00	0.00	0.00	0.00
Pt Care Spec.	$11.00	0.00	0.00	0.00
Total Variable		**$793,728.00**	**$127,563.43**	**$921,291.43**
Fixed Positions				
PSA	$10.00	$36,400.00	$5,850.00	$42,250.00
HN	$30.00	$62,400.00	0.00	$62,400.00
UC	$11.00	$43,472.00	$6,986.57	$50,458.57
CNS	$26.00	0.00	0.00	0.00
Total Fixed		**$142,272.00**	**$12,836.57**	**$155,108.57**
Total		**$936,000.00**	**$140,400.00**	**$1,076,400.00**

Differentials Variable	Rate	Hours	Total	
Charge	$1.00	5,824.00	$5,824.00	
Other	0.00	0.00	0.00	
Evenings	$2.00	14,560.00	$29,120.00	
Nights	$3.00	11,648.00	$34,944.00	
W/E	$2.00	13,312.00	$26,624.00	
		45,344.00	**$96,512.00**	

Differentials Fixed	Rate	Hours	Total	
Charge	$1.00	0.00	0.00	
Other	0.00	0.00	0.00	
Evenings	$2.00	1,768.00	$3,536.00	
Nights	$3.00	0.00	0.00	
W/E	$2.00	1,872.00	$3,744.00	
		3,640.00	**$7,280.00**	

the actual non-productive time in the previous 12 months generated this amount of non-productive time. The seniority of the staff, and the educational needs for the upcoming year, can change the non-productive factor. The spreadsheet can more realistically delineate the true staffing pattern needed to run this unit. The actual placement of staff by role and by shift considers the availability of staff and how they work. The goal of using these spreadsheet models is to achieve a direct HPPD that closely approximates the HPPD developed in the volume (statistics) budget seen in Exhibit 4-3.

This spreadsheet example also allows for projecting mix of staff, and allows for the calculation of salary dollars. The manager needs to use current salaries for each staff member, averaged by position, and then raised for increases planned for the following fiscal year. In some organizations, the manager gives the FTE distribution to Finance and then the projected budgeted salary is calculated. These spreadsheets can accurately provide the managers with a guideline for the average time off by position by shift. If managers hire based on the total FTEs needed, and plan vacation, holiday, sick time (VHS) within the modeled amounts, then there will be enough resources to staff the unit at the assumed census and acuity. This spreadsheet also calculates salary dollars if not done already by central Finance. It is advisable for the manager to roughly calculate these dollars for comparison when Central Finance calculates the salaries.

Comments Related to the Variable Salary Budgets

Staff Mix

Some acuity systems break the required hours down into professional (RN), paraprofessional (LPN), and assistant (CNA) categories. Using these as benchmarks for the most efficient *staffing mix*, the manager can accurately develop his or her recruitment plan. The manager must be cautioned here, as market forces and shortages must be factored into mix and type of staff used in calculating the variable dollars needed. It would be very dangerous to the financial health of the organization, or to the quality of patient care, if the wrong mix of staff calculations was used.

Prudent Budget Methodology

Often now, projected patient revenue is used to model variable dollars after overhead departments and capital needs are deducted. In other words, direct care (VL) receives the revenue dollars left. Rather, a prudent methodology should be used, such as the one illustrated in Exhibit 4-4, to create logical variable dollar budgets. These variable dollars are rolled up to match the projected revenue budget.

Budgetary Decision Making and Negotiation

The final budget is never completed today without cross-functional negotiation, strategic decision making and ultimately expense reduction. The Chief Nursing Officer must articulate the needs, assumptions, and critical decisions to be made. Decisions like cutting fixed and overhead positions to maintain direct care hours are often made. Or, the mix of staff, the size or configuration of units, and/or pharmaceutical/supply use must all be adjusted to meet the budget. Maybe, a low or negative margin program must close. Or more positively, a new profitable service can be offered.

Typically, nursing salaries are the largest component of an acute care hospital's variable expenses. Therefore, these hours and dollars meet tough scrutiny with each successive year of managed care and BBA (Balanced Budget Act) reductions.

Nurse managers and executives need to incorporate their lived experience and the current body of knowledge around staffing when creating the direct-care labor budget. Furthermore, JCAHO (2004) and each state department of health require a consistent policy and procedure surrounding how nursing assignments are completed on a shift-by-shift basis. These regulatory bodies review the annual and ongoing system employed by a given hospital to assess both the competency of nursing personnel and the adequacy of the nurse staffing. Many factors, such as the experience of the staff, the intensity of nursing care, and the size of the unit help to decide the acceptable percentage of RNs in the direct care mix—not the least of which is the heightening concern about errors in health care. JCAHO standards HR 1.10 and 1.30 require each organization to evaluate the effectiveness of staffing by selecting and measuring four screening indicators. See Exhibit 4-5. The *Principles for Nurse Staffing* (ANA, 1999) provides a comprehensive source of guidance when designing the nursing staffing budget.

One should not excessively rely on a standard or an historical average HPPD when designing the labor budget. The experience of the staff, turnover rates, need for orientation and education, new patient types, decreasing length of stay, support of other disciplines and departments, and the experience and quality of unlicensed assistive personnel all affect how the staffing model is developed.

Variable Non-Salary Line Items

To accurately flex a patient care unit's budget, the manager needs to determine the *other variable line items*. Typical examples are linen, floor stock, pharmacy charges, and dietary charges to the unit's "cost" (profit) center number. A historical average cost per day for each of these items is determined for the current fiscal year, calculated by dividing actual cost for the item by

Exhibit 4-5   JCAHO's Screening Indicators

Clinical/Service Indicators	Human Resource Indicators
• Family complaints	• Overtime
• Patient complaints	• Staff vacancy rate
• Patient falls	• Staff satisfaction
• Adverse drug events	• Staff turnover rate
• Injuries to patients	• Understaffing as compared to hospital's staffing plan
• Skin breakdown	• Nursing care hours per patient day
• Pneumonia	• Staff injuries on the job
• Postoperative infections	• On-call or per diem use
• Urinary tract infections	• Sick time
• Upper gastrointestinal bleeding	
• Shock/cardiac arrest	
• Length of stay	

JCAHO also set up a data system called ORYX to keep track of performance data. Eventually JCAHO is planning to expand the measure sets to include: clinical performance; patient perception of care, treatment and services; health status; and administrative or financial measures. For more information on this, see http://oryx@jcaho.org.

From: Dunham-Taylor, J., and Pinzcuk, J. (2006). *Health Care Financial Management for Nurse Managers: Merging the Heart with the Dollar.* Sudbury, MA: Jones & Bartlett, p. 85.

the number of patient days in the time period. Then a new variable dollar budget is calculated for each of these line items based on the new projected volume and any anticipated inflation. Typically, the purchasing department or finance will estimate an inflation factor to be used in this calculation. Exhibit 4-6, Non-Salary Variable Budget Calculation, provides an example of these calculations.

Fixed Supply Component

So far we have covered the following components of the acuity-based flexible nursing budgets:

- the labor components,
- variable labor and fixed labor,
- the variable supplies.

Exhibit 4-6   Non-Salary Variable Budget Calculation

Hospital A
Variable Line Item Budget Calculator
FY 200X

+3% Inflation

Item	Current Year 8 Mos. Actual	Current Year 8 Mos. Days	Cost per Day	FY 200X Projected Days	FY 200X Budget
Linen	$ 40,100.00	4,666	$ 8.59	7,300	$ 62,707.00
Pharmacy	$ 60,599.00	4,666	$ 12.99	7,300	$ 94,827.00
Dietary	$ 20,239.00	4,666	$ 4.34	7,300	$ 31,682.00
Med/Surg Supplies	$ 30,134.00	4,666	$ 6.46	7,300	$ 47,158.00
					$236,374.00

The final area of responsibility for the nurse manager is fixed supplies. *Fixed supplies* include items such as: office supplies, books and periodicals, continuing education, equipment rentals, repairs and maintenance, and miscellaneous. The estimated expense for these items is usually the YTD projection, plus inflation, minus any known decreases, plus any known additions.

For example, office supplies, Tele1 used $10,000 in office supplies last year. The hospital just negotiated a group contract that will reduce this year's expense by 20%. Thus, the requested amount for this line item would be $8,000. However, this year an important conference is being offered and two nurses are presenting posters. Their travel, hotel, and registration will cost $2,000. The continuing education line was $1,000 last year and will need to increase to $3,000, to accommodate the two nurses doing posters.

$8,000	Office supplies
$3,000	Educational costs
$11,000	Total

The Final Variable Budget

The budget worksheet seen in Exhibit 4-7 displays the combined projections of both the variable and the fixed line items. The statistic budget is also seen. The cost per unit or statistic, and in this case, a direct hour of care, is calculated. Use the formula:

$$\text{Variable Salary Dollars} + \frac{\text{Variable Supply Dollars}}{\text{Statistics for the same time period}} = \text{Cost per Statistic}$$

Remember, these statistics are derived from the products acuity adjusted patient days. The patient care unit in this chapter produced six products: Class 1, Class 2, Class 3, Class 4, Class 5, and Class 6. Each product has an established number of hours of care associated with it. The statistic (hours) is the lowest common denominator, and therefore it is used to break down and examine the variable cost component.

Creating variances with a percent change calculated is useful to test our assumptions and plan. In this example, the FY 2001 Variable Budget increases 10.4% over the previous year, while the planned increase in volume is 5.6%. When we actually look at the cost per statistic, we see the planned cost per statistic rose $1.17 or 4.6%. Does this match our cost for inflation and wage increases planned? If yes, and the organization can afford these assumptions, the budget will be acceptable. Hospitals undergoing reengineering may attempt to reduce the cost per statistic or patient day. The planned and actual cost per statistic then becomes a good ongoing metric of variable costs.

Conclusion

The variable budget is a useful tool for managing a patient care unit. Often, the manager is held accountable for the static budget, which is averaged evenly over 12 months. In the static budget, the assumptions used are developed before the start of the year and do not mirror the changing demands of the patients on a given unit. When the cost per statistic or hour is appropriately developed and adequately supported by administration, then the manager's monthly budget will reflect the agreed upon target. Knowing the components of cost that comprise the budgeted cost per statistic allows for a detailed analysis of variance and corrective action plan. Ongoing diligence to analysis of variance, record keeping, and maintaining a reliable and valid patient classification system are necessary elements toward achieving accurate fiscal control—a control that supports the needs of patients and nurses alike. Nursing administration and management has to methodically develop budgetary plans, gain approval of them and then be willing to manage staffing resources within these financial plans.

Exhibit 4-7 Variable Budget Worksheet

Example Tele 1
FY 200Y

	a	b	c	d	d – c		d – b	
	FY 200X 6 months Actual	FY 200X Projected Actual	FY 200X Budget	FY 200Y Planned	Planned-Budget Variance	Percent Inc/Dec.	Planned-Actual Variance	Percent Inc/Dec.
Variable								
Salary								
Productive	$365,114.88	$730,229.76	$725,789.00	$793,728.00	$67,939.00	9.3%	$63,498.24	8.7%
Non-Productive	49,479.18	98,958.36	95,099.00	107,563.43	12,464.43	12.6%	8,605.07	8.7%
Differentials	43,056.00	86,112.00	85,678.00	93,600.00	7,922.00	9.2%	7,488.00	8.7%
OT	13,800.00	27,600.00	24,984.00	30,000.00	5,016.00	18.2%	2,400.00	8.7%
Sub Salary	**$471,450.06**	**$942,900.12**	**$931,550.00**	**$1,024,891.43**	**$93,341.43**	**9.9%**	**$81,991.31**	**8.7%**
Non-Salary								
Pharmacy	$45,449.25	$90,898.50	$89,321.00	$100,327.32	$11,006.32	12.1%	$9,428.82	10.4%
Laundry	30,075.00	60,150.00	59,465.00	66,389.31	6,924.31	11.5%	6,239.31	10.4%
Dietary	15,179.25	30,358.50	27,500.00	33,507.56	6,007.56	19.8%	3,149.06	10.4%
M/S Supplies	22,600.50	45,201.00	46,000.00	49,889.66	3,889.66	8.6%	4,688.66	10.4%
Sub Non-Sal.	**$113,304.00**	**$226,608.00**	**$222,286.00**	**$250,113.84**	**$27,827.84**	**12.3%**	**$23,505.84**	**10.4%**
Sub Variable	**$584,754.06**	**$1,169,508.12**	**$1,153,836.00**	**$1,275,005.27**	**$121,169.27**	**10.4%**	**$105,497.16**	**9.0%**
Statistics	23,000.00	46,000.00	45,000.00	47,560.00	2,560.00	5.6%	1,560.00	3.4%
Cost/Stat	**$25.42**	**$25.42**	**$25.64**	**$26.81**	**$1.17**	**4.6%**	**$1.38**	**5.4%**
Fixed								
Salary								
Productive	$65,445.12	$130,890.24	$128,450.00	$142,272.00	$13,822.00	10.6%	$11,381.76	8.7%
Non-productive	4,064.82	8,129.64	8,100.00	8,836.57	736.57	9.1%	706.93	8.7%
Differentials	3,348.80	6,697.60	6,500.00	7,280.00	780.00	11.6%	582.40	8.7%
OT	2,760.00	5,520.00	4,000.00	6,000.00	2,000.00	36.2%	480.00	8.7%
Sub Fixed Sal	**$75,618.74**	**$151,237.48**	**$147,050.00**	**$164,388.57**	**$17,338.57**	**11.5%**	**$13,151.09**	**8.7%**
Non-Salary Fixed								
Office Supplies	$2,356.00	$4,712.00	$4,000.00	$4,200.00	$200.00	4.2%	$-512.00	-10.9%
Rental Equip.	1,800.00	3,600.00	3,600.00	3,600.00	0.00	0.0%	0.00	0.0%
Repairs/Maint.	233.00	466.00	500.00	500.00	0.00	0.0%	34.00	7.3%
Travel/Ed.	1,569.00	3,138.00	3,000.00	2,500.00	-500.00	-15.9%	-638.00	-20.3%
Books/Mags.	123.00	246.00	200.00	200.00	0.00	0.0%	-46.00	-18.7%
Sub Non-Sal.	**$6,081.00**	**$12,162.00**	**$11,300.00**	**$11,000.00**	**$-300.00**	**-2.5%**	**$-1,162.00**	**-9.6%**
Sub Fixed	**$81,699.74**	**$163,399.48**	**$158,350.00**	**$175,388.57**	**$17,038.57**	**10.4%**	**$11,989.09**	**7.3%**
Total budget	**$666,453.80**	**$1,332,907.60**	**$1,312,186.00**	**$1,450,393.84**	**$138,207.84**	**10.4%**	**$117,486.24**	**8.8%**

References

American Nurses Association (ANA). (1999). *Principles for Nurse Staffing*. ANA Publication PNS-1.

American Nurses Credentialing Center. (2003). *Magnet Recognition Program: Recognizing Excellence In Nursing Service*. Washington, DC: ANCC.

Joint Commission on Accreditation of Healthcare Organizations (JCAHO). (2004). *2004 Comprehensive Accreditation Manual for Hospitals: The Official Handbook (CAMH)*. Racebrook: Joint Commission Resources, Inc.

Mayo, A.M., & Van Slyck, A. (1999). Developing staffing standards: statistical considerations for patient care administrators. *Journal of Nursing Administration*, 29(10), 43–48.

PART II

Long-Term Care Issues

The modern nursing home is the result of many years of evolution and refinement. Approximately 2.4 million residents reside in long-term care facilities in this country, and these tend to be especially frail, fragile, vulnerable, and cognitively impaired. Chapter 5 describes the various kinds of long-term care facilities and ownership categories. Fast-moving changes that are driving the health care system today demand that the long-term industry look at it with "new eyes." Nurse administrators will learn about accountability, federal regulations, reimbursement issues, budgeting, and staffing and scheduling requirements from the perspective of an experienced long-term care nurse administrator.

To be effective in long-term care, the nurse administrator needs to understand the payment system. Chapter 6 explains the Resident Assessment Instrument (RAI) process and its core component, the Minimum Data Set (MDS). This information is vital in the reimbursement computation process for the resident stay. The MDS is a set of assessment and screening elements, forming the backbone of comprehensive resident assessment. One hundred eight MDS 2.0 assessment items serve to classify residents by their resource needs. This chapter will give you a history of this reimbursement mechanism, and exhibits and scenarios that affect resident care.

Within the world of the prospective payment system for long-term care, Medicare is the primary source of facility reimbursement. In long-term care, Medicare reimburses based on the results of assessments that are required at different times during a patient's stay. These assessments reveal specific services that are provided by the organization. Chapter 7 addresses the ways that Medicare assessments are tracked, completed, and used as indicators that produce reimbursement rates. In addition, the connection between these assessments and the patient's individualized care plan is addressed.

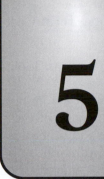

Managing Long-Term Care Resources

Frances W. "Billie" Sills, MSN, RN, ARNP, CLNC

Susie Hutchings, RN, C, CPHQ

> Yet somehow our society must make
> it right and possible for old people not to
> fear the young or be deserted by them,
> for the test of a civilization is in the
> way that it cares for its helpless members.
> —*Pearl S. Buck*

Introduction

Long-term care continues to be the fastest growing segment of the health care continuum. It is also one that finds itself caught in the middle of various state and federal regulations, punitive survey processes, and ongoing reductions in the various reimbursements, all of which result in additional budget constraints and staffing shortages. It is during, or because of, these turbulent times that new ideas can emerge. At this time, we must look at reshaping the future of long-term care.

This environment can offer nurse administrators an extraordinary personal and professional challenge. The image of the "county nursing home" of large patient wards; the smell of urine and other wastes; and death as a result of pressure ulcers, pneumonia, and dehydration is no longer valid. While some of the general public continues to view "nursing homes" this way, the truth of the matter is that the ongoing growth of this industry has demanded change. This growth is the result of many changes in the continuum of health care such as:

- the short length of stay in acute care hospitals;

- predictions that one in four individuals who have reached the age of 65 will spend some time in a long-term care facility; and

- the increasing need for "long-term or extended care" beds as patients are discharged from acute care earlier and are unable to care for themselves at home.

The modern nursing home is the result of many years of evolution and refinement. Approximately 2.4 million residents reside in long-term care facilities in this country, and these residents tend to be especially frail, fragile, vulnerable, and cognitively impaired.

Free-standing and single-function nursing homes are slowly disappearing. In their place are campuses designed to serve the elderly with a continuum of care that consist of retirement communities with assisted living apartments, and long-term care facilities that include rehabilitation, skilled nursing, and intermediate nursing care.

Long-term care facilities of today provide the foundation for a comprehensive, community continuum of care. With the range of services offered, care management principles provide the right service at the right time at the right cost. The nursing home should no longer be viewed as the "point of no return." It should be the "thinking person's choice" when the need for long-term care is apparent.

The challenge that is presented to the leaders in long-term care is best described by Marcel Proust, who said "The real voyage of discovery consists not in seeking new landscapes but in having new eyes." The traditional long-term paradigm that drives health care delivery, and the staff that delivers it, is one of predictability and control with regulations and policies.

Fast moving changes that are driving the health care system today demand that the long-term care industry look at it with "new eyes." The industry can only shape a better future if it collectively moves from the old traditional way of looking at things to a new one. The world today is changing from one of rigid hierarchies and bureaucracies to one of employee empowerment. Ideas for improving delivery of care are more likely to exist when employees are empowered to create new approaches. While we must deal with regulatory compliance because the system demands it, at the same time, we cannot allow it to be the only driving force in the delivery of care. The use of a new and emerging paradigm of change and transformation must be one that is less rigid. Ideas for improving care delivery come when employees feel empowered to look at new approaches to old problems. Then employees can work across boundaries, rather than being constrained by the hierarchies and bureaucracy that characterize so much of the long-term care industry.

Because of this, managing the long-term care organization presents one of the most unique challenges to both nursing and business administrators. The uniqueness of long-term care stems from the fact that these organizations or "facilities" are both social and clinical settings where residents and extended families are totally immersed as full-time members of a new community. For the residents this has become their home—where they live, work, play, grow older, and, in time, die. For families, it is a time filled with many feelings—guilt, sadness, love, and an ongoing effort to make their "space" be as much like home as possible.

This uniqueness also challenges the "regulatory mind set" of the leaders in long-term care to transform their organizations. One of the ways that this challenge is being met is through a radically different approach to the care of the older adults known as *The Eden Alternative*. This concept was developed by Dr. William Thomas, a Harvard-trained family physician.

The program's main mission is the elimination of the "three plagues of the long-term care institution—loneliness, helplessness, and boredom" and to show, "how companion animals, the opportunity to care for other living things, and the variety and spontaneity that mark an enlivened environment, can succeed where pills and therapies fail" (http://www.aalc.org/ltc.htm).

In a typical "Edenized" facility, family members and visitors will be surprised to see dogs and cats wandering around freely, sleeping in the rooms of residents, or in many cases, even on the beds with the residents. Many facilities also have birds and fish in many general areas of the environment. Some facilities let a resident keep the pet they have had for years when they enter the facility. This seems like a great concept. Studies and advocates of the concept claim that fewer antidepressant drugs are used, and both residents and employees are happier.

In this "humanized habitat" residents can also help care for the animals. As we have entered the new millennium, where 76 million baby boomers are on the brink of retirement, it is time for the industry to embrace the Eden concept. Older adults value independence, physical activity, intellectual curiosity, caring, and spirituality. The Eden concept provides not only a much more humanized environment, but variety and spontaneity during this time of their lives.

Long-term care facilities in the 21st century are most effective when they can provide an environment that promotes independence in decision-making and life styles suitable for their residents. This means that health care providers in this setting need to understand how to care for the elderly, and how to assess functional and cognitive impairment to determine if it is part of the "normal aging" process, and is the result of illness or a disease process. Caring for the elderly is not caring for an older version of a younger person. Health care needs vary tremendously as individuals age. Diseases present different symptoms in the elderly than in younger individuals, and the elderly person's condition can be much more complex. This complexity is also observed because the elderly often have more than one disease or chronic condition which can interact in ways that produce adverse effects that are not found in the younger individual who experiences fewer ongoing conditions.

Changes in metabolism, immune response, organ function, and the cumulative affects of multiple chronic conditions and diseases can certainly affect the course of any illness in an older individual. The overall condition of an older person also affects the progress of the disease process. Nutrition, level of impairment, availability of social supports, economic conditions, and the environment, all play an interrelated role in the severity and progression of illness. Health, functional status, and the quality of life are closely interrelated in the elderly and can be predictors of the level of care required to meet the needs of the individual.

Several factors can predict the need for long-term care. Living alone, loss of functional independence, inability to carry out activities of daily living, and cognitive impairment are prime indicators for the need of a stay in a long-term care facility.

One out of every five individuals living past the age of 65, and one out of three aged 85 or older, will spend some time in a long-term care facility. The "aging" of society and changes in our acute care settings have changed the character of the long-term care facility. Gone are the small, home-like facilities that provided a permanent home for the elderly, who for the most part, were in good health but unable to live alone independently in the community.

Several years ago the dominant concern with long-term care was the inappropriate placement of individuals in this setting. This has now been replaced by debate over whether the nation has enough facilities, resources, and funding to care for those elderly who truly need the services provided by long-term providers.

The continued growth of the aging population has presented us with needs that are diverse and multitudinous, and these needs fluctuate at different periods of time as the individual's capacities and life demands change. This has required a wide range of services essential to meet the complex and changing need of the elderly. Some of these services include but are not limited to:

- **Home Health Care/Community Support Services.** These services range from nursing care and specialized therapies to non-medical services such as meal preparation and homemaking.

- **Assisted Living.** This is a special combination of housing, personalized supportive services, and health care designed to meet the needs—both scheduled and unscheduled—of those who need assistance with activities of daily living (ADL), such as bathing, dressing, eating, and monitoring medications and some medical conditions such as hypertension. This particular type of setting is also referred to as Retirement Centers, and Independent or Supportive Living Centers.

- **Alzheimer Units.** This type of unit provides specialized care and supportive programs for persons with Alzheimer Disease, or with other forms of memory loss or cognitive impairment, whereby they present a threat to themselves or others. These units can be found in Assisted Living facilities or Long-Term Care centers in a designated, secure section of the facility.

- **Hospice Care**. This type of care can be provided in the home or in a facility setting such as long-term care. Its focus is to relieve suffering and to improve the quality of life for the persons and/or families living with a terminal disease. Services can include pain or symptom control, and an array of emotional, spiritual, and physical supportive services.

- **Long-Term Care Facilities.** The old "nursing home image" is changing into a complex, dynamic care site. At present there are three levels of long-term care. They are:

  - *Intermediate care,* in which the resident usually requires assistance with activities of daily living (bathing, dressing, grooming, transfer and ambulation, eating, and toileting) as well as medication administration, and/or treatment regimens. The U.S. Department of Health and Human Services definition of intermediate care is as follows:

    > An *intermediate care facility* (ICF) is . . . certified, . . . meets Federal standards, and provides less extensive health-related care and services. It provides nursing service, with limited licensed staff. The majority of 'on hands care' is provided by certified nursing assistants. Most intermediate care facilities carry on rehabilitation programs, but the emphasis is on personal care and social services. Mainly, these homes serve people who are not fully capable of living by themselves, yet are not necessarily ill enough to need 24-hour skilled nursing care . . . (Raffel and Raffel, 1994, p. 183).

  Intermediate care is further broken into two levels by Medicaid:

    - *Intermediate care I.* (ICF I), which provides licensed nursing services, supervision, and supportive services.

    - *Intermediate care II.* (ICF II), which is also called 'board and care.' This level provides room, board, and personal and daily maintenance care. The majority of the care is delivered by non-licensed staff and/family members with supervision and medications provided by licensed staff, i.e., LPNs.

- The *skilled care* resident requires skilled nursing care from a registered nurse on a daily basis. This care may include but is not limited to wound care, enteral feedings, intravenous therapy, respiratory treatment, careful monitoring of complex medical conditions, and/or rehabilitation. The U.S. Department of Health and Human Services definition of skilled care is as follows:

A *skilled nursing facility* (SNF) is a nursing home that has been certified as meeting Federal standards within the meaning of the Social Security Act. It provides the level of care that comes closest to hospital care with 24-hour nursing services. Regular medical supervision and rehabilitation therapy are also provided. Generally, a skilled nursing facility cares for convalescent patients and those with long-term illnesses (Raffel and Raffel, p. 183).

Who Needs Long-Term Care?

An estimated 12.1 million Americans need assistance from others to carry out everyday activities. Most, but not all, persons in need of long-term care are elderly. Approximately 53 percent are persons aged 65 and older (6.4 million); 44 percent are working age adults aged 18–64 (5.3 million); and 3 percent are children under age 18 (400,000).[1] Approximately 2.4 million residents reside in long-term care facilities in this country. When admitted into a long-term care facility, residents often are experiencing several chronic diseases, although a specific medical problem may bring about their need for long-term care.

A typical resident for long-term care is an 80+ female, with no surviving spouse, whose children are elderly themselves and unable to care for an elderly parent. There are fewer friends that are able to provide care because many friends have died. In the future there will be additional changes as studies show that individuals are not having as many children as in the past, and children are living further away. This leaves fewer people available to provide care. Thus, the elder may not be able to remain at home with family.

Residents are usually admitted to a long-term facility directly from the hospital with multiple diagnoses, including some evidence of impaired mental function. Whether the stay is for a short or a long term, the residents are sicker than in the past, and are more disabled than individuals who use home health services. This demands that the long-term care facilities must now provide unique services that are not duplicated in the hospital or other settings. Almost every individual in long-term care has at least one impairment, and the average is four impairments per resident. These impairments require some type of assistance: in carrying out activities of daily living, with medication administration and monitoring, and with overall assessment of medical status due to one, or more, chronic illnesses.

The leading diagnoses in long-term care are circulatory disease, cognitive impairment, and mental disorder. It is safe to say that all residents have more than one condition present at the time of admission, and more than half have three or more admitting diagnoses. The top conditions that are seen at the time of admission are:

---

[1]The Henry J. Kaiser Foundation (November, 1999). Long-term care: Medicaid's Role and Challenges (publication # 2172), Washington, DC.

- Cardiovascular diseases, including stroke, with its multiple effects, and hypertension, account for two-thirds of individuals entering the long-term care system;

- Mental and cognitive disorders, which are almost as common, include depressive disorders, anxiety disorders, and organic brain damage; and

- Disorders of the endocrine system, most commonly Type II diabetes or hypothyroidism (Sahyoun et al., 2001).

While these medical conditions are the most common diseases present at the time of admission, they are not necessarily the primary reason for the admission. Cognitive impairment, incontinence, and general functional decline are strong factors that result in an individual entering a long-term care facility. When cognitive impairment becomes moderate or severe, and the individual is exhibiting such behaviors as hitting, wandering, or being unable to keep oneself out of danger (e.g., turning the stove on and forgetting it, not remembering to take medication, or taking too much), they become too difficult to manage at home. Alternately, they may be living alone at home and be unable to care for themselves any longer. This results in a long-term care admission. It is important to understand that more than half of the residents in long-term care facilities are cognitively impaired to one degree or another. This creates an even more complex challenge to the nursing staff that cares for them.

Alzheimer's disease and cerebral vascular disease are two of the main sources of cognitive difficulties. Families of individuals that exhibit these types of behaviors often do not understand what is happening with their loved one, and are in need of ongoing education about the disease process; they do not understand why they are observing the various behaviors, and, most importantly, they do not know how to respond to these behaviors. This creates another challenge for a limited number of nursing staff.

Activities of daily living (ADLs) are a measure of functional ability in basic, self-care tasks. ADLs continue to be a major determinate in how much care an individual requires as well as their ability to live independently. These six basic tasks include:

- Bathing

- Dressing

- Eating

- Transferring from a bed to a chair

- Toileting, including the ability to take one's self to the bathroom and accomplish basic personal hygiene tasks

- Walking (mobility); the use of adaptive equipment is considered if it provides the ability to be mobile independently (Granger et al., 1987).

Bathing and dressing are often the first ADLs in which individuals will require assistance. In 1985, 92 percent of residents needed assistance, and in 1997 this number remained at 92 percent. Eating is generally the one ADL that individuals can do the longest, and yet studies have shown that in 1985 the number of individuals in long-term care requiring assistance was 40 percent, and by 1997 this number had risen to 45 percent. The number of ADLs with which residents need help has generally been a good measure of the level of care that is required. That number continues to rise, and as of 1997, the mean number was 4.4 ADLs (out of 6). While ADLs continue to be used as a predictor for the amount of care a resident will require, it is not an accurate one. This number does not assign an amount of time each task requires, which will vary with the individual resident based upon the present status of other medical and cognitive problems. Additionally, this number does not consider that this population also experiences difficulty in seeing and hearing. Approximately 60 percent of the residents use eyeglasses, while 11 percent require hearing aides. This adds to the time necessary to assist the resident to go about their daily activities.

The increase in the level of disability is certainly reflected in the ongoing change of the case mix in long-term care. Because of new medical technology and home health care, individuals have been able to remain at home longer. Patients are being discharged from acute care to a "skilled unit or transition unit" housed within the acute care hospital for further treatment and rehabilitation, and then discharged back to the community.

Therefore a total transformation of the old "nursing home" has occurred. Long-term care facilities now have embraced what is known as *subacute* or *skilled care*. They have developed special units that meet the Medicare criteria for skilled nursing care, aggressive rehabilitation programs, extensive wound care programs, and hospice. Long-term care facilities have been renamed *healthcare and rehabilitation centers*. There is a belief that the residents that are in the skilled unit within the hospital are somewhat *sicker* and *are more complex*; they are perhaps patients that need closer monitoring of their complex medical status. However, there are those facilities with a skilled unit that are able to manage more acute and medically complex patients that are stable. The facility must have the personnel and resources necessary to care for any patient that is admitted. This is one of the many areas where the clinical expertise and judgment of a registered nurse is a MUST.

Once residents have successfully completed the program, many are discharged home, or have experienced a more peaceful death. When residents are unable to successfully complete a program and are unable to return home, they are then considered for placement in "intermediate care." Most long-term care facilities today have both "skilled and intermediate care units."

These changes will have a special impact on women as they live longer, yet generally have lower incomes than men. Today, women in the workforce—and 92.5 percent of nurses are women—continue to be paid approximately 75 cents to every dollar a man makes. Retirement incomes will continue to reflect this problem. At retirement, women are usually paid lower monthly annuity benefits because they live longer than men. Thus incomes for older women actually average 55 percent of what older men make. This could be further compounded if there is not enough money to pay Social Security benefits. "It is estimated that by 2032, payroll taxes will cover only 70% to 75% of promised benefits" (Meier, 2000, p. 168). To make matters worse, Medicare continues to raise premiums; and Medicare eligibility may be raised to 67 years or higher.

Types of Long-Term Care Facilities

Long-term care may be provided in either a long-term care unit within a larger facility, or in a free-standing long-term care facility. A *long-term care unit* is a specific unit or number of beds that reside within the walls of an acute care setting such as a hospital. The skilled unit provides nursing care to individuals who require *more extensive monitoring* of the existing medical problems resulting in a longer length of stay than a hospital can provide under the present Prospective Payment System. These hospital-based skilled units usually range from 20 to 60 beds.

Skilled care may also be provided in a *free-standing long-term care facility*. These free-standing facilities are typically 120-bed facilities that provide a range of services which may include intermediate care, skilled care, and hospice care. As of 1999 in the United States, there were 18,000 nursing homes with 1,879,600 beds. Many facilities are part of large multisystems, the largest long-term care multisystem being Beverly Enterprises.

Ownership

Facility ownership in long-term care varies. It can be proprietary, government owned, institutional based, jointly owned, a partnership, a limited partnership, corporate owned, or franchised.

Proprietary. A proprietary long-term care facility is held under patent, trademark, or copyright by a private person or company. This can be for-profit, or not-for-profit. The sole proprietorship is the oldest and most common type of long-term care facility. In general, the proprietor may operate his business in any manner he chooses so long as he does not interfere with the legal rights of others. He must, however, observe the provisions of federal, state, and local laws relating to taxation, minimum wage, sanitation, and other matters. The sole proprietor either makes his own contracts with others, or engages agents to do it on his behalf. He retains all profits and bears the full loss from business operations. His liability to creditors for business debts extends to his personal fortune.

Government Owned. Another type of not-for-profit ownership is held by a governmental body such as the federal, state, county, or city government. They may directly manage the facility although usually a governmental employee, board, or agency hires an administrator to manage the facility. The administrator answers to the designated person or board. The government, and the courts, is obligated to protect rights and to help clarify ownership.

Institutional Based. A third type of ownership occurs when the facility is connected with another institution such as a hospital. Here the institution is responsible for the management of the facility. In this case the institution could be either not-for-profit or for-profit.

Jointly Owned. A long-term care facility can be jointly owned. Here an enterprise is entered into by two or more people for profit and for a limited purpose, such as purchase, improvement, and sale; or for leasing of real estate. A joint venture has most of the elements of a partnership. However, unlike a partnership, a joint venture anticipates a specific area of activity and/or period of operations, so after the purpose is completed, bills are paid, and profits (or losses) are divided, the joint venture is terminated.

Partnership. A long-term care facility can be owned by a partnership. Here the for-profit or not-for-profit business is owned by more than one person, each of whom is a "partner." A partnership may be created by a formal written agreement but may be based on an oral agreement or just a handshake. Each partner:

- Invests a certain amount (money, assets, and/or effort), which establishes an agreed-upon percentage of ownership.

- Is responsible for all the debts and contracts of the partnership even though another partner created the debt or entered into the contract.

- Has a share in management decisions.

- Shares in profits and losses according to the percentage of the total investment.

Limited Partnership. Another type of for-profit ownership is called a "limited partnership." Here responsibility for debts is limited to the managing "general partners." The invested "limited partners" cannot participate in management, and are limited to a specific profit percentage.

Corporate Owned. A long-term facility can be owned by a specific corporation. The corporation is responsible for the operation and financial management of the facility. Although this is generally for-profit, it can include non-profit facilities.

Franchise Agreement. A franchise agreement can be granted by the government to a person or corporation to operate a business. Examples can include such things as a taxi permit, a bus route, an airline's use of a public airport, a store to sell specific goods or services, or a long-term care facility. Here the franchise agreement, or business contract, is in place between the individual or corporation providing the goods or services, and the government.

Accountability in Long-Term Care

Long-term care is the most highly regulated industry in this country. The never-ending changes in regulation present additional challenges. This offers nurse administrators in long-term care the challenge of working in an environment where validating processes is a very important part of management. Performance improvement processes are essential.

There are two main routes to public accountability for long-term care facilities: licensure and certification. Each state grants the facility owners (regardless of for-profit or non-profit status) a license to operate.

Certification, although granted by the federal government, is determined in a state process. Certification is needed for Medicare reimbursement. The federal government reimburses facilities for providing covered services to Medicare recipients, and also partially funds the state-administered Medicaid programs. Each state must conduct the Omnibus Budget Reconciliation Act (OBRA) survey process used to certify that the facility qualifies to receive federal funds every 9 to 15 months.

Ultimately the surveys determine whether the facility will continue to qualify for continued licensure; and reimbursement from public funds are indirectly based on how their staff and practitioners provide care. The care does invariably reflect how well an organization functions.

There are five critical ingredients for providing successful care. They ensure that care is:

1. Based on sound principles and evidence;

2. Accommodated but does not focus primarily on regulations;

3. Supplied via a proper care delivery process;

4. Provided by qualified individuals who perform their functions and know their roles; and

5. Guided by effective management, following basic management principles.

Patient care in this setting has become more and more complex; therefore the delivery of competent personal care is no longer sufficient. The demands for the management of common clinical situations is now the norm. Long-term facilities must support evidence-based practices for common conditions and problems, including the risks and limits of medical care in the frail elderly and for those with an end-stage or terminal condition.

Nursing, with the full support of administration, must ensure that all staff have been given, and use, the information. Most relevant interventions that staff must face in long-term care are relatively straightforward and inexpensive. For example, it is vital to identify and address the special needs of residents that are at high risk for falls and/or skin breakdown. This can be accomplished by admission assessments that include special skin/fall assessments scales that determine the risk level of the resident. Specific care protocols are then determined for the individual to prevent breakdown, or to avoid a fall that results in an injury such as a fracture.

Patient-focused care—not discipline-centered, regulatory-centered, or reimbursement-centered care—must always be the goal. Effective management focuses the staff of all disciplines on appropriate care as the route to regulatory compliance, and not the other way around.

The Federal Long-Term Care Survey and Regulation Process

In 1987 Congress past the Nursing Home Reform Act as part of OBRA. The Act had five major components that would forever change how things were done in the nursing home industry. They ensured resident rights, quality of life, and quality of care; required specified staffing; required regular resident assessments; and set up federal standards and survey procedures, as well as enforcement procedures.

Resident Rights, Quality of Life, and Quality of Care

The Nursing Home Reform Act states that residents have:

- The right to be free from physical and mental abuse;
- The right to be free from physical and chemical restraints;
- The right to privacy; and
- The right to voice grievances.

The new focus is on quality of life as well as quality of care. The Act specifies that facilities must care for residents in a manner, and in an environment, that promotes the maintenance and enhancement of the highest level of quality possible for the individual. Facilities must also provide services that assist the resident to attain and/or maintain the highest practicable physical, mental, and psychosocial well-being.

Staffing and Services

The Act recognized the importance of staff and services required in this setting. RN minimum staffing requirements were increased to one RN Director of Nursing, one RN eight hours per day seven days a week, and one licensed nurse (RN or LVN/LPN) 24 hours per day. Overall, facilities are required to provide sufficient staff to provide adequate care. This becomes increasingly complex and challenging because no acuity system has been developed for long-term care, so staffing ratios are based on staff per beds, rather than staff to meet needs of the resident population.

It is expected that many changes will be seen in long-term care's future as the medical needs of the elderly increase in number and complexity, requiring an increase in the number of RNs for assessment and clinical problem solving.

There are now minimum training standards for nursing assistants. These include not less than 75 hours of training, and successfully passing a competency evaluation, before they can be employed as a nursing assistant.

The act also specified that there are minimum services that the facilities must provide. These include: nursing services and specialized rehabilitation, social services, pharmaceutical services, dietary services (including a dietitian), an ongoing activities program, and dental services.

Resident Assessment

Perhaps one of the most important components of the act is the new Resident Assessment requirement. It requires that facilities complete a resident assessment on each resident. The assessments are comprehensive, follow a standardized and uniform format, and must be completed and signed by an RN. The resident assessment tool called the MDS (Minimum Data Set) was developed in 1990. Its components include: background information, cognitive patterns, communication and hearing, mood and behavior, physical functioning, and other components. (Full details regarding the MDS are in Chapters 6 and 7.)

The MDS has been tested and re-tested. It continues to have high reliability and validity, and is generally recognized as having made a major contribution to improving resident assessments and the care provided by the nursing facilities. The MDS must be completed within the first 14 days of admission.

On the day of admission nursing completes an assessment using the appropriate MDS screens. An interim care plan is printed out and used until the final one is completed by all disciplines on the 14th day. The MDS must be completed by a multidisciplinary team, where each discipline documents that their section is complete and correct, and it is nursing's responsibility to review the document and sign stating that the information contained in the entire document is correct.

It goes without saying that, in theory, open and ongoing communication occurs between the disciplines. In reality, while the disciplines struggle to communicate with each other, case load and time constraints result in inaccurate information being documented.

An example of this can occur in the section, Mood and Behavior, which is the responsibility of Social Service to fill out. The section of the MDS of Mood and Behavior is divided into 5 sections. One of the sections deals with behavior. Sub-categories in the section include wandering, verbally abusive behavior symptoms, physically abusive symptoms, socially inappropriate/disruptive behavioral symptoms, and resisting care. Scoring in this section is divided into 4 responses:

- Behavior not exhibited past 7 days.

- Behavior of this type occurred 1–3 times past 7 days.

- Behavior of this type occurred 4–6 times but not daily past 7 days.

- Behavior of this type occurred daily (Heaton Resources, 2002).

Because the social workers see the resident only two or three times a week, they may rate the resident one way, i.e., "behavior not exhibited past 7 days," when for the other 23-and-a-half hours of the day the nursing staff deals with very different behavior or mood changes and would say, "Behavior of this type occurred 4–6 times but not daily past 7 days." The social worker must rely on what the nursing staff has documented, or communicated to them in some other way, or the social worker will rate the resident the way in which they observe the resident.

This holds true for all the disciplines that are involved in documenting on the MDS. Conflicting information on the MDS, medical record, and discussions with the clinical staff, will result in the state surveyors citing the facility with a deficiency of some type. Creativity, open communication, and respect between the disciplines are essential to avoid the consequence of cited deficiencies.

Federal Standards and Survey Procedures

A set of 30 Quality Indicators (QIs) were developed using the MDS data. These include: accidents, behavioral/emotional problems, clinical problems, elimination and continence problems, infection, nutrition, physical functioning, psychotropic drugs, quality of life, sensory/communication problems, and skin care. The QIs can be used by the facilities to monitor quality of care, and by state survey agencies to:

- Identify residents that should be reviewed during the survey process, and

- Identify potential problem facilities.

Enforcement Procedures

Many changes were established in the survey process. These procedures included:

- Mandating that regular surveys of facilities occur about every 9–15 months and after any change of ownership;

- Investigation of any complaints about the facility, and ongoing monitoring to ensure compliance with the regulations;

- Surveys must be unannounced, and must include registered nurses as members of the survey team;

- State surveyors must not have conflicts of interest with the facilities they survey, and they must have completed comprehensive training in the survey process; and

- Findings from the surveys must be made available to the public, and as of this writing they are available online at www.cms.hhs.gov/quality/mds20.

There are two types of surveys that occur in long-term care facilities:

1. Standard surveys that include a case mix-stratified sample of residents. These surveys use the indicators of medical, nursing, rehabilitative care, dietary, activities, sanitation, infection control, physical environment, qualifications and experience of staff, and ongoing education of staff to examine care the patient received. There are approximately 185 separate standards that facilities must meet (excluding the life safety standards which are separate).

2. Extended surveys are done in those facilities that are found to be providing substandard care under the standard survey. The extended survey uses an expanded sample of residents in the facility to identify the causes of substandard care (Medicare, Nursing Home Compare. *Collecting and Updating Nursing Home Data*. 2004).

The survey process is a detailed one and can take three to four days to complete. It includes the following tasks:

1. **Off Site Preparation:**

- Identifying areas of concern;

- Identifying residents for sample; and

- Identifying special survey needs.

2. **Entrance Conference/On Site Preparation:**

- Confirm any special resident populations; and

- Asks for information about the facility

3. **Initial Tour of the Facility.**

4. **The Sample Selection of Residents (a rule of thumb is 12 residents per 100 beds) should include:**

- A mix of heavy and light care residents;

- Interviewable and non-interviewable residents;
- Residents with special problems;
- New admissions;
- Residents under age 55; and
- Other choices (such as recent fractures, or multiple falls).

5. **Information Gathering:**

- Observations of the facility and residents;
- Informal and formal interviews with residents;
- Resident record reviews;
- Group interviews with resident council members; and
- Interviews with families and friends.

6. **Information Analysis for Deficiency Determination:**

- Review and analyze all information to determine whether the facility has failed to meet one or more requirements; and
- Determine whether to conduct an extended survey.

7. **Exit Conference:**

- Discussion of findings with management group.

8. **Writing the Statement of Deficiencies.**

9. **Deficiency Categorization.**

10. **Post Survey Revisit and/or Follow-up** (www.cms.hhs.gov/quality/mds20):

The determination of the *severity of a deficiency* is based on four levels:

1. *No actual harm with a potential for minimal harm;*

2. *No actual harm but a potential for more than minimal harm;*

3. *Actual harm that is not immediate jeopardy; or*

4. *Immediate jeopardy to resident health and safety* (www.cms.hhs.gov/quality/mds20).

The *scope of deficiencies* are categorized as:

1. *Isolated;*

2. *Consistent pattern; or*

3. *Wide-spread* (www.cms.hhs.gov/quality/mds20).

Deficiencies are rated both by *scope* (is it an isolated event or wide-spread?) and by *severity* (no actual harm or immediate jeopardy).

If the survey team determines that the resident's health or safety is in immediate jeopardy, immediate action must be taken to remove the jeopardy and correct the deficiency through specified remedies, such as temporary management, or termination of the facility's participation in Medicare and Medicaid.

If the deficiency does not jeopardize the health and safety of residents, then other remedies may be imposed. These can include: denial of Medicare and Medicaid payments for all residents, or newly admitted residents; civil money penalties (up to $10,000 dollars); transfer of residents; state monitoring; a directed plan of correction; and other remedies. The survey team can also decide to close the facility to new admissions until it corrects the stated deficiency.

As the survey process has become so comprehensive, and has a significant element of subjectivity, the Centers for Medicare and Medicaid Services (CMS) continues to issue survey guidance to the agency's regional offices to clarify ongoing survey issues. Although the State Operations Manual does give instructions regarding the survey process, the guidelines should also assist facilities in responding to deficiencies related to care issues, such as helping residents maintain a practicable level of functioning, determining an avoidable/unavoidable decline in functioning and/or skin breakdown, or inappropriate restraint use.

Avoidable or Unavoidable Issues

Two of the most difficult determinations to make in the long-term care population are: 1) If a decline in the condition of a resident has occurred, or if there are indications that the resident is not at the highest practicable level of functioning, and 2) Is this an avoidable or unavoidable situation? In order to determine if this outcome is avoidable or unavoidable, several activities for information gathering must occur including:

- On-site observations;
- Ongoing dialogue with the direct-care giving staff, resident, and family members; and
- A recorded review to clarify and validate information.

It is also important to determine if the facility:

- has a continuous on-going process that consistently provides individualized care for the resident. Ongoing observations, such as talking with residents, families and staff, are a good way to gain this information.

- completes a comprehensive assessment that identifies the resident's baseline status and potential for improvement.

- identifies and assesses risk factors that were/are present, and which may have contributed to the decline or failure to improve, including the individual's ongoing medical conditions.

- develops appropriate care plans, and consistently implements the appropriate interventions to ensure the individual resident is at the highest level of functioning, and addresses any high risk indicators that have been identified for this individual.

- conducts ongoing evaluation of the outcomes of the care provided to the resident population, such as: has the resident reached his/her goals, declined or improved, and have appropriate interventions been tried and/or adapted? (www.cms.hhs.gov/quality/mds20)

The *avoid* ability of "decline and failure to improve" must be evaluated against the resident's baseline functional status and disease states. It is important that both surveyors and providers *not* assume that age inevitably results in a resident's decline or failure to maintain the level practical level of functioning.

If, during information gathering, any of the following are found, one would suspect that the decline was likely **AVOIDABLE**:

- Assessments are incomplete, and/or not accurate.

- There is evidence that they have not been done in an individualized, comprehensive manner.

- Interventions are not ongoing, or completely implemented, or provided according to the standards of care.

- There is no evidence of an ongoing process of evaluating the resident's response to their plan of care, such as stated interventions with reassessments and revision of interventions if appropriate.

Decline is likely **UNAVOIDABLE** when one or more of the following is present:

- Progression of the underlying disease process, and/or other factors such as: medical conditions; psychosocial factors; activity level; medication toxicity has been identified and assessed; all with the implementation of interventions continuously evaluated.

- There is a steadfast refusal of care despite ongoing efforts to provide alternative treatments (www.cms.hhs.gov/quality/mds20 and www.thompson.com/libraries/healthcare/home/special_reports/homeguidance.html).

Investigating Resistants Use

The use of restraints, both physical and chemical, has become a major concern in the long-term care setting. While federal regulations and the Social Security Act do not ban the use of restraints, there are regulations that prohibit their use except under certain circumstances. The overwhelming evidence demonstrates that the use of restraints contributes to the downward spin in the overall condition of the long-term care residents. It is important to note that medical symptoms alone do not justify the use of restraints. The facility must identify how the restraint will protect the individual from injury and/or prevent the individual from removing essential medical devices providing treatment. To determine compliance with the restraint regulation, it is critical to understand both what encompasses restrictive behaviors as well as the selection and application of restraint. Another key element is to understand whether or not the particular restraint will effectively treat the presenting symptoms, either by improving the condition, or by contributing to the worsening of the condition.

The Future of Governmental Guidance Regarding Surveys

In 1998 the Federal Administration announced a national initiative to "crack down" on perceived deficiencies in long-term care facilities. Since that announcement substantial state and federal government resources have been directed at identifying and correcting alleged problems in the long-term care industry.

Long-term care facilities continue to struggle to comply with federal and state directives. More and more facilities are realizing the adverse impact that a negative survey has on current business and liability exposure (from civil cases), future certificate of need reviews, and future ability to attract residents. In addition, there are the immediate perils of licensure and certification status, and the imposing of civil monetary penalties (CMPs), which can be as much as $3,050 to $10,000 per day of immediate jeopardy, or $1,000 to $10,000 per instance of deficiency (not to exceed $10,000 per day).[2] According to 42 C.F.R. (Code of

---

[2]42 C.F.R. & 488.438(a)(1)(i). From: *Navigating Survey and Certification Issues for Long-Term Care Facilities: What You Need to Know About Appeals, Governmental Guidance and the Future*, RTP 41152X2. (May 2001). Atlanta: Health Care Practice Group at Womble Carlyle Sandridge & Rice, PLLC.

Federal Regulations) and 489.53, a provider who has had an enforcement remedy imposed against it must be given the opportunity to appeal that imposition. The number of cases that challenge remedies or enforcement tools that have been imposed by CMS after negative certification surveys have grown tremendously since 1998. Greater numbers of cases are expected in the 21st century.

The decision to challenge CMS' determination and imposition of an enforcement remedy, in cases where a long-term care facility can establish substantial compliance and reasonable conduct in light of all the circumstances, cannot be over-emphasized. Too often, facilities fail to appeal adverse surveys even though they believe they have not received a full review by the surveyors, or they know of additional facts which would change the interpretation of an event. A challenge of the assigned penalty is especially appropriate where the facility can demonstrate that it acted with reasonable care and followed current protocols.

An example of this follows:

In Koester Pavilion v. HCFA (HHS DAB), Doc. No.C-97-554, Dec. No. CR650 (Feb. 29, 2000), the ALJ (Administrative Law Judge) rejected HCFA's[3] determination that a facility's use of a Posey waist restraint on a resident along with side rails that were not full-length placed its residents in immediate jeopardy because the facility followed instructions more current than those used by the State surveyors. The totality of the circumstances revealed that no accident hazard was posed (the requisite quality of care was satisfied) because the facility followed the most current cautionary instructions for the restraint,[4] positioned the resident in the middle of the bed, and provided substantial monitoring of the resident. The ALJ also found the facility to be in substantial compliance with quality of care requirements for the prevention and treatment of pressure sores because the provider promptly identified sores caused by new shoes of several residents and properly treated them.[5] Based on these findings, the ALJ held that HCFA was not authorized to impose a CMP (civil monetary penalty) against the facility. On October 18, 2000, the HHS DAB (Health and Human Services Department Appeals Board) affirmed the ALJ's determination that the facility did not commit an immediate jeopardy violation using resistants, preventing pressure sores. Therefore, while the DAB agreed that that the $3,050 CMP for the day of restraint usage was unauthorized, the DAB reinstated the $50 per day

---

[3]HCFA (Health Care Finance Administration) is now called CMS (Centers for Medicare and Medicaid Services).

[4]Cautionary instructions issued the year before had warned facilities not to use the resistant without full length or continuous bed rails. These were the instructions relayed to the State surveyors in determining that the facility allowed an accident hazard to exist. The facility, on the other hand, had the current instructions and had followed them. The ALJ noted that the failure to heed a manufacturer's cautionary instructions is a factor in determining whether an accident hazard exists, but does not create one per se. Failure to follow such instructions may prevent the manufacturer from being held liable, and therefore might expose the facility to greater liability if an accident occurs.

[5]The ALJ found that the facility did all that it could to prevent pressure sores and treat any that were identified. Therefore, the ALJ found HCFA's citation of the provider for failure to provide adequate care to several residents was erroneous and did not support a CMP.

CMP for the fifty-day period cited by HCFA for a non-immediate jeopardy deficiency (*Navigating Survey and Certification Issues for Long-Term Care Facilities: What You Need to Know About Appeals, Governmental Guidance and the Future*, RTP 41152X2. (May 2001). Atlanta: Health Care Practice Group at Womble Carlyle Sandridge & Rice, PLLC).

While guidelines provide some guidance to State surveyors, significant decisions remain within the exclusive discretion of the surveyors, who may or may not have uniform or standardized training to identify potential deficiencies, or to interpret standards from their individual perceptions. A finding of immediate jeopardy is very serious for a facility in terms of public relations, immediate sanctions, and potential decertification, not to mention seriously affecting the "bottom line" in an industry that is already under-financed.

Because the long-term care industry is the most regulated segment in health care and undergoes, at a minimum, yearly certification surveys, cases challenging surveyors' findings will continue to increase. As federal and state pressure on long-term care facilities continues to strengthen, more facilities need to appeal enforcement remedies, and the underlying factual assumptions supporting the cited deficiencies. Cases occurring since 2000 have demonstrated that facilities can prevail during an appeal, showing that appeals are not a futile endeavor.

It has been my experience over the years that any kind of a survey or inspection (as is done frequently in the military) brings on a certain amount of stress. However, the most stress-producing survey has to be Medicare State surveys. It is not so much that they are unannounced, but that from the moment that the team of surveyors enters the front door, the demands on your time can be overwhelming. While they are in a facility, many of the staff are constantly running to get "this or that" leaving no time for them to do their routine jobs. Patient care can suffer in this kind of environment.

Surveyors come into a facility with their survey plan decided. The plan is based on the data the long-term care facility has provided to them. The data is rooted in the facility's past surveys, complaints from residents or family members received during the past year, and/or OSCAR reports. The OSCAR's CMS' Online Survey, Certification, and Reporting database, and CHSRA reports are the Center for Health Systems Research and Analysis. This database includes the long-term care characteristics and health deficiencies issued during the three most recent state inspections and recent complaint investigations. The information on the facility's characteristics derived from OSCAR is prepared by each facility at the beginning of the regular State inspection. This information is reported by the facility themselves through the MDS data reporting system. The OSCAR data contained on the Nursing Home Compare website is updated on a monthly basis and the MDS[6] data is updated quarterly. The team will also concentrate on various, but selected, OBRA and state codes.

---

[6]The MDS is explained in Chapters 6 and 7.

Because of the number of rules and regulations placed upon the long-term care industry, the surveyors cannot possibly concentrate on all of the rules at any one visit. Therefore, a survey conducted in one facility is totally different, or inconsistent from, surveys done in other facilities. Because of these inconsistencies, the surveyors, or the facility, have no data that can be used to see if there is ongoing improvement, or whether changes have been positive or negative. For example, you can have a perfect survey for 4–5 years, and then have one with ten or more deficiencies of varying scope and severity. What this tells us is that the focus of the surveys may have changed that year, and/or you have a different survey team with varying years of surveyor experience.

While the present survey system is being "sold" as "outcome-based," this does not appear to be the case. Surveys still focus on paperwork. The age-old statement of, "If it isn't charted, it wasn't done" continues to be the battle cry of the surveyors. Common sense appears to be left at the door when the survey begins.

For example, a resident is in a terminal state from end stage renal disease and could no longer feed herself. The staff documented every hour exactly what she accepted from them in the form of fluids. However, it was not documented in the Care Plan that the woman was at the "end of life" stage. A citation could be issued for failure to plan care. The lack of the documentation in the care plan did not alter the fact that the staff had, indeed, met the resident's needs.

Another example is when the patient has been assessed as a high-fall risk. A common nursing standard would be to have the least restrictive restraint (such as a lap buddy) that would prevent the patient from falling. If the care plan, the RAP, and all documentation does not follow the restraint protocol, the facility will be cited for improper usage of restraints. This places the nursing staff in a no-win situation because you get cited if the patient falls, or you get cited if the patient is restrained.

For those of us who have experienced such incidents, it has become very clear that new and innovative methods must be developed to identify the poor quality facilities, and separate them from the good quality facilities that strive day-by-day to provide compassionate care to their residents.

To present the long-term care industry in a poor light does the industry a grave injustice, and the individuals that suffer are the very ones that require our services. The industry provides an invaluable service to communities, and, in return, deserves to be recognized and commended for the good that is done. The long-term care facility is an important component of a comprehensive continuum of care. With its range of services, it can use care management to provide the right service at the right time for the right cost.

Ethical Decision-Making in Long-Term Care

Ethical issues are an important part of health care. Long-term care facilities are redefining ethical principles to match the issues in the long-term environment. With the availability of technology and more skilled staff, long-term care facilities now provide higher levels of care. This means that we have to reexamine at many of the ethical decisions that will need to be made by individuals and/or families.

In hospitals, medical treatment focuses on acute illness and recovery. If there is an order of "Do Not Resuscitate," it is for a brief period of time. Autonomy issues are dealt with according to a traditional model. If the patient has the ability to make decisions, he/she makes the decision. If not, a surrogate makes decisions on behalf of the patient, using either substituted judgment, or the best interest standard.

The situation is totally different in long-term care. Patients/residents are admitted with the underlying understanding that this will become their home. The care is based on medical treatment, rehabilitative, or palliative care, rather than equipment and procedures. Many residents have varying degrees of diminished mental capacity so there may need to be decisions made involving autonomy, and other issues. It is important to respect individual variations, and not base decisions on a simple categorization of the resident as having, or not having, that capacity.

There are two basic principles of biomedical ethics that have to be considered. They are:

- *Autonomy*—each individual should be in control of his or her own person, both body and mind. A competent individual has the right to accept or refuse medical treatment. The doctrine of informed consent grew out of this.

- *Beneficence*—what is best for each person's welfare should be accomplished. It incorporates two obligations. The first is to do that which is for the good of the individual, and the second is to do no harm to the individual. In some cases the two obligations must be balanced against each other. In other words, the amount of good must be balanced against the amount of harm.

The principles of autonomy and beneficence come into conflict when an individual wishes to refuse a treatment that others believe would be beneficial. Generally, the principle of autonomy has been accepted as primary in medical ethics, and the principle of beneficence as secondary. However, in the long-term care setting, where state and federal regulatory policies to provide care must be complied with, the principle of beneficence may override the principle of autonomy.

Autonomy in long-term care is measured differently than it is in an independent living situation. When placement of an individual occurs, it is because of age, illness, dependent behaviors or dementia, or because the person requires personal and medical support. The long-term care facility, to meet both state regulatory standards and provide care in a cost-effective manner, has routines and schedules for eating, bathing, dressing, medications, activities, and bedtime that deprive residents of choices they would have made had they been in independent living.

An ethical goal for the long-term care facility should be to maximize the autonomy of all the residents. Residents should be given an opportunity to demonstrate their highest level of functioning. To protect the rights of the residents, facilities must develop guidelines to assist the clinical staff in assessing a resident's capacity to give informed consent. Four standards that should be considered are:

- The ability to communicate choices;

- The ability to understand information about treatment decisions;

- The ability to appreciate the situation and grasp the relevant consequences; and

- The ability to manipulate the information provided in order to compare the benefits and risks of the various options (Goldsmith, 1994, pp. 30–31).

The Use of Agents and Directives

Autonomy for the resident can be encouraged by assisting the competent resident to appoint an agent to make future medical decisions when they are no longer able to do it themselves. Making advanced directive decisions is a difficult thing to do and there is no good time to approach this topic. There are many documents and planning tools that are available: health care proxies, durable powers of attorney, advance or medical directives, living wills, and value statements. The documents vary according to state, and any documents completed by residents must conform to state law. With the use of a combination of one or more or these documents, the resident can designate a surrogate and provide the information necessary to make the surrogate's decision reflective of the resident's wishes. Because of current HIPAA regulations, all facilities, pharmacies, and so forth must have their clients sign forms that state who can receive information. It appears to be an overreaction to the HIPAA regulations. I suspect that there will be some revision and/or clarifications.

Withholding or Withdrawing Medical Treatment

Perhaps the most critical and difficult ethical decisions in long-term care are whether to administer or to withhold treatment that is in the scope of usual medical care. This is only considered when an individual is suffering, beyond hope of recovery, unable to respond to therapy, or living a life that the individual would not want to live. Withholding a necessary treatment might allow death to occur naturally and with dignity.

In order to make this decision, certain data must be compiled. This includes:

- Assessment of the individual's physical and emotional status;
- Prognosis with and without treatment;
- Risks and burdens of treatment;
- The individual's level of intellectual functioning;
- Assessment of the individual's quality of life;
- Previously expressed wishes of the individual and family; and
- Recommendations of caregivers, family, and physician.

There should be consensus among the resident's family, physician, and other health care workers. Data and decisions must be documented in the resident's medical record.

"Do Not Transfer" and "Do Not Hospitalize" Decisions

Hospitalization is required for evaluation and treatment when an individual's condition worsens. The decision to hospitalize needs to be made in accordance with the treatment objectives for the individual. This is a very difficult decision for families and/or significant others to make. It must be made on a situation-by-situation basis, always taking into consideration the individual's own wishes.

There are many ethical issues that will need to be resolved in the long-term care setting. As the resident population becomes more acutely ill and more cognitively impaired, families and staff will have to confront these issues. The facilities must have policies and/or guidelines related to these issues. Staff will particularly need educational programs and case reviews to assist them in understanding and carrying out clinical decisions based on bioethical principles.

Reimbursement in Long-Term Care

Long-term care has experienced constant change in the reimbursement arena. As of 1999, 9 percent of the $4,358 per capita (per person) spent on health care in the United States was spent on nursing home care. Long-term care expenses have become such an issue that in 1996, the Health Insurance Reform Act was passed, making long-term care expenses, including home care, tax deductible. There are basically three methods of reimbursement in long-term care: private pay, Medicare, and Medicaid.

Private Pay

Private pay means that the individual and/or his family are responsible for the overall cost. Long-term care insurance, a new option, is now available but it is expensive and many people do not have it. In the last decade, more than a hundred long-term care insurance policies became available. These insurance plans are for both in-home care and for institutional care.

Medicare

Medicare is a health insurance program for:

- People 65 years of age and older;

- Some people under 65 years of age with disabilities; or

- People with end-stage renal disease (permanent kidney failure requiring dialysis or a transplant) (www.medicare.gov).

Medicare[7] has two parts:

- Part A (Hospital Insurance)—Most people 65 years or older do not have to pay for Part A.

- Part B (Medical Insurance)—Most people 65 years or older pay monthly for Part B.

The majority of the skilled nursing care in long-term care facilities is paid for, or reimbursed by, Medicare Part A. There are very specific criteria that must be met when a resident is admitted to a long-term care facility under Medicare Part A. For example, the resident must have a three-day hospital stay previous to their admission to the long-term care unit, they must have a diagnosis or a condition which requires skilled services, and they must have an order for admission to skilled services from a physician.

There are also very specific guidelines relating to the documentation of skilled services that are being provided in the facility. For instance, the Minimum Data Set (MDS)[8] has very specific guidelines as to how it should be completed for a skilled resident. Daily documentation relating to skilled care must meet the Medicare requirement not only for the consistency in resident care, but also to meet the requirements for reimbursement.

---

[7]Further explanation of Medicare and Medicaid is provided in Dunham-Taylor, J. and Pinczuk, J. (2006). *Health Care Financial Management for Nurse Managers: Merging the Heart with the Dollar.* Sudbury, MA: Jones and Bartlett.

[8]See Chapters 6 and 7 for more explanation about the MDS.

As the prospective payment system evolved in the long-term care arena, the assessment and documentation of clinical care became very closely related to reimbursement. The amount of reimbursement from the Medicare system is actually determined by the data that is entered in the MDS.

Long-term care is only covered for the first 20 days under Medicare. The patient must then make a co-payment for the next 80 days. After 100 days, there is no long-term care coverage. Custodial care of more than 100 days for the elderly does not exist in Medicare. So how does the patient pay for custodial care? Medicaid may pay, if the patient is below the poverty level established by the state. If the patient is above the poverty level, the patient's income, property, and other assets are "spent down" until the patient is below the poverty level. Then Medicaid benefits will begin.

When a person does not choose to spend down, other caregivers, such as relatives, may care for the person in the home. This can often be a burden, especially when there is no one else available to relieve the caregiver. This often creates financial burdens for both the caregiver and for the person receiving the care.

Medicaid

Federal legislation mandates the states to share costs for Medicaid with the federal government. Medicaid has various names in each state, and is a health insurance program that has criteria that are state specific. State legislators were faced with having to find money to fund this program, and funding worsens each year as Medicaid costs continue to rise. Many of the residents in our long-term care facilities, sometimes as many as 80 percent in a given facility, are covered by Medicaid. Some states pay designated amounts for all Medicaid residents in our facilities, while some states have designated a skilled and an intermediate level of care for reimbursement. Many states are now providing reimbursement through the Medicaid system that is similar to the Medicare system, based on specific resident assessments.

Veterans Administration (VA)

If a veteran, the Veterans Administration provides funds for the care of long-term care residents either within the environment of the Veterans Administration or by contractual agreements with long-term care facilities.

Other Models

Some nice models for community-based long-term care have been developed. One example is the Program for All-Inclusive Care for the Elderly (PACE), and the Social Health Maintenance Organization (S/HMO) projects. These two demonstration projects are important as HCFA (CMS) has invested years of thought and effort into providing community-based long-term care. Both PACE and S/HMO emphasize home- and community-based services. Integrating acute and long-term care involves coordinating and integrating the Medicare and Medicaid benefits. Integration and coordination should address both financing and service delivery.

The goal of the PACE and S/HMO projects is to reduce fragmentation of services, contain costs, and effectively integrate acute and long-term care into a single, seamless system. These projects were established based on the need for a beneficiary-centered continuum of care for people who need long-term care, and recognizes that individuals in long-term care have significant acute and chronic care needs. Since Medicaid and Medicare represent over half of the long-term spending, these programs can play a central role in the development of a more beneficiary-centered system.

PACE has already shifted from a demonstration project to a permanent program and is available in many states. It is a capitated benefit that features a comprehensive service delivery system. PACE combines medical, social, and long-term care services for frail individuals in states that have chosen to offer it under Medicaid.

The Budgetary Process

One of the most serious problems facing long-term care facilities is the continuous acceleration of costs. Long-term care facilities are functioning in a demanding and often hostile regulatory environment. The increasing complexity of the industry is the result of the demands being placed on the facilities to provide a broad array of services to residents meeting basic personal care up to what is now being classified as "subacute" hospital care.

Regulatory demands range from those that have a broad application, such as the Americans with Disabilities Act, to those that are more targeted at nursing home reform, such as sections of the OBRA of 1987. The problem with well-meaning legislative initiatives is that they cost the long-term facility money that is simply not reimbursed.

This situation requires a strong and informed management team that can read and understand financial statements, deal with the reimbursement issues, and work with the finance team to develop creative and effective mechanisms to track all revenues due to the facility, generate new sources of revenue, and control expenses, without compromising the quality of care provided to the residents. In the long-term care setting most of the financial decisions are made by the corporate level of the organization. This level is not involved in the day-by-day financial management of the facilities, but exerts its control by allocating funds through annual capital and operating budgets, approving new positions, and establishing approval levels for any purchases over a certain amount.

Simply stated, in most cases the annual budget is sent down to the various facilities with little input from the "grass root" level of the corporations. It is important that those on the management team understand the budget process so they can correctly interpret the budget and its ramifications.[9]

Staffing and Scheduling

Staffing is the most critical and persistent concern facing long-term care facilities. Many staffing studies have been done over the years regarding staffing, and they are starting to provide evidence that quantity, quality, and staff mix can affect patient outcomes. For instance, Dunham-Taylor and Pinczuk (2006) cite three studies:

- Bliesmer, Smayling, Kane, and Shannon (1998) found that greater use of licensed nurses in the first year of admission resulted in improved functional ability, increased probability of discharge home, and decreased probability of death. There was no difference found with chronic patients who had been in long-term care over a year.

- Hendrix and Foreman (2001) found that, "NAs have substantially more impact than RNs on minimizing long-term care decubitus costs, but both were significant. This study shows that the average nursing home operator would need to spend approximately $380 per resident for RNs and $569.98 to $1,820.32 per resident for nurse aides to achieve this staffing ratio. Increased LPNs did not achieve fewer decubiti so this study advocated reducing or eliminating LPNs. *When staffing was not at the minimum suggested by this study, the researchers found that the nursing homes spent $84,085,167 within the industry on decubiti—a cost that could have been eliminated with inadequate staffing.*

- After doing 8 years of research on nursing home patient care levels, federal health officials (Pear, 2000) have found that 54 percent of all nursing homes fall below minimum nurse staffing standards and further said that patients were endangered with low staffing levels. They found out staffing levels were much higher in not-for-profit nursing homes compared with for-profit nursing homes. In their study results, federal officials advocated that minimum staffing standards for all care facilities would be 2 hours per day per patient of nurse aide and 12 minutes per day per patient of RN time. Outcome measures in this study included: decubiti, malnutrition, weight loss, dehydration, need for hospital admissions, and possible death. When there were low staffing ratios the staff turnover rate increased (p. 172).

---

[9]Dunham-Taylor, J. and Pinczuk, J. (2006). *Health Care Financial Management for Nurse Managers: Merging the Heart with the Dollar*, Sudbury, MA: Jones and Bartlett, provides detailed information on budgets and staffing that will be a helpful reference.

There has also been some research about nurses' perceptions about the patient care.

> Many RNs have become frustrated, stressed, and disillusioned with hospital and long-term care inpatient nursing. Studies are finding that nurses report the quality of their care is not as high as it used to be—or needs to be (2001 ANA Staffing Survey). Nurses are saying that the work is too hard and thankless. . . . This dissatisfaction with nursing [is] caused by inadequate staffing, heavy workloads, increased use of overtime, and not enough support staff (Dunham-Taylor and Pinczuk, 2006, p. 785).

As one reviews the literature one comes to the conclusion that it is a combination of the three—quality, quantity, and staff mix. There are many other factors that affect staffing which include but are not limited to: turnover of staff; expansion of health care facilities; the knowledge explosion; the technology explosion; and the decrease in acute care hospital stays.

The staffing model a facility uses is a reflection of the facility, and of nursing departments' philosophy and goals. Ideally, the staffing budget should not drive or define the organization's purposes. The reality, unfortunately, is that a resource-driven environment will direct and constrain the mission and goals that can be achieved.

Therefore, we are challenged to be creative and efficient managers. I am always reminded of what was told to me as a young second lieutenant in the USAF by my first Chief Nurse: "Remember when it comes to patient care, God gave nurses a special gift and that is the ability to make do with what we have whether it is equipment or people." Over the years I have found her to be absolutely right.

One method to retain staff is to develop a "clinical ladder," similar to ones that have been developed for nurses, only for nursing assistants. A model that can be used is one of Mentorship or Leadership. This program prepares experienced nursing assistants to act as a "mentor" or preceptor for new nursing assistants. A suggested curriculum for this mentorship/leadership program is given in the Appendix at the end of this chapter. Candidates receive 80 hours of classroom instruction, have weekly meetings with the course instructor to discuss progress, dialogue about problems, and complete forms that are needed. These nursing assistant mentors receive additional pay as well as a different title.

The mentors then act as preceptors, helping to orient new nursing assistants. At the end of the orientation period, the mentors recommend, or do not recommend, the new nursing assistant's continued employment. The mentor is also involved if the new nursing assistant is counseled. This program provides an excellent growing experience for the mentor, and the new employee builds a relationship with the mentor that gives him/her more confidence. The leadership part can also be helpful to the facility because many of the nursing assistants have leadership capabilities that can be used to determine orientation and training needs of peers, to set up job descriptions, to teach others about good techniques to use to better serve residents, and so forth.

Nursing's Role in Long-Term Care

The nurse managers in long-term care are pioneers in a profession that has a continuous increase in the number of people who require the services. Long-term care is a challenging environment that offers incredible rewards for those who accept the challenge.

The central mission of a long-term care facility is *NURSING CARE*. Administrators in long-term care need to appreciate the centrality of the nursing care function in the facility and organize the operations of the facility to support the nursing function. Most long-term care facilities have in their mission statements something that refers to the quality of care provided. In order to provide that "quality" care the nursing department must be given the resources to do the job—resources including personnel, equipment, and supplies.

This begins with the appointment of a Director of Nursing as a top management position in the organization. This individual must be educationally and experientially qualified for the position. Because of the importance and scope of responsibilities, the director of nursing should be educationally prepared at the master's level in nursing and experienced in the care of the elderly.

The responsibilities of the director of nursing in long-term care settings include: implementing extensive and complex federal and state regulations; operationalzing the concept of *resident*, instead of patient; operationalizing the concept of home; developing services with the capability of caring for elderly persons, whose presentation of illness is unique and very different from younger persons; and focusing on residents' potential capabilities rather than limitations.

The long-term care setting also requires a nursing leader who clearly understands the differences between acute and long-term care, and is able to administer a department responsive to the differences. One of the many challenges facing the nursing leader is that of staff retention. The majority of staff in this setting are certified nursing assistants, and the turnover numbers of this group of staff is overwhelming—anywhere from 30–400 percent. The ongoing training, orientation, and recruitment takes a large amount of the nursing department's budget.

Bureaucracy has taken hold in the long-term care setting, which can make it easy to lose sight of the caring and nurturing environment that should determine outcomes and services delivered to the residents. In the ongoing demands to meet both the federal and state regulations, a facility may become obsessed with the tasks to be accomplished rather than the outcomes.

One must not forget that TIME, ENERGY, PERSONNEL, and RESOURCES are required to manage the documentation and forms that must be completed on a shift-by-shift and daily basis. The ability of the nursing department to perform assessments, establish priorities, develop appropriate plans of care, and deliver and monitor care (making adjustments when indicated) ensures that the long-term care facility will be able to manage resources and achieve effective productivity, as well as reduce the risk of liability from negligence. The most important goal is to provide an environment where residents enjoy a quality of life that is respectful of his/her capabilities, and where staff members are able to grow.

Because patients are often in the facility longer, there are some unique opportunities for nursing staff. One of the most beneficial is the opportunity to provide "holistic care," care that meets the needs of the residents from a physical, mental, and spiritual arena. Relationships that are established with both residents and family members during their stay in the long-term care facility gives nursing staff the opportunity to care for, and care about, the resident and the family members. In many cases members of the nursing staff become "members" of the family. This has proven to be a great comfort at the time of the resident's death. Nursing staff has the opportunity to assess the residents' total needs and work with others to meet those needs in the most compassionate and efficient manner.

The knowledge that each of these participants brings to the table in the triangle of care (see Exhibit 5-1) is very valuable and can enhance the care of the resident in long-term care. *Residents* are the people that we must assess in order to identify their needs. Their involvement in the care planning process is crucial to best meet their needs. The *family* brings a lifetime of experiences with the resident, plus the ability to encourage and support them. The *staff* has the experience and knowledge that has been attained through years of experience in caring for the elderly. The degree to which the people represented in this triangle of care collaborate together for the good of the resident will dictate the consistent quality of care which the resident receives.

Exhibit 5-1   Triangle of Care

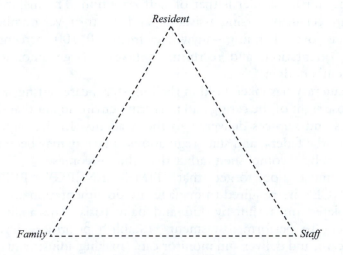

Source: American Hospital Association, personal communication.

American Nurses Credentialing Center (ANCC) Magnet Program: Recognizing Excellence in Nursing Services

The Magnet Recognition Program was developed by the ANCC to recognize health care organizations that provide the very best in nursing care and uphold the professional practice tradition within nursing. The program also provides a vehicle for disseminating successful practices and strategies within nursing systems. In an industry that depends on the provision of nursing care, achieving this magnet recognition seems to be a natural. ANCC has recently extended the program to include long-term care facilities. For the long-term care industry to ignore this opportunity is foolish, as it has been proven that regardless of the healthcare organization's size, setting, or location, achieving Magnet designations serves to attract and retain quality employees. Magnet designation helps consumers locate health care organizations that have a proven level of excellence in nursing care. In the present environment, rife with controversy about patient safety in facilities, medical error rates, and nursing shortages, consumers need to know how good the care is at the facilities.

The Magnet Recognition Program is based on quality indicators and standards of nursing practice as defined in the American Nurses Association's Scope and Standards for Nurse Administrators (2004). The Magnet designation process includes the appraisal of both qualitative and quantitative factors in nursing. Recognizing quality patient care and nursing excellence, the program provides consumers with the ultimate benchmark to measure the quality of care that they can expect to receive. Imagine the state survey results in a facility that holds the Magnet designation.

Key Players in Long-Term Care Facilities

There are many key interdisciplinary managers in the long-term facility that contribute to the quality of care provided to the residents. Those key managers are:

- Executive Director of Nursing
- Rehabilitation Services Manager
- Health Information Manager
- Business Office Manager
- Social Services Director
- Dietary Manager
- Activity Director
- MDS Coordinator, and
- Staff Development Coordinator

This list includes all the individuals on the interdisplinary management team to provide the comprehensive care that is required in long-term care. Open, honest, and constructive communications must occur between all disciplines. The relationship between the nurse executive and the other department heads must be one of mutual respect. As mentioned before, regarding the MDS, these individuals must talk and/or have a way of communicating information with each other so the information recorded on the MDS is consistent with the medical record. Documentation of the individual disciplines is required to provide the comprehensive care to the residents who reside in our facilities.

Conclusion

The winds of change are swirling around us and it up to us to take up the challenge to "break the mold" or we will find ourselves "back in Kansas" and left behind wondering what happened.

References

American Nurses Association. *Nurse Competence in Aging.* Retrieved March 29, 2004 from www.nursingworld.org/nca/.

American Nurses Association. (2004). *Scope and Standards for Nurse Administrators.* Washington, DC: ANA.

American Nurses Association. (2001). *2001 ANA Staffing Survey.* Washington, DC: American Nurses Publishing.

Bliesmer, M., Smayling, M., Kane, R., & Shannon, I. (August 1998). The relationship between nursing staffing levels and nursing home outcomes. *Journal of Aging & Health,* 10(3), 351–372.

Credentialing Center American Nurses. (2003). *ANCC Magnet Program-Recognizing excellence in nursing services.* Retrieved March 29, 2004 from www.nursingworld.org/ancc/magnet.html.

Chenitz, C., Stone, J., Salisbury, S. (1991). *Clinical Gerontological Nursing, a Guide to Advanced Practice.* Philadelphia: W.B. Saunders Company.

Dunham-Taylor, J., & Pinczuk, J. (2006). *Health care financial management for nurse managers: Merging the heart with the dollar.* Sudbury, MA: Jones and Bartlett.

Eliopoulos, C. (1993). *Gerontological Nursing 3rd Edition,* Philadelphia: J.B. Lippincott Company.

Family Caregiver Alliance. (2001). *Selected Long-Term Care Statistics.* Retrieved March 28, 2004, from www.caregiver.org/caregiver/jsp/content_node jsp? nodeid=440.

Goldsmith, S. (1994), *Essentials of Long-Term Care Administration.* Gaithersburg, MD: Aspen.

Granger, C., Seltzer, G., Fishein, C. (1987). *Primary Care of the Functionally Disabled.* Philadelphia: J.B. Lippincott Company.

Hendrix, T., & Foreman, S. (July–August 2001). Optimal long-term care nurse staffing levels. *Nursing Economic$*, 19(4), 164–175.

Medicare, Nursing Home Compare. *Collecting and Updating Nursing Home Data.* Retrieved March 3, 2004 from www.medicare.gov/NHCompare/Static/Related/DataCollection.asp?dest==NAVHom.

Meier, E. (May–June 2000). Medicare, social security, and competitive benefits are neglected nursing issues. *Nursing Economic$*, 18(3), 168–170.

Mitty, E. (1998). *Handbook for Directors of Nursing in Long-Term Care.* New York: Delmar.

Navigating Survey and Certification Issues for Long-Term Care Facilities: What You Need to Know about Appeals, Governmental Guidance and the Future, RTP 41152X2. (May 2001). Atlanta: Health Care Practice Group at Womble Carlyle Sandridge & Rice, PLLC.

New York State Department of Health, Managed Care, *About Managed Long-Term Care.* Retrieved March 25, 2004 from www.health state.ny.us/nysdoh/mancare/mltc/.

Pear, R. (July 23, 2000). U.S. recommends strict new rules at nursing homes: Concern over staffing: Officials say patients may be endangered by shortages of both nurses and aides. *New York Times.*

Polich, C., Parker, M., Hottinger, M., Chase, D. (1993). *Managing Health Care for the Elderly.* New York: John Wiley & Sons.

Raffel, M., & Raffel, N. (1994). *The U.S. Health System: Origins and Functions,* 4th ed. New York: Delmar.

Sahyoun, N., Pratt, L., Lentzner, H., Dey, A., Robinson, K. (2001). The changing profile of nursing home residents: 1985–1997. *Aging Trends,* No. 4. Centers for Disease Control and Prevention: National Center for Health Statistics.

The Senior Alliance Area Agency on Aging 1-C. (2004). *Eden Alternative,* Retrieved March 25, 2004 from www.aaalc.org/ltc.htm.

Simms, L., Price, S., Ervin, N. (1994). The *Professional Practice of Nursing Administration, 2nd Edition.* New York: Delmar Publisher, Inc.

Tavormina C.E. (2003). Embracing the Eden Alternative in long-term care environment. *Geriatric Nursing 20*(3), 158–161.

Vladeck, B. and Department of Health and Human Services. (1996). *Testimony on Long-term Care Options: PACE and S/HMO, Before the House Ways* and *Means, Subcommittee on Health April 18, 1996.* Retrieved March 25, 2004 from www.hhs.gov/asl/testify/t960418a.html.

Helpful Websites

Agency for Health Care Policy and Research—www.ahcp.gov/
Aging—DD..listserve@uky.edu
American Nurses Association—www.ana.org
American Nurses Credentialing Center—
    www.nursingworld.org/ancc/magnet.html
Centers for Disease Control and Prevention (CDC)—www.cdc.gov/

Gerisource—www.gerisource.com/
HCFA (CMS): The Medicare and Medicaid Agency—www.hcfa.gov/
Health Information Research Unit—http://hiru.mcmaster.ca/
Long-Term Care Survey Guidance—www.thompson.com/libraries/
   healthcare/home/special_reports/homeguidance.html
Medscape—www.medscape.com/
National Health Information Center (NNIC)—http://nhic-nt.health.org/
National Institutes of Health—www.nih.gov/
National Institute of Nursing Research (NINR)—www.ninds.nih-gov/
WebMedLit—www.webmedlit.com/

Appendix
Nursing Assistant Mentor Program Curriculum

The mentoring program consists of six educational modules with the following objectives.

MODULE ONE: WHAT MAKES A MENTOR?
Mentors will:

Learn about their mentoring program;

Learn the definition of a mentor;

Understand their responsibilities as mentors;

Define the characteristics of an ideal caregiver.

MODULE TWO: MENTOR AS TEACHER
Mentors will:

Understand the characteristics of adult learners;

Discuss different learning styles;

Learn how to evaluate the learning of the new CNA;

Appreciate the value of self-evaluation.

MODULE THREE: MENTOR AS LEADER
Mentors will:

Learn the definition of leadership;

Understand two primary leadership styles;

Gain insight into their own leadership style;

Learn how to be leaders to their mentees.

MODULE FOUR: COMMUNICATION SKILLS
Mentors will:

Gain an understanding of the basic elements of communication;

Understand and learn to practice active listening skills;

Understand and learn to practice giving good feedback.

MODULE FIVE: STRESS MANAGEMENT
 Mentors will:
   Learn to identify and practice effective ways to reduce stress;
   Understand and avoid unsuccessful ways of dealing with stress;
   Learn to help their mentees cope with stress;
   Recognize and check themselves for signs of stress;
   Learn to reduce stress by managing time more effectively.

MODULE SIX: YOUR JOB AS A MENTOR
 Mentors will:
   Understand the duties and responsibilities of a mentor;
   Learn what is expected of them during the new CNA's critical "break-in" period and beyond;
   Be able to administer the evaluation forms;
   Learn about providing ongoing support to the mentee.

Source: Pillemer, K., Meador, R., Hoffman, R., & Schumacher, M. (2001). *CNA Mentoring Made Easy*, Somerville: MA: Frontline Publishing Corporation.

6

The Resident Assessment Instrument (RAI): The Minimum Data Set (MDS)

Steven B. Littlehale, MS, APRN, BC, RN

Cheryl Field, MSN, CRRN, RN

Diane L. Brown, BC, RN

The key to understanding the operation of the nursing home is a thorough knowledge of the Resident Assessment Instrument (RAI), and its core component, the Minimum Data Set (MDS). The MDS, a geriatric functional needs assessment tool, offers direct links between regulatory oversight, payment, quality monitoring, and care. Indeed, it electronically informs the federal and state survey certification process. A subset of MDS items drives all Medicare, and much of the Medicaid reimbursement, and the MDS supports all care-giving processes and outcome monitoring.

Historical Background

In 1965 the U.S. Government enacted Social Security Amendments that established the Medicare and Medicaid programs (Title 18 and Title 19, respectively). Medicare is a two-part program to help the elderly and disabled pay for their costs of health care. Medicare Part A covers most hospital, skilled nursing, and home care. Part B pays for physician services, outpatient services, diagnostic tests, laboratory services, cancer screening, home health services not covered in Part A, along with medical equipment costs. Medicaid, a cost-sharing program involving both state and federal funds, provides services for medically indigent people, including children, and for people with severe and permanent disabilities that are under age 65, and for elderly over 65 receiving welfare.[1]

Because these health care costs began to rapidly climb, the federal government entered into a prospective payment system[2] for hospitals in 1983. This system was based on a per-episode classification system called diagnosis-related groups (DRGs). Long-term care providers, however, continued to receive cost-based reimbursement (Kovner et al., 1995).

Then, in 1986, in response to reports of elder abuse and poor quality in nursing homes, the Institute of Medicine (IOM) investigated, and found, a lack of standards and wide variation in quality of care across the nursing home continuum, regardless of facility size, ownership, or location. Findings focused on the value of a uniform needs assessment tool and the need for strong Federal regulation.

This report was coupled with the 1987 General Accounting Office's (GAO) confirming report stating that nursing homes were operating under Federal minimum standards, and that nursing home conditions were variable. These reports led Congress to pass the Omnibus Budget Reconciliation Act in 1987 (OBRA 1987). One part of OBRA '87, the comprehensive Nursing Home Reform Act (P.L. 100-203), expanded the requirements for Medicare or Medicaid certification. This Act mandated the implementation of a standard and comprehensive *resident assessment system.*

The majority of states required nursing homes to implement the RAI in December 1990. Before beginning work on the development of the RAI, the Health Care Finance Administration (HCFA)[3] realized the dynamic nature of the nursing home industry, the growth of the frail elderly population, and the increasing complexity of the residents being cared for, and set forth the expectation that instrument revisions would be ongoing. As version 1.0 was intro-

---

[1]Medicare and Medicaid are further explained in the book, Dunham-Taylor and Pinczuk (2006) *Health Care Financial Management for Nurse Managers: Merging the Heart with the Dollar.*

[2]Prospective payment is where the payer determines the cost of care before the care is given, telling the provider the amount to be paid for the care.

[3]Health Care Finance Administration, now the Centers for Medicare and Medicaid Services (CMS).

duced, the Office of Research and Development, under a separate HCFA contract, authorized a demonstration project in six states to begin linking assessment to quality and reimbursement. Feedback from version 1.0, and the demonstration project, fueled the next version. Work on version 2.0 of the RAI began in 1993, and was implemented in January 1996. This version is still in use, with version 3.0 well into development and expected to be released sometime in 2006. While this date will probably be extended, the Centers for Medicare and Medicaid Services (CMS) has released several MDS v2.0 manual updates.

In 1996, uncontained and rapidly increasing costs in Post Acute Care Medicare prompted Bruce C. Vladeck, then HCFA administrator, to propose the implementation of the RUG-III case mix system to the Subcommittee on Health of the House Committee on Ways and Means. This resulted in the Balanced Budget Act of 1997 (BBA-97). Section 4432(a) of the Balanced Budget Act of 1997 (BBA-97), public law 105-33, required the implementation of a per-diem Prospective Payment System for Medicare A reimbursement in any licensed Skilled Nursing Facility (SNF) for cost reporting periods beginning on or after July 1, 1998. This new *per diem* PPS for SNFs intended to cover all costs (routine, ancillary, and capital-related) of covered SNF services furnished to beneficiaries under Medicare Part A. This single act changed the traditional cost-based system that had existed for over 40 years.

In 1998 The Resident Assessment Instrument (RAI) became the foundation of the first Prospective Payment System (PPS) in long-term care. The PPS for long-term care was based on the outcomes of a Health Care Finance Administration funded project, called The Multi-State Nursing Home Case Mix and Quality Demonstration (NHCMQD). The purpose of this project was to design, implement, and evaluate a combined Medicare and Medicaid nursing home payment and quality monitoring system that used assessment data collected in Minimum Data Sets (MDS). This case mix system, Resource Utilization Group (RUG-III), measured intensity and types of services required by the resident and grouped them into 44 payment categories.

Each category reflected similar resource use with the highest resource use correlated to the highest payment level. *Resource use* included the amount of nursing staff required to care for groups of residents over a 24-hour time period, amount and type of therapy services provided, and time allocated by patient specific activities.

The relationship of resident characteristics and resources used was analyzed to identify characteristics that were significant predictors of resource expenditure. Clinical diagnoses and conditions, activities of daily living, the amount and frequency of skilled services, staff time, and support needed to complete care were identified as predictors of resource use. These predictors served as the framework around which the RUG-III groups were defined.

Then Section 1888(e)(4) of the Social Security Act was passed, establishing the RUG-III case mix system that measures the intensity of care and the services that are required for each resident and then translates that measurement into a payment level. The total rate paid per group is a result of a calculation that looks at each RUG category and adjusts it by a geographic wage index, a weighted nursing index, a weighted therapy index, and a non-case mix component for both urban and rural locations.[4]

Under the old cost-based system, a facility could bill for three major categories of care: routine, ancillary, and capital-related costs. Routine provider charges covered those costs encountered in daily care, including the cost of a semi-private room, meals, nursing services, minor medical supplies, medical social services, psychiatric social services, and so forth. Ancillary costs covered specialized service. Examples include diagnostic tests, medications, and therapies. Capital-related costs include those costs associated with building maintenance, land fees, or equipment needs.

However, as of July 1, 1998, prospective payment (PPS) for long-term care began a four-year transition period and required facilities to manage all three types of costs under a single daily reimbursement rate. The BBA of 1997 also attempted to reduce Medicare and Medicaid payments by $100 billion over a 10-year period. This aggressive program unintentionally exceeded its savings goals by an estimated $80 to $90 billion, leaving many facilities unable to cope with the extensive changes and reduced payments.

Providers of skilled services struggled to evaluate the costs of care for their patient populations compared to the potential reimbursement under the new PPS methodology. In its development, staffing and administrative costs were incorporated for reimbursement. No provisions were made for respiratory services, durable medical supplies, specialty beds, wound supplies, medications, laboratory, and radiology costs—often the highest percentage of true cost in caring for complex medical and rehabilitative patient needs.

The Medicare Payment Advisory Commission (MedPAC) has evaluated these outliers within the present RUG-III PPS system and has documented, clearly, these uncompensated resource variables. The under-funded cost of care for certain types of patients (i.e., respiratory patients, especially those requiring IV antibiotics and isolation measures) was so expensive that facilities stopped providing those services. Those patient groups remained longer, or returned, to the acute care settings because of placement difficulties. In addition, some small nursing homes stopped participating in Skilled Medicare programs, or simply closed their doors. Several large chains filed for bankruptcy under Chapter 11, asking for time to reorganize themselves financially, and better prepare for PPS.

The full impact of PPS in long-term care took the industry by surprise. Yet, it seems probable that the MDS 2.0, or future versions of this assessment (MDS 3.0), will most likely remain the primary assessment tool, and be tightly woven into regulatory and reimbursement programs.

The Balanced Budget Act of 1997 (BBA) required the Secretary to publish the annual update to the Skilled Nursing Facility (SNF) prospective payment

---

[4]These tables can be viewed in the *Interim Final Rule* published in the Federal register Vol. 63, No. 91, May 12, 1998/ Rules and Regulations.

system (PPS) 60 days prior to the beginning of the next fiscal year (October 1) to which the rates apply. In addition, under the BBA, CMS is required to develop refinements to the RUG-III methodology.

On April 10, 2000, a Notice of Proposed Rule-Making (NPRM) (65 FR 19188) was published. It contained a proposal for the RUG-III refinements to the case-mix system for federal fiscal year 2001. These refinements allowed the case mix model to better predict the costs of medically complex patients by identifying indicators of non-therapy ancillary costs (e.g., drugs, or respiratory therapy.) A new rehabilitation sub-category that captured beneficiaries with extensive clinical needs who also required rehabilitation services was added. In addition, a separate rate component was proposed for non-therapy ancillary services.

This proposal was halted in July of 2000 because CMS failed to design a "refined" RUG system that could accurately predict the cost of providing post-acute care due to a poor validity and reliability in the data.

In January 2001 the Medicare Payment Advisory Commission (MedPAC) recommended HCFA explore a new SNF Medicare Payment System and abandon its efforts to fix the present Medicare payment system for skilled nursing facilities. The eleven-member federal advisory panel concluded that the federal agency should focus all of its attention to develop a new Medicare patient classification system to be used across all post-acute care settings. Med PAC post acute care research director, Sally Kaplan, explained, "The commissioners believe that a post acute case-mix classification system should have core elements, yet as few as possible so that it can be completed accurately and with minimal effort" (SNF Payment & Strategy Advisor).

Accuracy and time for completion of the current MDS 2.0 remain an issue. Through the Benefit Improvement and Protection Act of 2000 (BIPA), Congress required HCFA to research and study a new or revised prospective payment system and report findings to Congress by 2005. To meet this mandate, CMS contracted with the Urban Institute in July of 2001 to assist in making incremental refinements to the case mix classification and begin the study to develop a new or revised system. This move could signify a second major change in the way Medicare pays for post-acute care.

The present system, described in the following sections, is a case-mix system called Resource Utilization Group, or RUG-III. Meanwhile future revisions to the system have been mandated to improve the accuracy of predicting and matching accurate resource utilization with financial reimbursement.

The Resident Assessment Instrument (RAI)

The RAI, by design, identifies residents' strengths, weaknesses, preferences, and needs in key areas of functioning. This instrument, developed by a consortium of research centers under contract to the Centers for Medicare and Medicaid Services (CMS), provides structure and framework for care-giving staff in nursing homes to thoroughly evaluate residents. The RAI was designed to provide an accurate, standardized, comprehensive, and reproducible assessment of the resident. It consists of three main parts:

- The Minimum Data Set (MDS)—a set of assessment and screening elements, forming the backbone of the comprehensive resident assessment.

- The Resident Assessment Protocols (RAPs)—protocols for care for 18 conditions.

- And the utilization guidelines or instructions—these determine whether the care was reasonable and necessary.

The Minimum Data Set

One-hundred-eight MDS 2.0 assessment items serve to classify residents into homogenous resource utilization groups by their resource needs. The likeness of patients in one particular group was measured by the case-mix demonstration study. The SNF enters the individual MDS data into a grouper program. A grouper software program, embedded in the clinical software of each nursing home, assigns residents into one of the current 44 RUG groups, based upon coded MDS items. (See Exhibit 6-1.)

Although RUG groups are displayed in hierarchical format (Exhibit 6-1), the grouper algorithm assigns a RUG category based on an index maximizing classification for Medicare PPS. In other words, Medicare payment categories rank in order by their case mix index or CMI, not their hierarchical position or dollar value. The grouper's inclusion criteria are weighted or indexed and, therefore, mutually exclusive. The current system uses two indices: one for urban areas (A02), and one for rural areas (A01). To index-maximize, determine all RUG groups into which the resident classifies, rather than assigning the resident into the first qualifying group. When you finish, record the CMI for each of these groups and select the group with the highest CMI (Exhibit 6-1). That group is the index-maximized classification for the resident.

The MDS 2.0 contains a set of essential assessment items that identify current resident function, areas of recent decline, diseases and conditions, measures of well being, needs, and preferences. Completed MDS assessments are encoded and transmitted by each facility, in accordance with a specified timetable, to a federal data repository, establishing a basis for regulatory scrutiny.

Upon admission, the nursing home completes an assessment on every resident in order to gain a holistic picture of the resident—their strengths and weaknesses, as well as care needs. This process ultimately leads to an individualized plan of care designed to meet the identified care needs. The admission assessment must be completed by the 14th day of nursing home residency.

In addition to this first look, the law requires a "comprehensive" or complete analysis of the resident annually, and any time a significant change of status

Exhibit 6-1   RUG-III Classification Elements

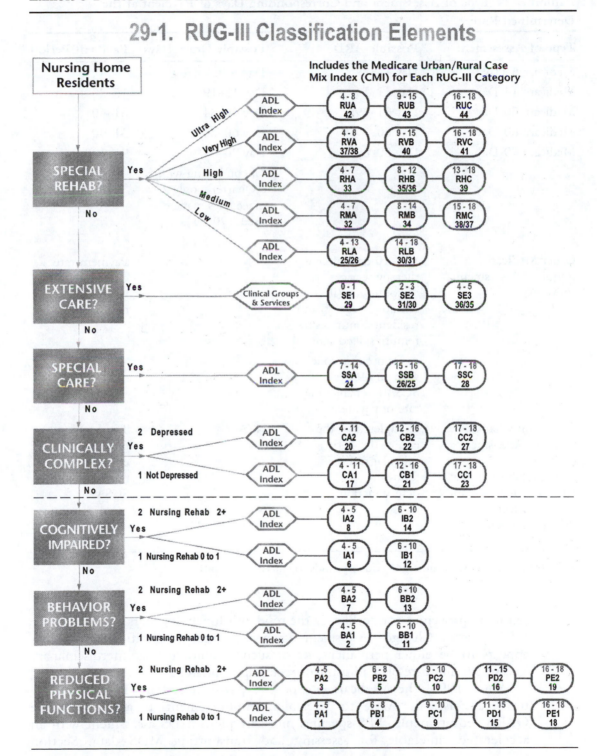

29-1. RUG-III Classification Elements

Nursing Home Residents

Includes the Medicare Urban/Rural Case Mix Index (CMI) for Each RUG-III Category

Source: 1997 Version, 44-Group Model based on work of Brant E. Fries, PhD.

Exhibit 6-2   Type of Assessment and Corresponding Days of Payment at the Determined Rate

Type of Assessment	Possible ARD	Possible Grace Days	Payment Period
Medicare 5-Day	Day 1–5	Day 6–8	1–14
Medicare 14-Day	Day 11–14	Day 15–19	15–30
Medicare 30-Day	Day 21–29	Day 30–34	31–60
Medicare 60-Day	Day 50–59	Day 60–64	61–90
Medicare 90-Day	Day 80–89	Day 90–94*	91–100
		*if combining with a Quarterly only 2 grace days may be used. (90–91).	
Other Medicare Required Assessment (OMRA)	• 8–10 days after all therapy services are discontinued (if in a Rehab Category) and resident continues to require skilled care • Or use this code with an off-cycle SCSA to change the rate of payment		Payment rate changes effective with the ARD of the OMRA.
Significant Change in Status Assessment (SCSA) Could establish a new RUG classification and remains effective until the next assessment	Completed by the end of the 14th calendar day following determination	N/A	The payment rate changes effective with the ARD of the SCSA

Adapted from: www.cms.hhs.gov/quality/mds20/rai1202ch2.pdf.

(either improvement or decline) in the resident's function occurs. Staff complete a "Significant Change" assessment when a change of condition occurs that appears to be either permanent, or of such magnitude that interdisciplinary assessment and care plan adjustment seems appropriate.

Since 1998, the Medicare prospective payment system (PPS) for long-term care uses the MDS to determine reimbursement. In addition to the OBRA requirements, PPS specifies more frequent MDS assessment with an accelerated timetable for assessing and transmitting MDS data. Section

1888(e)(6) of the Social Security Act defines the schedule of required MDS assessments and corresponding payment period for each assessment. Exhibit 6-2 displays the schedule. Because one MDS assessment establishes the daily rate of reimbursement for a specific period of time (14, 16, or 30 days), errors in data accuracy impact the appropriate RUG assignment (positively or negatively) over that time period. Assignment into an inaccurate higher RUG category (based on an inaccurate MDS assessment) may appear to be fraudulent to scrutinizing parties.

In addition to comprehensive assessment, federal regulation requires interim assessments, which vary state-by-state from a brief subset of MDS items to a full MDS. This assessment ensures the care plan accurately addresses identified resident needs. The completion of a quarterly MDS assessment followed by adjusting the resident's care plan (explained below), as needed, assures the goal is achieved. During the quarterly assessment, interdisciplinary care teams may identify a significant change in the resident's function. If so, a comprehensive assessment (full MDS assessment and Resident Assessment Protocols or "RAPs") replaces the interim assessment. Exhibit 6-3 identifies the different types of MDS assessments.

Assessment Reference Dates and Corresponding Dates for Payment

Under PPS, facility payment is determined from current functional condition, presence of diseases and conditions, and procedures received, as represented by the MDS assessment and resulting RUG. The facility receives the associated rate over a predetermined time. The MDS assessment projects patient resource use, therefore the provider is paid a rate forward in time, based on current and past data collection. Much like managed care systems that have guidelines for contracted levels and required communication, Medicare PPS determines daily rates within certain specified time parameters.

Within these time frames, the provider chooses an *assessment reference date* (ARD) within regulated guidelines. The assessment reference date is selected by the provider and all disciplines complete the MDS based on that date. The SNF transmits the completed MDS to the state, and when that MDS is accepted into the state's database, the facility may then complete and transmit a claim form (UB-92) to the Fiscal Intermediary (FI) for payment of the Medicare A beneficiary's stay. The claim form specifies the ARD, diagnoses, hospital qualifying stay, and other information necessary to process the claim.

Facilities attempt to set an ARD to capture the clinical data elements that completely describe the greatest needs of the resident, translated to the highest acuity. The selection of the ARD impacts care planning decisions as well as the SNF reimbursement system. Setting an ARD that accurately captures the clinical needs, that reflects high resource use, and that results in an accurate case mix reimbursement category are all coding goals. For example, a weak and medically complex resident with multiple co-morbidities and no current rehabilitation

Exhibit 6-3   Type of AssessmentDetermined Rate

Type of Assessment	Elements	Completion Requirements
Admission (Initial) Assessment (Comprehensive)	Full MDS and RAPs using Utilization Guidelines (referred to as comprehensive assessment)	Must be completed by the 14th day of resident's stay.
Annual Reassessment (Comprehensive)	Full MDS and RAPs using Utilization Guidelines (referred to as comprehensive assessment)	Must be completed within 366 days of the most recent comprehensive assessment.
Significant Change in Status Reassessment (Comprehensive)	Full MDS and RAPs using Utilization Guidelines (referred to as comprehensive assessment)	Must be completed by the end of the 14th calendar day following determination that a significant change has occurred.
Quarterly Assessment Medicare Post Acute Form (State-Mandated Subset or MPAF)	Subset of MDS or full MDS assessment or MPAF	Set of MDS items, specified by state (contains at least CMS established subset of MDS items). Must be completed no less frequently than once every 92 days.
Significant Correction of a Prior Full Assessment (Comprehensive)	Full MDS and RAPs using Utilization Guidelines (referred to as comprehensive assessment)	Completed no later than 14 days following determination that a significant error in a prior full assessment has occurred.
Significant Correction of a Prior Quarterly Assessment (State-Mandated Subset or MPAF)	Subset of MDS or full MDS assessment or MPAF	Completed no later than 14 days following determination that a significant error in a prior quarterly assessment has occurred.

Adapted from: www.cms.hhs.gov/quality/mds20/rai1202ch2.pdf.

needs will probably be sickest early in the admission. Selecting an early ARD accurately reflects that early high resource use and results in a higher, but accurate rate of payment. Conversely, a patient with few co-morbidities, but requiring intense therapy for a short duration would need to set the ARD to capture the therapy. The most complicated ARD selection situations are those where patients have both medical complexities and therapy needs and each situation must be considered on an individual basis.

Triggers and Resident Assessment Protocols

Some MDS items, when coded, are built-in "triggers" that automatically target problem areas which need further assessment. There are four different types of triggers: potential problems, broad screening, rehabilitation potential, and prevention. Triggered items, or a combination of triggered items, necessitate a review of a specific Resident Assessment Protocol (RAP)—a structured, problem-oriented framework for thinking about a triggered condition. RAPs provide a critical link to care planning decisions. There are 18 RAPs currently in use, though the CMS is developing additional RAPs. Each RAP contains the following: a brief summary of the triggered condition and the care goal, assessment items that suggest the need for additional assessment, and the guidelines for further assessment and care planning.

Federal guidelines require that RAPs be completed with the admission assessment, significant change assessments, significant correction assessments, and annual assessments. It is part of the comprehensive assessment. Exhibit 6-4 identifies all existing Resident Assessment Protocols.

Exhibit 6-4   Resident Assessment Protocols

RAP 1 – Delirium

RAP 2 – Cognitive Loss

RAP 3 – Visual Function

RAP 4 – Communication

RAP 5 – ADL Function/ Rehabilitation Potential

RAP 6 – Urinary Incontinence and Indwelling Catheter

RAP 7 – Psychosocial Well-being

RAP 8 – Mood State

RAP 9 – Behavioral Symptoms

RAP 10 – Activities

RAP 11 – Falls

RAP 12 – Nutritional Status

RAP 13 – Feeding Tubes

RAP 14 – Dehydration/ Fluid Maintenance

RAP 15 – Dental Care

RAP 16 – Pressure Ulcers

RAP 17 – Psychotropic Drug Use

RAP 18 – Physical Restraints

Adapted from: www.cms.hhs.gov/quality/mds20/rai1202ch4.pdf.

The Current 44 RUG-III Categories

At time of print, there are 44 resource utilization payment categories (see Exhibit 6-1). There are seven major categories that are based on clinical characteristics and functional abilities. After being assigned into a major category, additional parameters such as functional abilities (Activities of Daily Living—ADLs), clinical signs of depression, restorative nursing, and level of main category resource intensity, can be split into several subcategories. The final category is the resident's RUG group. The major categories are underlined in Exhibit 6-5.

Determination of Facility-Specific Per Diem Rates

The actual dollar amount paid to each facility per RUG group varies based on the geographic location of the facility. Health Insurance Prospective Payment System (HIPPS) Codes are used on the UB-92 (or SNF bill) to indicate the rate of payment. The HIPPS code is a five-digit alphanumeric code where the first three digits represent the RUG classification from the MDS and the last two digits represent the type of assessment. Each HIPPS code links to the revenue code 0022 on the SNF bill. The system multiplies the rate of payment by the number of days (units) associated with the HIPPS code during the specified period. The standard system then sums the amount payable for each HIPPS code and determines the proper reimbursement.

President Clinton signed additional legislation that increased reimbursement to Medicare Part A and Medicare Part B spending. In 1999, the Balanced Budget Refinement Act (BBRA) added a temporary four percent increase to all RUG categories and an additional 20 percent to 15 selected RUG categories. CMS sought to revise the RUG-III system that would address the higher medical acuities and ancillary costs experienced by the facility. On July 31, 2000, the Health Care Financing Administration published a final rule in the *Federal Register* (65 FR 46770), continuing the temporary rate increases for another year after a failed revision of RUG-III.

In December 2000, Congress passed the State Children's Health Insurance Program (SCHIP) Benefits Improvement and Protection Act of 2000 (BIPA 2000), which mandated adjustments to the SNF PPS rates effective from April 1, 2001 through September 30, 2002. These adjustments increased the nursing component of the rate calculation by 16.66%, retained the 4% add-on, dropped the 20% add-on to the three rehabilitation rates, but then increased all rehabilitation rates by 6.7%. A Program Memorandum, A-01-08, highlighting these changes was published on January 16, 2001. On average, this legislation increased providers' Medicare reimbursement by more than $44.00 per patient per day (www.cms.hhs.gov/providers/snfpps/snfpps_rates.asp).

Exhibit 6-5   Seven Major RUG-III Classification Groups

Major RUG Group	Split	End-Split	Characteristics Associated with Major RUG-III Group
Rehabilitation	5 subcategories based on # of minutes, disciplines	ADL Index	Residents receiving physical, speech, or occupational therapy
Extensive Services	ADL Index (minimum)	Clinical Indicators	Residents receiving complex clinical care or with complex clinical needs such as IV feeding or medications, suctioning, tracheostomy care, ventilator/respirator, and co-morbidities that make that resident eligible for other RUG categories.
Special Care	ADL Index	Clinical Indicators	Residents receiving complex clinical care or with serious medical conditions such as multiple sclerosis, quadriplegia, cerebral palsy, respiratory therapy, ulcers, stage III or IV pressure ulcers, radiation, surgical wounds or open lesions, tube feeding and aphasia, fever with dehydration, pneumonia, vomiting, weight loss, or tube feeding.
Clinically Complex	ADL Index	Depression Indicators	Residents receiving complex clinical care or with conditions requiring skilled nursing management and interventions for conditions and treatments such as burns, coma, septicemia, pneumonia, foot/wounds, internal bleeding, dehydration, tube feeding, oxygen, transfusions, hemiplegia, chemo-therapy, dialysis, physician visits/order changes.
Impaired Cognition	ADL Index	CPS, Nursing Rehab	Residents having cognitive impairment in decision-making, recall and short-term memory. (Score on MDS 2.0 cognitive performance scale >=3.)
Behavior Problems	ADL Index	Nursing Rehab	Residents displaying behavior such as wandering, verbally or physically abusive or socially inappropriate, or who experience hallucinations or delusions.
Reduced Physical Function	ADL Index	Nursing Rehab	Residents whose needs are primarily for activities of daily living and general supervision.

Adapted from: www.cms.hhs.gov/quality/mds20/rai1202ch6.pdf.

Fiscal year 2003 saw two temporary rate add-ons (16.66% increase in the nursing component and the 6.7% increase in rehabilitation rates) "cliff" or "discontinue," even though CMS did not refine the RUG system to better account for higher acuities and costly ancillary services. The temporary 4 percent across the board add-on and 20 percent add-on to the three major medically complex categories remain in effect at the present time.

During that time frame CMS sought to reevaluate the RUG system, and to submit a new plan for Medicare reimbursement along the post-acute continuum. To reach that goal, several groups proposed additional studies. Then CMS awarded a contract to the Urban Institute as described previously.

Inpatient Rehabilitation Post-Payment System

The Minimum Data Set for Post Acute Providers (MDS-PAC) was the data set originally proposed to be used in *Independent Freestanding Rehabilitation facilities* and *long-term care located within acute hospitals*. The implementation date of this tool remains undetermined. Instead, the tool mandated for use by the inpatient rehabilitation facilities is the Inpatient Rehabilitation Form—Patient Assessment Instrument (IRF-PAI). The IRF PPS was effective for cost reporting periods beginning on or after January 1, 2002. Payments under the IRF PPS are made on a per discharge basis.

A patient classification system is used to classify patients in IRFs into case-mix groups (CMGs). The IRF PPS uses Federal prospective payment rates across distinct CMGs. A majority of the CMGs are constructed using rehabilitation impairment categories (RICs), functional status (both motor and cognitive), and age (though in some cases, cognitive status and age may not be a factor in defining a CMG). Special CMGs account for very short stays, and for patients who expire in the IRF. Each CMG accounts for a patient's clinical characteristics and expected resource needs.

Development of MDS 3.0—Original Timeline 2005

As of this printing, CMS has announced revised goals for the development of the MDS 3.0, but has not set a new implementation date. CMS intends to:

- Update clinical relevance of the instrument,

- Improve ease of use,

- Use standard scales language,

- Increase resident voice, and

- Create electronic health record (EHR) completion.

Many factors have delayed the original timeline for the development and implementation of the updated version, including funding for expanded validation work, stakeholder and industry requests to ensure coordination with new payment system, and new government initiatives and partners. For example, the President's e-Gov initiative includes the Consolidated Health Informatics (CHI) Initiative. The goal is to work in sync with the health industry to adopt CHI standards that enable inter-operability in federal health care enterprise. This applies to the following agencies: HHS, VA, and DoD, and requires clear, unambiguous data that can be encoded as well as data that can be sent through electronic messaging.

CMS has contracted with RAND Health and Harvard University to evaluate MDS 3.0. At the end of this five-phase project, the evaluation team expects to improve MDS content and utility, improve wording and instructions, identify problems and offer solutions, review results, and identify need for additional care planning tools. They will also evaluate item performance, validity, and the impact on functions.

The Care Plan

OBRA '87 requires that every nursing home resident have a comprehensive plan of care. This care plan is tailored by the MDS assessment process and, therefore, unique to the resident. Federal guidelines require that care plans include measurable objectives to meet the resident's needs as identified by the MDS and RAPs. The care plan must help the resident attain or maintain the highest practicable physical, mental, and psychosocial well-being, regardless of level of impairment. To ensure accuracy and effectiveness using a dynamic clinical model, the MDS, RAPs, and Care Plan link in an ongoing process of evaluation of needs, planning of care, delivery of care, and reassessment.

Utilization Review

Medical review criteria instruct reviewers to determine if care was reasonable and necessary, as well as supported by documentation. Initially, under the new system, medical reviewers were also instructed, by Program Memorandum A-99-20, to assign the patient into one of the top 26 RUG-III categories. This would meet the Medicare skilled criteria, and thus reduce the burden of utilization review.

However, the physician's order for skilled care (certification and recertification) was (and is) still a requirement. Those categories (shown above the dotted line in Exhibit 6-1) were presumed Medicare skilled, and any resident grouped into these categories was considered skilled throughout the reimbursement period identified by the specific type of assessment.

This status was updated in March 2000 in Program Memorandum A-00-08, which narrowed the "deemed" status concept to apply to the number of days between admission, and the Assessment Reference Date (ARD) to the first (5-day) MDS. In other words, when a facility completes an MDS resulting in a prospective rate of payment for 14 days, the *presumption* of skilled care applies only to *some*, but not all, of those 14 days. The patient's skilled needs must be ordered and documented as defined by the guidelines in the Medicare CMS Online Publication 100, and the Level of Care requirements as defined in 42 CFR 409.31.

It was hoped that the MDS and RUG-III system alone would fulfill the skilled needs utilization review (UR) process, thereby offering efficiency to a burdensome system. This goal was not achieved.

Key Elements for Accurate Assessment

Despite the fact that many nursing home operations are driven by MDS assessment, the MDS has been implemented with varying success. Anecdotally at best, clinicians view the RAI as an excellent clinical tool that brings the interdisciplinary care team together to focus on the resident's needs; at worst, it is seen as an egregious violation of the Paperwork Reduction Act. This wide range of reactions can be understood by examining how clinicians first learned about the MDS, the attitudes of the people who taught them (though education was often absent), and the way the RAI was supported (or not supported) in their facility. Initial educational and operational barriers, high staff turnover in today's marketplace, and financial viability demand a "back to basics" approach to ensure adherence to the utilization guidelines.

Turning to the *User's Manual for MDS 2.0* provides the structure for accurate assessment, as summarized in Exhibit 6-6. The key to understanding the RAI process, and successfully using it, is in believing that its structure is designed to enhance resident care and to promote the quality of a resident's life. This success occurs not only because it follows an *interdisciplinary* problem-solving model but also because

Exhibit 6-6   Key Elements for Accurate Assessment

- Interdisciplinary involvement in MDS/RAP assessment and care plan process
- 24 hour caregiver input into assessment
- Initial and ongoing education in MDS/RAP assessment
- Ongoing internal and external audits for MDS accuracy
- Access to most current manuals
- Internet access for CMS updates and industry support

Source: User's Manual for MDS 2.0.

staff, across all shifts, are involved in its "hands-on" approach. Thus, the process flows smoothly from one component to the next and allows for good communication and uncomplicated tracking of resident care (*v2.0 User's Manual MDS 2.0*).

Reliability and Validity of the MDS v2.0

While few would argue the value of systematic assessment of nursing home residents, concerns regarding the reliability and validity of the MDS continue to proliferate despite the substantial improvements made when the instrument was revised (v2.0). Numerous systematic studies support the reliability and validity of the MDS assessment instrument, and numerous evaluative studies support the idea that the RAI is responsible for key improvements in several process and outcome quality areas.

However, reliability and validity in systematic studies is not the same as reliability and validity in routine clinical use. Simply put, clinicians who receive training in the MDS (usually at the facility's cost) and follow the utilization guidelines tend to achieve high reliabilities. Any compromise to the education and implementation process weakens reliability and clinical meaningfulness of the RAI. Researchers, including some federal agencies and clinicians, who deviate from the proscribed RAI assessment process report lower reliabilities than those that follow the guidelines.

The Consequences of Inaccurate Assessment

As stated, the MDS is central to nursing home reimbursement, to survey and certification status, and to the measurement of quality (Quality Indicators and Quality Measures). Most clinicians and industry experts can readily identify which MDS items are the driving forces in the clinical, regulatory, and financial algorithms; however, the primary purpose of the RAI is missed when one's focus is solely on these items.

When the focus remains solely here, false positives and false negatives in the evaluation of quality go unnoticed, and valuable resources are inappropriately expended to deal with false improvement opportunities. Provided care isn't fairly reimbursed under the Prospective Payment System (PPS) because MDS inaccuracies frequently classify residents into lower paying groups.

At the same time, cases of fraud are unwittingly created because residents are placed into higher payment groups due to misunderstandings in the MDS assessment process. Sadly, true opportunities for clinical improvement are missed as the interdisciplinary team responds to the realities of working in one of the most regulated industries.

Congress began debate, in 2001, for global Medicare reform and the search for a more equitable payment system for nursing homes. Reliability and integrity of the next reimbursement system depend on accurate clinical data collection with management tools that will distinguish poor assessment from fraud and abuse. Research and analysis of nursing home data, based on poor coding practices, offer skewed results.

One way to ensure accuracy of MDS data is through data integrity audits. Data integrity is the completeness, logical consistency, and clinical and statistical reasonableness of MDS data. For example, integrity would be questioned if a resident was reported to have diabetic retinopathy yet no diagnosis of diabetes. The MDS contains over 500 assessment items that describe the resident. Because the assessment is a holistic assessment, functional areas should complement each other.

To gain quantitative insight into the magnitude of the issue, an analysis of data integrity was completed by LTCQ, Inc. of Lexington, Massachusetts. This analysis used 250,000 MDS assessments conducted at more than 150 nursing homes in fifteen states between January 1999 and June 2000. More than 200 tests of data integrity were applied to this data set.

The pie chart in Exhibit 6-7 illustrates that 68 percent of analyzed MDS records contained at least one data integrity issue. Of the 68 percent, there was an average of 2.7 data integrity issues per assessment, meaning that if an MDS assessment had errors, it was likely to have more than one. This is shown in the bar chart, which quantifies the number of assessments with multiple issues. This analysis was again repeated in 2003 using a nursing home sample size of 1,000. The same results were demonstrated.

Exhibit 6-7   Number of MDS Data Integrity Issues Found in 250,000 MDSs

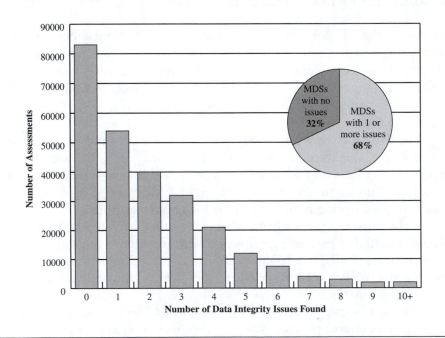

Source: LTCQ, Inc. Q-Metrics Data Integrity Audit Provider Service Database.

Data integrity issues impact care planning, financial reimbursement, and the evaluation of quality. These outcomes are woven into the RAI process quality indicators (QI), quality measures (QM), and prospective payment system (PPS). The impact of one error is demonstrated by the following example.

Most residents with short-term memory impairment would not be expected to have totally intact decision-making skills, since many daily decisions require a person to refer to recent information or experience to make a rational choice of what to do. Most completed MDS assessments support this relationship, however, some do not. MDS assessments submitted from facilities to the right of the line on the graph in Exhibit 6-8 accurately reflect the relationship between short-term memory and decision-making skills. Facilities to the left of the line missed the relationship.

The consequence of not understanding this relationship affects care planning when the resident with early cognitive impairment is not adequately cared for and opportunities for preventing further decline are missed. Improper assessment of these items affects the quality indicators when residents who are high risk for functional decline due to cognitive impairment are inaccurately classified as low risk. Furthermore, and of financial significance, an appropriate classification of a resident into the Cognitively Impaired RUG-III group may not occur when a valid relationship between short-term memory and decision-making ability is not noted by the assessment team. This results in a lower paying RUG-III group.

Exhibit 6-8   Short-Term Memory Impairment with Impaired Decision-Making Skills

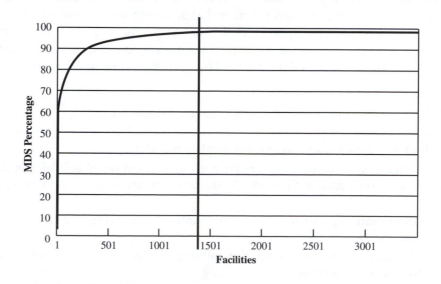

Source: LTCQ, Inc. Q-Metrics Provider Service Database.

Implications for Nurse Administrators

Nurse administrators play a critical role in the overall financial success of SNF units. Communication, timely and accurate completion of the MDS, and effective interdisciplinary team function are integral components of the RAI system that the nurse administrator controls. The nurse administrator should consider the core objectives shown in Exhibit 6-9 for successful PPS management, and determine his/her role in managing and improving the systems needed to meet these objectives.

Any analysis of the unit operations should consider the RUG groups the unit-specific population will most probably fall into. Specialty units (i.e., wound care units) can expect a high rate of clinically complex, or special care, RUG scores. A unit that has many orthopedic patients should expect a high percentage of rehabilitation RUG scores. Knowing the daily RUG rates and occupancy projections can help predict unit revenue. These predictions can then be considered against the cost of providing care to specific populations of patients.

Strategies for PPS Operations Management

Finding strategies to balance the business operations of the unit with the clinical needs of the populations it serves is the greatest challenge for health care leaders. Health care is a business, and the individuals that it serves should be sheltered from this fact as much as possible, and treated as if they were the only patients on your unit. What a challenge this sets forth!

To achieve success, nurse administrators must see their many roles contained in a middle management position. These roles generally include advocate, leader, educator, mentor, and team member. Nurse administrators are asked to advocate for a number of "customers." Their nursing license requires that they act as a patient advocate at all times, while their position as administrator requires that they advocate for the needs of their staff. Their position as team member(s) on a man-

Exhibit 6-9 Strategies for Successful PPS Nursing Management

- Ensure all staff understand and accurately complete the MDS.
- Establish formal communication patterns for both written and verbal information sharing. This needs to be formalized both within the nursing staff, and between interdisciplinary departments.
- Assure MDS software is performing accurately, hardware is available, and staff has adequate computer training.
- Consider Medicare a managed care product and train staff to communicate with the nurse manager just like a case manager.
- Provide ongoing education and ensure compliance with policies and procedures.
- Review and establish per diem contracted rates with vendors to reduce costs, and educate staff of these cost-saving approaches.

agement team requires that they advocate for the needs of the nursing department, and the facility as a whole. Their role as educator means that they advocate for the needs of compliance, competency, and future program development. Balancing the components of the advocacy role alone, on a daily basis, yet being able to make decisions that result in smooth unit management, is an amazing challenge![5]

Get Smart with ARD Dates!

One strategy administrators can implement involves the assessment reference dates (ARD). Current law allows some flexibility in setting these dates. This flexibility allows the facility to select the date which yields the highest paying RUG group (and therefore, captures the resident's highest acuity), ultimately being sensitive to the patient's need for service and clinical fragility upon admission. Attention to patient-specific details will give the nurse administrator all the information needed to help establish the "best" assessment reference date. The date chosen should accurately reflect the patients needs and yield the highest RUG rate for the facility. The most advantageous date may be when most nurses are not scheduled to work, or may occur when the least number of admissions are predicted. In this role the nurse administrator must educate and support staff, and help them to understand the need to adjust other facets of their caseload to assure timely and accurate completion of the MDS, based on an assessment reference date (ARD) which yields the best reimbursement.

Put Expectations in Writing

It is important that all team members understand and support the mission of the unit. All team members have an active role in achieving that mission. The nurse administrator needs to articulate the model for completing the MDS. This model may be either interdisciplinary or multidisciplinary. The *interdisciplinary* model directs members of the interdisciplinary team to complete sections of the MDS prior to a team review of every item. All clinicians provide input to all sections of the assessment. In a *multidisciplinary* model, clinicians complete their assigned sections, and review the care plan together. Instead of each team member reviewing all sections, one person, usually the RN Assessment Coordinator, reviews the assessment for completeness and cohesion of assessment. Whichever model is practiced the process needs to be observed, supported, and reinforced by the nurse manager.

Policies that state how work will be shared are important to have in writing. All team members need clear direction in their roles. When new policies are written, even seasoned staff must learn new ways to accomplish the work. Nursing units tend to "grow" their own set of informal rules, which are carefully planted

---

[5]You will find additional excellent information that will help to achieve this goal in Dunham-Taylor and Pinczuk (2006) *Health Care Financial Management for Nurse Managers: Merging the Heart with the Dollar.*

in the minds of new employees and cultivated for many years in the history book titled, "*Because we have always done it this way*," by "Ms. This is how we do things." Prospective payment management is new; it requires a new attitude for "doing things," and requires written support to sustain the needed changes.

Check and Change Documentation Systems

Consider all the documentation completed in a 24-hour day and look at the pieces that are repeated, across all disciplines. Nursing leaders need to reduce and streamline the documentation demands placed on the staff whenever possible. The MDS 2.0, RAPs, and Utilization Guidelines demand specific information from every member of the Interdisciplinary team.

Using documentation forms that follow the coding definitions set forth by the Utilization Guidelines will reduce error, improve MDS accuracy, and decrease documentation time. Daily narrative notes should focus on the skilled needs of the patient and their functional, medical, and emotional response to treatments aimed at meeting those needs.

Often the contents of a RAP summary are the same information needed to support billing of skilled services. Teaching documentation efficiency can reduce the time needed for RAP summaries, as the author of the RAP can simply refer the reader to the daily note that contains the supporting information for both skilled services and the RAP.

For example, a resident who is admitted with a pressure ulcer should have a detailed assessment of the wound, and should summarize interventions to treat and prevent further skin breakdown. This information might be contained in an admission assessment and the initial care plan, or in the narrative notes. Either way, if done well, this work can be referred to when completing the Pressure Ulcer RAP.

Communication

The nurse administrator is an integral player involved in interdisciplinary communication. Interdisciplinary team members need to interact and communicate on a daily basis to assure patient related information is both shared, and considered, on the MDS. An accurate interdisciplinary care plan then results. In SNF settings, communication is a team challenge. Team members will look to the nurse administrator to role model, support, and reinforce patterns of open, honest communication between departments.

Communication is a key function of effective team performance. How the team functions in daily interaction, shared meeting space, family education, determining rehabilitation intensity goals, and so forth should be an essential component to the nurse administrator's role, and will determine the success of the prospective payment model. All team players need to know the plan of the rehabilitation department, and the rehabilitation department needs to know the plan for medical management.

Interdisciplinary Team (IDT) Function

It is when the team functions *together* for the patient that they are most successful. This teamwork enhances the best of every member on the health care team. Coordinating this level of involvement is challenging, and requires a dedication to the idea that interdisciplinary team function impacts patient outcomes, and when the team functions well, patients benefit. Conversely when the interdisciplinary team functions poorly, patient care is negatively impacted.

Conclusion

It is essential for the long-term care nurse administrator to both have a thorough knowledge of the Resident Assessment Instrument (RAI), and to communicate this effectively with staff. This needs to be linked with effective interdisciplinary teamwork on a daily basis.

References

Descriptive Documentation Is Key to Proper Reimbursement. October, 2000. *PPS Alert for Long-Term Care,* Vol. 3 (10).

Dunham-Taylor, J., & Pinczuk, J. (2006). *Health care financial management for nurse managers: Merging the heart with the dollar.* Sudbury, MA: Jones and Bartlett.

Frost, B., in *Legislative Issues Related to Postacute Care* in Nathenson, P., Ed. (1999) *Integrating Rehabilitation and Restorative Nursing Concepts into the MDS.* Association of Rehabilitation Nurses. Health Care Financing Administration Federal Register. July 31, 2000.

Kovner, A.R., Jonas, S., Banta, H.D., Kovner, C., Salsberg, E., Richardson, H., & Brecher, C. (1995). *Jonas health care delivery in the United States.* New York: Springer Publishing.

Models of excellence: Providers share their strategies for success under PPS. November–December 2000. *Subacute Care Today,* Vol. 3(4)

SNF Payment & Strategy Advisor. February 1, 2001. Vol. 14(3).

Vladeck, B.C. (1996). *Medicare payment for home health agency and skilled nursing facility services: Statement before Subcommittee on Health, House Committee on Ways and Means.* Available at www.cms.hhs.gov/scripts.

Revised Long-Term Care Resident Assessment Instrument User's Manual, version 2.0. December 2002. Available at www.cms.hhs.gov/medicaid/mds20/default.asp.

www.cms.hhs.gov and www.cms.hhs.gov/medlearn/matters offer a wide variety of publications and resource information on this topic and are recommended for site surfing.

7

An Interdisciplinary Approach to the MDS

Amy M. Cripps, MSN, BSN, RN

Within the world of the prospective payment system (PPS), Medicare is the primary source of facility reimbursement, especially in long-term care. In this setting, Medicare reimburses based on results of assessments required during a patient's stay. These assessments reveal specific services that the organization provides. This chapter addresses the ways that Medicare assessments are tracked, completed, and used as indicators that produce reimbursement rates. Additionally, this chapter addresses the connection between these assessments and the patient's individualized care plan.

Brief History

In 1997, Congress passed the Balanced Budget Act in an attempt to control federal health care spending. A major component of the federal budget is Medicare. Medicare is Title XVIII of the Social Security Act and is also known as "Health Insurance for the Aged and Disabled." Approximately 95 percent of the elderly population in the United States is covered by Medicare (Baker and Baker, 2000, p. 25). Before the Balanced Budget Act was passed, skilled nursing facilities (SNF) were paid for costs allocated and incurred during a patient's stay at the facility. The ruling to change to a prospective payment system was given by the Health Care Financing Administration (HCFA) (Hawryluk, 1998c). HCFA has since changed its name to the Centers for Medicare and Medicaid Services (CMS).

Under PPS, skilled nursing facilities are paid a specific per diem rate based on patient acuity and services provided. Since the change in payment method has taken place, skilled nursing facilities have been cautiously accepting high acuity patients because they risk losing money. Some providers say that prospective payment system (PPS) rates are inadequate for more medically complex patients. When high acuity patients are admitted to skilled nursing facilities, the key to receiving proper payment is efficiency. "Inefficiency will be penalized with a loss" (Fisher, 1998b). According to Wagner (1999), PPS is the "ultimate intersection for cost efficiency and quality." She also states that the three key objectives of providers under PPS are enhanced clinical review, effective cost containment through utilization review, and close consultation among all staff members involved in patient care. PPS was put into effect in July 1998. A study conducted by the American Health Care Association (AHCA) revealed that between the first quarter of 1998 and the first quarter of 1999, the Medicare per diem payment dropped 15 percent, approximately 50 dollars per day (1999).

Overview of the Minimum Data Set

Medicare reimburses facilities participating in prospective payment system (PPS) programs only when assessments are done at specific times during the stay of the Medicare patients. These assessments provide indicators that allow for different reimbursement rates, and must be done during distinct times throughout the patient's stay as well as cover distinct days of a patient's stay (see Exhibit 7-1). If the assessments are not done during these times, the facility may receive a default rate of payment instead of the full payment that it is entitled to receive. Medicare has identified specific services as being eligible for reimbursement. Therapy (physical, occupational, or speech) is the highest reimbursable skill under Medicare guidelines.

When a patient enters a skilled nursing facility, Medicare typically covers all or part of the first 100 days of the patient's stay. Medicare pays 100 percent of the first 20 days and continues to pay a large portion of incurred patient expenses for the next 80 days. Facilities must perform assessments, known as Minimum Data Sets (MDS), to give an overall picture of the patient (see chapter appendix). The MDS is "a core set of screening, clinical, and functional status elements, including common definitions and coding categories that form the foundation of the comprehensive assessment for all residents of long-term

Exhibit 7-1   Medicare Required Assessments

Medicare Required Assessment	Assessment Window (including grace days)	Payment Period
5-day assessment	Days 1–5 (6–8)	Days 1–14
14-day assessment	Days 11–14 (15–19)	Days 15–30
30-day assessment	Days 21–29 (30–34)	Days 31–60
60-day assessment	Days 51–59 (60–64)	Days 61–90
90-day assessment	Days 81–89 (90–94)	Days 91–100

From: www.cms.hss.gov/quality/mds20/rai1202ch2.pdf on pages 2–27. Retrieved on 1/28/05.

care facilities certified to participate in Medicare" (Lovvorn, 1998, pp. 1–4). MDSs are required at specific times throughout the first 100 days of a patient's stay when covered by Medicare.

Five different assessments are required. They are: 5-day assessment, 14-day assessment, 30-day assessment, 60-day assessment, and 90-day assessment. These assessments each have a certain number of days in which to be completed. In addition, each assessment has "grace days" that provide an extension for completion. Each assessment completed provides a code that Medicare uses when reimbursing skilled nursing facilities. Each assessment covers specific days of the patient's stay. Exhibit 7-1 identifies each assessment, the assessment window (including grace days), and the payment period.

As shown in Exhibit 7-1, the first assessment is referred to as the 5-day assessment, even though the assessment window is days one through day eight. After the assessment is completed, a code is provided that corresponds to a reimbursement rate. This per diem rate covers days 1 through 14 for the 5-day assessment, as shown in the chart. If an assessment is not done within the correct time period, Medicare will pay a default rate of reimbursement, instead of the payment that the skilled nursing facility is entitled to receive (Harris, 1998). Assessments can include any information from the seven days prior to and including the assessment date. These seven days are referred to as the assessment reference period, or ARP. The more complex the patient's care during the ARP, the higher the reimbursement rate will likely be. The MDS also serves to provide data that measures quality of care and to "improve clinical practice guidelines" (Fisher, 1998a). The connection to quality indicators will be discussed later in this chapter.

Skillable Services

In order to be covered under Medicare, patients must require what providers call "skillable services." Long-term skilled nursing facilities usually admit new Medicare patients with an order for some type of therapy. Therapy can include one or more of the following: physical therapy, occupational therapy, and/or speech therapy. Therapy is the skillable service that provides the highest reimbursement rates. Other services may be provided in addition to therapies or may be provided as a stand-alone skillable service.

There are seven broad categories of services that consist of criteria that a patient must meet in order to be included in those categories. The seven categories are rehabilitation, extensive services, special care, clinically complex, impaired cognition, behavior problems, and reduced physical function (Harris, 1998). Only placement in the first four of these seven categories guarantees Medicare reimbursement. Assignment in the category of impaired cognition, behavior problems, or physical function may or may not result in reimbursement depending on the need for daily skilled nursing care.

Any patient receiving a certain amount of therapy will fall under the rehabilitation category. Other skillable services will fall under different categories. These seven categories correspond to different reimbursement levels (see Exhibit 7-2). Examples of other skillable services under Medicare include tube feeding, tracheostomy care, intravenous medications or feedings, suctioning, ventilator or respirator needs, certain types of wound care, and sliding scale insulin injections. The complexity and cost of the care provided determines which of the seven categories a service belongs to and will therefore determine the reimbursement rate. Failure to include reference to any skillable service on the MDS may result in a decreased reimbursement rate.

As stated before, reimbursement is given on a per diem basis that is effective for each day throughout the remainder of the current assessment period (Hawryluk, 1998a). If skillable services are erroneously left out of the MDS, the payment will be decreased for every day remaining in the assessment period.

The MDS coordinator, who is a registered nurse, typically attests to the completion of the assessments. The information that is included within an MDS comes primarily from the staff members who care for the patient and the documentation in the patient's chart. Documentation is extremely important and provides an accurate picture of the patient's health status at a specific point in time. Information to be included in the assessments may come from any area of the patient's chart, including, but not limited to, activities, medication administration record (MAR), nurses' notes, dietary, rehabilitation, social services, and physician progress notes and orders (Shephard, 2001). For example, the MDS coordinator can only reference injections in an assessment if injections are addressed within the patient's record, most likely on the MAR.

The MDS also requires that changes in a patient's bed mobility, eating, transferring, toileting, and cognitive status be addressed (Hoffman, 1999). If the patient's record fails to show these changes, the MDS coordinator may fail to include them on the MDS. Aside from inadequate documentation, improper payment could also be a result of medical unnecessity, noncovered services, or outright Medicare fraud (Hawryluk, 1998b).

Exhibit 7-2   Clinically Complex Categories

Special Rehabilitation

Ultra high	720 minutes of therapy per week At least 2 types of therapy 1 therapy = 5 days per week 1 therapy = 3 days per week
Very high	500 minutes of therapy per week At least 1 type of therapy = 5 days per week
High	325 minutes of therapy per week At least 1 type of therapy = 5 days per week
Medium	150 minutes of therapy per week At least 1 type of therapy = 5 days per week
Low	45 minutes of therapy per week 1 therapy = 3 days per week in addition to 2 areas of nursing rehabilitation/restorative care = 6 days per week for 15 minutes each

Extensive Services

ADL score =/> 7 and 1 or more of the following services:

In the last 7 days:

- Parenteral/IV feeding

In the last 14 days:

- Suctioning
- Tracheostomy
- Ventilator/respirator
- IV medications

Special Care

ADL score =/> 7 and 1 or more of the following services:

- Fever with vomiting, weight loss, pneumonia, dehydration, or tube feeding
- Pressure ulcers–stage 3 or 4 *or* 2 or more sites at any stage
- Tube feeding and aphasia
- Respiratory therapy 7 days per week
- Surgical wounds with treatment
- Open lesions with treatment
- Radiation therapy
- Cerebral Palsy with ADL score =/> 10
- Multiple Sclerosis with ADL score =/> 10
- Quadriplegia with ADL score =/> 10

Exhibit 7-2   Clinically Complex Categories *(continued)*

Clinically Complex

1 or more of the following:

In the last 7 days:

- Dialysis
- Dehydration
- Internal bleeding
- Pneumonia
- Chemotherapy
- Oxygen use
- Burns
- Coma
- Septicemia
- Tube feeding
- Transfusions
- Foot wounds with treatment
- Hemiplegia with ADL score =/> 10
- Diabetes with 7 days injections & MD order changes =/> 2

In the last 14 days:

- MD visits =/> 1 and order changes =/> 4 or
- MD visits =/> 2 and order changes =/> 2

Impaired Cognition

Cognitive Performance Score of =/> 3:

- Short term memory loss
- Daily decision making impaired
- Making self understood
- Dependence with eating

Behavior

1 behavior =/> 4 times per week:

- Inappropriate behavior
- Physical abuse
- Verbal abuse
- Wandering
- Resists care

in addition to hallucinations or delusions.

Reduced Physical Function

Patients who do not meet the criteria of any other group

(No clinical variables used)

Data from: www.cms.hhs.gov/quality/mds20/rai1202ch6.pdf.Retrieved on 1/28/05.

For the MDS to be accurate, it is vital that all disciplines involved in a patient's care be actively involved in the completion of the MDS. Typically, each department head is responsible for gathering information and completing specific sections of the MDS. For example, the dietician may be responsible for completing information regarding any weight changes, as well as other pertinent information such as tube feeding and the patient's caloric intake and requirements. The recreation coordinator is typically responsible for inclusion of involvement in activities and other related information. A member of the social services team plays a vital role in MDS completion because a significant amount of information revolves around mood, behavior, cognition, and other psychosocial factors. The MDS coordinator usually completes the remaining sections related to communication, vision, physical functioning, continence, disease diagnoses, current health conditions, skin conditions, medications, and any other special treatments or procedures.

Each person who completes any portion of the MDS must sign the document to certify the accuracy of the section or sections completed by that person. Clinical disagreement among members of the MDS team does not constitute fraud. Instead, this interdisciplinary effort results in the most accurate representation of the patient's condition, and allows for both proper reimbursement and better patient care. The completion of the MDS may seem very subjective at times. For this reason, it is extremely important that patient documentation is thorough and accurate. Additionally, this information provides the general public with standards of patient care based on comparison of different long-term care facilities.

Specifics of Resource Utilization Groups

Until now, each level of reimbursement has been referred to generically. Each reimbursement level is actually referred to as a Resource Utilization Group, or RUG level. A higher RUG level corresponds to a higher use of resources by the skilled nursing facility, and therefore results in a greater reimbursement level. After an assessment is completed, a patient will fall into one of the 44 RUG levels. Therapy results in a higher RUG level. Skillable services without therapy result in lower RUG levels (see Exhibit 7-3). A patient's ability to perform his or her own activities of daily living (ADLs) also contributes to the RUG level (Harris, 1998). ADLs consist of activities such as bathing, toileting, dressing, and personal hygiene. If a patient requires extensive assistance with ADLs, more time is required of the nursing staff, which is why ADL dependency increases RUG levels. A combination of extensive ADL assistance and a high level of therapy results in the highest RUG levels possible.

As previously discussed, skillable services fall into one of seven categories. Each of these categories can be further divided into different levels related to a patient's ADL dependence. Currently, four specific ADLs are taken into account when calculating RUG levels. These are bed mobility, toileting, transfer, and eating. Patients are scored from zero to four for each specific ADL based on the

Exhibit 7-3 Pre-Admission RUG-III Screening Worksheet

Pre-Admission RUG-III Screening Worksheet

Resident Name			Date of Birth	Sex	Hospital		Hospital Admission Date
Hospital Phone		Medicare Days Used				SNF Days Used	
Primary Diagnosis						DRG	
Completed on:		Potential Admission Date:				Completed by:	

Instructions: Using information gathered from the client's clinical record, complete Sections 1 through 4 in sequence. Once the client's assessment indicates a "YES" answer in a section, then skip to Section 5-Functional Physical Performance. As indicated, specify the location in the resident's clinical record where supporting documentation can be found.

Section 1-Special Rehabilitation (If total number of therapy minutes <45 min. skip to Section 2)

During the first 7-day period in the facility, the client will have received:	Circle Y/N
720 minutes or more (total) of therapy per week in at least two disciplines, one for at least 5 days, AND a second for at least 3 days **(Ultra High Intensity) or**	Y / N
500 minutes or more (total) of therapy per week in at least one discipline for at least 5 days **(Very High Intensity) or**	Y / N
325 minutes or more of therapy in at least one discipline for at least 5 days **(High Intensity)** or If this is a Medicare 5 day or Readmission/Return Assessment, then the following may apply: In the last 7 days the client received 65 minutes or more of therapy AND In the first 15 days from admission 520 minutes or more of therapy is expected with Rehabilitation services expected on 8 or more days.	Y / N
150 or more minutes or more of therapy in any combination of the 3 disciplines for at least 3 days **(Medium Intensity)** or If this is a Medicare 5 day or Readmission/Return Assessment, then the following may apply: In the first 15 days from admission 240 minutes or more of therapy is expected with Rehabilitation services expected on 8 or more days.	Y / N
45 or more minutes or more of therapy in any combination of the 3 disciplines for at least 3 days **(Low Intensity)** and 2 or more nursing rehabilitation services for at least 15 minutes each with each administered 6 or more days, **or If this is a Medicare 5 day or Readmission/Return Assessment, then the following may apply:** In the first 15 days from admission 75 minutes or more of therapy is expected with Rehabilitation services expected on 5 or more days; 2 or more nursing rehabilitation services received for at least 15 minutes each with each	Y / N

* Nursing Rehabilitation includes:
- Passive or active range of motion (P3a,b);
- Amputation/prosthesis care (P3i);
- Splint or brace assistance (P3c);
- Dressing or grooming training (p3g);
- Eating or swallowing training (P3h)
- Bed mobility or walking training (p3d,f);
- Transfer training (p3e);
- Communication training (P3j);
- Any scheduled toileting program or bladder retraining program (H3a, b)

If **YES** is indicated in this section, the client's case mix category is probably **Special Rehabilitation**

Section 2-Extensive Services (If ADL Score <7, skip to Section 3)

Client must have an ADL Score of > 7			Circle Y/N
In the 7-day period ending with the Assessment Reference date, did the client receive: Parenteral / IV feedings (K5a)			Y / N

In the 14-day period ending with the Assessment Reference date, did the client receive:	Last Date	Location of Re-	Circle Y/N
IV Medication (does not include fluids without medication) (P1ac)			Y / N
Suctioning (P1ai)			Y / N
Tracheostomy Care (P1aj)			Y / N
Ventilator or Respiratory Treatment (P1al)			Y / N

To determine specific "Extensive Care" RUG Grouper (i.e. SE1, SE2, SE3) assign one (1) point for the following:
- Parenteral / IV feeding (K5a)
- IV Medication (P1ac)
- Criteria met in "Special Care" section (max of 1 pt)
- Criteria met in "Clinically Complex" section (max of 1 pt)
- If client meets the criteria of being cognitively impaired (refer to Cognitive Performance Scale)

If **YES** is indicated in this section, the client's case mix category is probably **Extensive Services**

Assessment Reference Date: This date refers to the specific endpoint in the MDS assessment process. The date sets the designated endpoint of the common observation period, and all MDS items refer back in time from this point

Proposed ARD (MM/DD/YY):

Section 3-Special Care

Does the client currently have one of the following with an ADL score of at least 7:	Circle Y/N
Multiple Sclerosis and ADL > 10 (I1w)	Y / N
Quadriplegia and ADL > 10 (I1z)	Y / N
Cerebral Palsy and ADL > 10 (I1s)	Y / N

During the 1st 7-day period in the facility, the client will have/received treatment for:	Circle Y/N
Ulcers (pressure or stasis) 2= sites over all stages with 2 or more skin treatments (M1a, M1b, M1c, M1d, M5a, M5b, M5c, M5d, M5e, M5g, M5h)	Y / N
Any Stage III or IV pressure ulcer with 2 or more skin treatments (M2a, M5a, M5b, M5c, M5d, M5e, M5g, M5h)	Y / N
Surgical wounds or open lesions with skin treatments (M4c, M4g, M5f, M5g, M5h)	Y / N
Fever (j1h) with one or more: - Tube Fed* (K5b, K6a, K6b) - Vomiting (J1o) - Dehydration (J1c) - Pneumonia (I2e) - Weight Loss (K3a)	Y / N
Tube Feeding* (K5b) and Aphasia (I1r)	Y / N
Respiratory therapy for 7 days in the facility (P1bda)	Y / N

In the 14-day period ending with the Assessment Reference Date, did the client receive:	Last Date	Location of Record	Circle Y/N
Radiation therapy (P1ah) or implant			Y / N
Meets criteria in Extensive Services, but has ADL score < 6, then client classifies Special Care (SSA).			Y / N

If YES is indicated in this section, the client's case mix category is probably **Special Care**

Section 4- Clinically Complex

Does the client currently have :	Circle Y/ N
Comatose condition (B1) and not awake (N1) and completely ADL dependent	Y / N
Hemiplegia/Hemiparesis (I1v) and ADL > 10	Y / N
Pneumonia (I2e)	Y / N
Septicemia (I2g)	Y / N
Diabetes Mellitus (i1a) and injections for 7 days (o3) and at least 2 days with MD order changes (P8)	Y / N

In the 14-day period ending with the Assessment Reference Date, did the client receive:	Last Date	Location of Record	Circle Y/ N
Chemotherapy (P1aa)			Y / N
Dialysis (P1ab)			Y / N
Oxygen Therapy (P1ag)			Y / N
Transfusions (P1ak)			Y / N

During the last 14-day period (or since admission if less than 14 days ago) did the client receive :	Circle Y/ N
At least 4 MD order changes (P8) and 1 or more visit (P7)	Y / N
At least 2 MD order changes (P8) and at least 2 visits (P7)	Y / N

During the 1st 7-day period in the facility, the client will have/received treatment for:	
Dehydration (J1c)	Y / N
Internal Bleeding (J1l)	Y / N
Tube Feeding* (K5b)	Y / N
Burns (2nd or 3rd degree) MM4b	Y / N
Infection of foot (M6b) or open lesions on foot (M6c) and application of dressing foot (M6f)	Y / N
Meets criteria in Special Care but has an ADL Score < 6.	Y / N

If YES is indicated in this section, the client's case mix category is probably **Clinically Complex**

*Tube Feeding Note: Tube feeding calories > 51% (K6a) or tube feeding with total calories > 26% (K6a) and fluid parenteral or enteral intake of > 501cc/day (K6b) in the last 7 days

Exhibit 7-3   Pre-Admission RUG-III Screening Worksheet *(continued)*

Section 5- ADL FUNCTIONAL PERFORMANCE ASSESSMENT

INSTRUCTIONS: 1. Complete this section to ESTIMATE THE ADL SCORE VALUE for RUGS Code ESTIMATION only.
2. Estimation is based on ADL functional self-performance **during** the hospital stay.
NOTE: An ADL Score > 7 is required for a client to be placed in Extensive Services

ADL SCORING

G.1.a. BED MOBILITY		
How client moves to and from lying position, turns side to side, and positions body while in bed.	Supervision or Independent	1
	Limited Assist	3
	Extensive Assist	4
	Dependent	5
	Estimated Score	

G.1.b. TRANSFER		
How client moves to and from lying position, turns side to side, and positions body while in bed.	Supervision or Independent	1
	Limited Assist	3
	Extensive Assist	4
	Dependent	5
	Estimated Score	

G.1.h. EATING		
How client eats and drinks (regardless of skill). Includes intake of nourishment by other means (e.g., tube feeding, total parenteral nutrition)	Supervision or Independent	1
	Limited Assist	2
	Dependent or Extensive Assist	3
	Estimated Score	

G.1.i. TOILET USE		
How client uses the toilet room (or commode, bedpan, urinal); transfers on/off toilet, cleanses, changes pad, manages ostomy or catheter, adjusts clothes.	Supervision or Independent	1
	Limited Assist	3
	Extensive Assist	4
	Dependent	5
	Estimated Score	

Estimated Pre-Admission ADL Value

ADL SELF-PERFORMANCE GUIDE:

INDEPENDENT   - No help or oversight

SUPERVISION   - Oversight, encouragement or cueing provided

LIMITED ASSIST   - Client highly involved in activity; received physical help in guided maneuvering of limbs or other non-weight
bearing assistance

EXTENSIVE ASSIST - While client performed part of activity, help of the following type(s) were provided:

** Weight Bearing Support

** Full Staff Performance

DEPENDENT   - Full Staff Performance of Activity

Continue to Next page for RUG Classification

Exhibit 7-3 Pre-Admission RUG-III Screening Worksheet *(continued)*

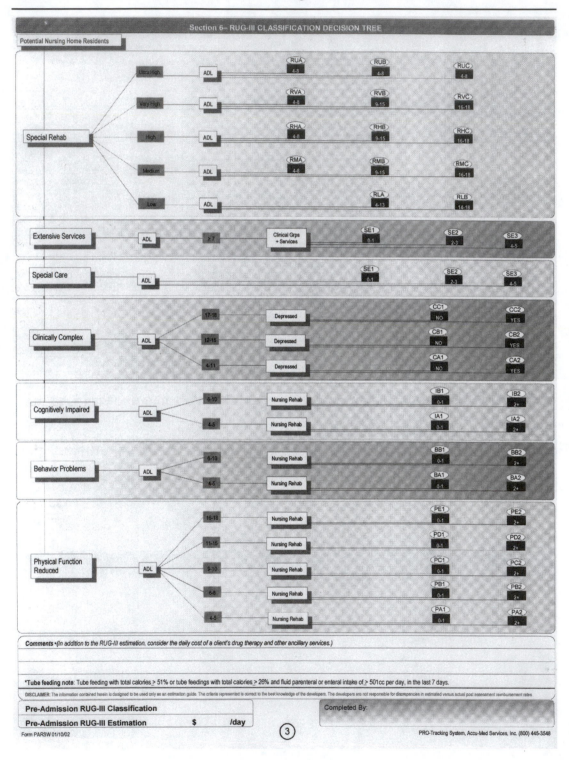

patient's ability to independently perform these ADLs. These scores are assigned as follows:

0—Independent performance.
1—Supervised performance.
2—Limited assistance.
3—Extensive assistance.
4—Total assistance.

These scores are typically assigned by certified nursing technicians or the nurses assigned to each patient. After the ADL scores for each of the four areas are totaled, they are used to calculate the RUG level for each particular assessment. Typically, the software program that is used to enter the MDS data automatically calculates the RUG level after the assessment is completed. For more information on manually calculating ADL scores, please refer to the CMS website at www.cms.gov.

The seven categories, along with their corresponding RUG levels, may be found in Exhibit 7-3. The first of these categories is called *special rehabilitation* and typically includes any type of therapy or combination of therapies provided (physical, occupational, and/or speech). The special rehabilitation category can be further broken down into subcategories. These are as follows: ultra high, very high, high, medium, and low. These subcategories are determined by the number of minutes and days that a patient receives therapy, as well as the number of therapy services provided during the assessment reference period.

- "Ultra high" consists of at least two types of therapy for a total of 720 or more minutes. One of these types must be delivered at least five days weekly and the other must be provided at least three days.

- "Very high" consists of 500 or more minutes of at least one type of therapy for five or more days during the ARP.

- "High" consists of 325 or more minutes of at least one type of therapy for five or more days during the ARP.

- "Medium" consists of 150 or more minutes provided five days by one type of therapy or five days of therapy across three disciplines.

- "Low" consists of 45 minutes of therapy for three days per week in addition to two areas of nursing restorative care for six days at a minimum of 15 minutes per area each day (www.cms.hhs.gov/quality/mds20/rai1202ch6.pdf).

The next broad category is called *extensive services*. A patient's ADL score must be at least seven to fall into this grouping. This category contains specific treatments that a patient may have recently received. These treatments include parenteral or intravenous (IV) feedings in the past seven days, or any of the following in the past 14 days: suctioning, tracheostomy care, ventilator or respirator requirements, or IV medications. Any one or more of these treatments combined with an ADL score of seven or greater automatically places a patient into the *extensive services* category. These treatments may have been received before admission to the long-term care facility. However, to be captured in the MDS, the transferring facility must provide sufficient documentation and the information must remain on the patient's permanent medical record. This is but one example of the importance of documentation related to completion of the MDS.

The next category is referred to as *special care*. A patient must have an ADL score of seven or greater in addition to having specified diagnoses or receiving specific treatments. Some of the treatments include the following: tube feeding in addition to the presence of aphasia, surgical wound treatments, open lesion treatments, radiation therapy, or respiratory therapy seven day per week. Some of the diagnoses or conditions that place a patient in this category include certain stages of pressure ulcers; fever with accompanying symptoms such as vomiting, weight loss, pneumonia, or dehydration; cerebral palsy, multiple sclerosis, or quadriplegia. These last three diagnoses must be in addition to an ADL score of at least ten.

The *clinically complex* category contains a number of conditions or treatments that may qualify a patient for this level of reimbursement. Some of these include dialysis, dehydration, pneumonia, chemotherapy, burns, septicemia, transfusions, and oxygen therapy. Please refer to Exhibit 7-3 for a complete list (Williams, 2003). A patient may have any ADL score and remain eligible for reimbursement at this level. The clinically complex category uses what is referred to as an *end-split*. If a patient exhibits at least three signs and/or symptoms of depression as listed in section E1 on the MDS, in addition to the previously mentioned conditions, the patient is classified as "depressed" and receives a slightly higher rate of reimbursement.

An eligible patient who is placed in any of the previous categories automatically receives Medicare reimbursement. The remaining three categories may or may not result in reimbursement, based on documentation and individual review. The fifth category is known as *impaired cognition* and primarily revolves around the presence of some type of cognitive deficit. Some of the conditions that may place a patient in this category include short term memory loss, impaired daily decision making, inability to make self understood, and dependence with eating.

The next category is *behavior*. For a patient to fall into this category, either hallucinations or delusions must accompany other specific behaviors. These include such behaviors as inappropriate behavior, physical or verbal abuse, wandering, and resisting care. It should be noted that a patient who is cognitively able to refuse care based on an informed decision should not be coded as being resistant to care.

The final category is referred to as *reduced physical function*. Residents who do not meet the criteria of any other group may fall into this category because the resident still needs assistance with ADLs at any level. No clinical variables are used as requirements for placement in this category. These last three categories— impaired cognition, behavior, and reduced physical function—also use an end-split, referred to as nursing rehabilitation. If at least two or more areas of nursing restorative care are provided for six days per week and at least 15 minutes per day, the end-split results in a slightly higher rate of reimbursement.

Note that the conditions given as requirements for these categories do not constitute an exhaustive list and should not be used to calculate RUG scores for individual patients. Please refer to the CMS website or contact your local fiscal intermediary for updates or changes related to reimbursement requirements. It is important to remember that regardless of what level of care a patient receives, reimbursement is not possible without extensive documentation of that care.

Other Medicare-Required Assessments

Along with the required assessments previously discussed, an additional assessment should be completed when a patient stops receiving in-patient therapy, but continues to be skilled for a different service. This assessment is referred to as an "Other Medicare Required Assessment," or OMRA. If this assessment is missed, the resulting loss could be devastating to the facility. In this section, the OMRA is analyzed for its fiscal worth within the PPS and the monetary losses that could occur if the OMRA is incomplete or not completed at all.

As stated before, a RUG level obtained from an assessment is applied to the remaining days of the assessment period. If a high RUG level is produced due to therapy, that RUG level is applicable to each day following until the next assessment is due. One exception to this rule is if a patient stops receiving therapy, but continues to receive other skillable services under Medicare, an additional assessment is required. Therapy (physical, occupation, or speech) is the highest reimbursable skill under Medicare.

When a patient stops receiving therapy but continues to be covered under Medicare, an OMRA assessment is required to decrease the reimbursement level at which Medicare makes payment. If this particular assessment is missed, the results could be a loss of thousands of dollars. Because therapy contributes to the highest RUG levels, Medicare views the reimbursement as being excessive if therapy is discontinued.

The OMRA assessment must be done eight to ten days after therapy is discontinued so that no amount of therapy is reflected in the new assessment or the new RUG level. Additionally, if therapy remains in the current physician orders, but a patient does not participate in therapy for ten or more days, the OMRA must be completed. The ten days may or may not include weekends. For example, if a patient participates in therapy on a Friday, is sick Monday through Friday of the next week, and refuses on Monday of the next week, the total of ten days without therapy requires an OMRA to be completed. At this point, communication is vital. The MDS coordinator must complete the OMRA so the facility does not simply receive Medicare's default reimbursement rate.

When the OMRA is completed, a new RUG level is obtained, which gives a lower reimbursement level. In the example just given, when the patient continues participating in therapy, the required assistance and acuity of the patient once again increase, yet the new RUG level is set until the next assessment is due. In the case in which therapy continues, but the patient does not participate, the MDS coordinator may not know until day ten that an OMRA is required and is due to be completed. If an OMRA is not done as required, Medicare pays out a default rate of reimbursement. For this reason communication is very important.

To avoid default payment in lieu of a higher RUG level resulting from a required OMRA, communication must be effective and ongoing among the MDS coordinator, rehabilitation coordinator, director of nursing, and social work director. Level-of-care meetings should be held at least weekly to discuss progress in therapy, refusals, last day of therapy for a patient, and skillable services other than therapy. Upon admission, information regarding a patient's skillable services should be given to the MDS coordinator. He/she should also verify completion of the therapy evaluation with the rehabilitation coordinator so that the maximum number of therapy days and minutes can be included in the initial MDS. A daily exchange of e-mails or other type of routine communication between the MDS coordinator and the rehabilitation coordinator can easily accomplish this. The MDS coordinator should verify therapy days and minutes before the assessment is locked and transmitted to the fiscal intermediary for approval. This is done by having the rehabilitation coordinator review original therapy records and compare days and minutes to the MDS assessment information.

Case Study

To combine all of the information regarding assessments, RUG levels, default payments, and ADLs, examples with numbers inserted are given to provide a clearer understanding of how Medicare PPS works in long-term care skilled nursing facilities. (Please refer to Exhibit 7-4 for RUG levels and payment rates at the time of this printing.)

Example 1. A patient is admitted to a skilled nursing facility on January 1. After learning that the patient will be receiving physical therapy, occupational therapy, and speech therapy, the MDS coordinator e-mails the rehabilitation coordinator to verify that the therapy evaluation has been completed. When setting the assessment date, the maximum number of therapy days and minutes should be taken into account. With the admission date (January 1) being day one, the assessment date is set for January 7 so that the seven prior days of therapy are included. The patient also requires extensive assistance with all of his ADLs. For the five-day assessment, a RUG level of RUC is obtained, which provides a $457.51 per diem rate of reimbursement. As noted in Exhibit 7-1, the five-day assessment covers the first fourteen days and would, therefore, provide a gross revenue of $6,405.14 for the first two weeks of this patient's stay.

Exhibit 7-4   RUG Levels with Reimbursement Rates

RUG Category	Nursing Component	Therapy Component	Non-case mix Component	Total Per Diem Reimbursement Rate
RUC	$168.99	$227.90	$60.62	$457.51
RUB	**$123.49**	**$227.90**	**$60.62**	**$412.01**
RUA	$101.39	$227.90	$60.62	$389.91
RVC	**$146.89**	**$142.82**	**$60.62**	**$350.33**
RVB	$135.19	$142.82	$60.62	$338.63
RVA	**$105.29**	**$142.82**	**$60.62**	**$308.73**
RHC	$163.79	$95.21	$60.62	$319.62
RHB	**$137.79**	**$95.21**	**$60.62**	**$293.62**
RHA	$113.09	$95.21	$60.62	$268.92
RMC	**$175.49**	**$77.99**	**$60.62**	**$314.10**
RMB	$141.69	$77.99	$60.62	$280.30
RMA	**$124.79**	**$77.99**	**$60.62**	**$263.40**
RLB	$144.29	$43.55	$60.62	$248.46
RLA	**$103.99**	**$43.55**	**$60.62**	**$208.16**
SE3	$220.98		$72.98	$293.96
SE2	**$180.69**		**$72.98**	**$253.67**
SE1	$152.09		$72.98	$225.07
SSC	**$146.89**		**$72.98**	**$219.87**
SSB	$136.49		$72.98	$209.47
SSA	**$131.29**		**$72.98**	**$204.27**
CC2	$145.59		$72.98	$218.57
CC1	**$128.69**		**$72.98**	**$201.67**
CB2	$118.29		$72.98	$191.27
CB1	**$109.19**		**$72.98**	**$182.17**
CA2	$107.89		$72.98	$180.87
CA1	**$97.49**		**$72.98**	**$170.47**
IB2	$89.69		$72.98	$162.67
IB1	**$87.09**		**$72.98**	**$160.07**
IA2	$74.09		$72.98	$147.07
IA1	**$68.89**		**$72.98**	**$141.87**
BB2	$88.39		$72.98	$161.37
BB1	**$84.49**		**$72.98**	**$157.47**
BA2	$72.79		$72.98	$145.77
BA1	**$62.40**		**$72.98**	**$135.38**
PE2	$102.69		$72.98	$175.67
PE1	**$100.09**		**$72.98**	**$173.07**
PD2	$93.59		$72.98	$166.57
PD1	**$90.99**		**$72.98**	**$163.97**
PC2	$84.49		$72.98	$157.47
PC1	**$83.19**		**$72.98**	**$156.17**
PB2	$66.29		$72.98	$139.27
PB1	**$65.00**		**$72.98**	**$137.98**
PA2	$63.70		$72.98	$136.68
PA1	**$59.80**		**$72.98**	**$132.78**

(www.cms.hhs.gov/providers/snfpps/snfpps_rates.asp)

Example 2. When the 14-day assessment is due, speech therapy has discontinued, and the number of minutes of occupational therapy provided has decreased. Physical therapy continues as before. The RUG level to cover days 15 through 30 is RVB, or $338.63 per day. The total reimbursement for this assessment period is $5,418.08.

Example 3. When the 30-day assessment is completed (which can be done any day from days 21–29), occupational therapy has been discontinued, and physical therapy continues at a lower level; this produces a RUG level of RHB, or $293.62 per day. This is a total of $8,808.60 for this assessment period.

Example 4. On day 27 of the patient's stay, all therapies are discontinued. This particular patient receives tube feeding and therefore continues to be coded as skilled under Medicare. An OMRA is required between days 35 and 37 (eight to ten days after therapy is discontinued). In this case, the OMRA is completed on day 35 with a resulting SE3 RUG level, which is $293.96 per day. The total reimbursement for the remainder of the assessment period is $7,642.96.

For a patient with a high reimbursement rate covered by Medicare, what would be the facility's lost revenue if a required OMRA was executed late or not at all? The answer to this question seems to be quite simple at first glance, but as it has been shown, Medicare PPS is a very difficult concept which requires in-depth discussion and explanation in order to even begin in answering the posed question. Let's continue with this example to determine lost revenue due to a missed or incomplete OMRA.

Example 5. Lost revenue is a simple calculation of the difference between what the RUG level should be and the default rate of payment. In this example, the correct RUG level, as stated in *example four*, is SE3, for a total reimbursement of $7,642.96. During the week that therapy is discontinued for this patient, the level-of-care meeting has been cancelled due to inservice scheduling. The MDS coordinator is unaware that an OMRA is required to change the reimbursement level. Instead of receiving a payment of $293.96 per diem, the skilled nursing facility receives a default payment of $132.78 per diem for the remaining of the assessment period because of the missed OMRA. This results in a $3,452.28 total reimbursement, which is a difference of $4,190.68, or almost 55 percent.

Net revenue is expressed as gross revenue minus revenue deductions. Exhibit 7-5 displays the numbers pertaining to net revenue for the previous example. Because net revenue is actual revenue for the facility, it is easy to see, even without knowing costs, how contribution margin and operating income may be affected. The negative impact is increased if more than a bare minimum of required OMRAs are not completed in a timely manner or if they are not completed at all.

Resident Assessment Instrument

The Resident Assessment Instrument (RAI) is the process of using information gathered in patient assessment to individualize care for these patients. The RAI

Exhibit 7-5   Revenue Loss Related to Other Medicare-Required Assessment (OMRA)

	OMRA completed	OMRA not completed
Gross Revenue	$7,642.96	$7,642.96
Revenue Deductions	0	(4,190.68)
Net Revenue	$7,642.96	$3,452.28

involves completion of the patient assessment, resident assessment protocols, and the patient care plan. Each of these segments of the RAI will be further discussed in this section.

Minimum Data Set

In addition to the Medicare-required MDS, each state regulates the completion of assessments that often coincide with the Medicare MDS. The purpose of these assessments is to provide a method to individualize and compare patient care. A full state assessment must be completed annually for every long-term care patient. In addition, quarterly assessments must also be completed for each patient. A quarterly assessment is a slightly shorter version of the full state assessment. Many software programs combine the MDS and state assessments so that they may be completed simultaneously, if they are due at the same time. If a patient exhibits a major change, an additional assessment is required. This change may either be an improvement or a decline and is referred to as a *Significant Change of Status* (COS).

A COS is a full, comprehensive assessment that addresses changes which affect a patient's quality of life. As stated before, these changes may constitute either an improvement or a decline in the patient's condition. A COS is defined as "a major change in the resident's status that is not self-limiting, impacts on more than one area of the resident's health status, and requires interdisciplinary review or revision of the care plan" (Lovvorn, 1998). The COS meets a facility's continuing responsibility to provide quality of care and quality of life for its patients. A COS can be completed at any time during the patient's set schedule of state required assessments.

A full assessment is also referred to as a *comprehensive assessment*. A comprehensive assessment involves all aspects of the RAI, including completion of the resident assessment protocols and formulation of a patient care plan. Quarterly assessments merely necessitate a review of the existing patient care plan. Because a COS should involve a change in overall holistic patient care, it is based on a comprehensive assessment, and therefore requires a completion of the RAI, resulting in a new patient care plan.

Resident Assessment Protocols

Information from the comprehensive assessment may trigger certain areas of focus to identify in the patient's plan of care. These areas are known as resident assessment protocols (RAPS). For example, a patient who receives psychotropic medications or has a history of wandering may be at an increased risk for falls. A patient who has peripheral vascular disease or is incontinent may be at increased risk for developing pressure ulcers. The information gathered for the assessment reveals specific areas in which a patient may require intervention to maintain or improve quality of life. The RAPS are then used to create a patient's individualized plan of care. A total of 18 different RAPS are used to guide the creation of the patient's care plan. Please refer to Exhibit 7-6 for a complete list.

Plan of Care

A patient's plan of care (POC) is a document that reveals patient problems, goals, and interventions to meet those established goals. A single POC may contain sev-

Exhibit 7-6   Resident Assessment Protocol (RAPS) Summary

1. Delirium
2. Cognitive loss
3. Visual function
4. Communication
5. ADL functional/rehabilitation potential
6. Urinary incontinence and indwelling catheter
7. Psychosocial well-being
8. Mood state
9. Behavioral symptoms
10. Activities
11. Falls
12. Nutritional status
13. Feeding tubes
14. Dehydration/fluid maintenance
15. Dental care
16. Pressure ulcers
17. Psychotropic drug use
18. Physical restraints

From: www.cms.hhs.gov/quality/mds20/rai1202ch4.pdf, p. 4–14. Retrieved 1/28/05.

eral patient problems identified through the RAI process. In the example given above, a patient's POC may reveal that a patient is at risk for falls related to psychotropic medication use, history of wandering, and episodes of dizziness as evidenced by a history of falls resulting in injury. The goal for this patient may be that the patient will remain free from injury due to falls. The POC lists interventions the facility uses to reach established goals. For this specific problem, interventions may include a pharmacy review of all medications, including side effects and interactions, placing the patient on a secured unit of the facility, and investigating possible causes of dizziness. The interventions are the specific point at which the POC becomes individualized. If the patient has a history of falls at home due to an unstable walker, the POC should address removing, repairing, or replacing the walker. In short, the RAI is the use of the patient assessment to identify patient problems and establish interventions to improve a patient's quality of life.

Connection to Quality Indicators

All long-term care facilities are subject to state surveys that revolve around patient care, conditions, and outcomes. During the survey process, the facility is required to provide a roster of current patients. This roster represents a "snapshot" of patient conditions. These conditions are taken from the patients' most recent MDSs. A few of the established conditions, or quality indicators, are:

- New fractures,
- Prevalence of falls,
- Symptoms of depression,
- Use of nine or more medications,
- Incontinence,
- Indwelling catheter,
- Weight loss,
- Physical restraints, and/or
- Prevalence of little or no activity.

This is a brief list of the quality indicators that exist. In addition, three additional indicators represent a sentinel health event. These are prevalence of fecal impaction, dehydration, or pressure ulcers. A sentinel health event provides enough concern that a further investigation may be warranted.

It is easy to see how the information that is entered into the MDS can be used during the survey process. The importance of the quality indicators revolves around proper patient care and documentation. The process may resemble the following scenario.

A surveyor notes that a patient has a pressure ulcer (a trigger), reported on the patient's last MDS. The surveyor then reviews any documentation pertaining to the care of that condition. This may include progress notes by nurses and doctors, treatment records, and the patient's care plan. If the surveyor finds documentation that reveals different treatment methods, communication with family members and physician, patient education, proper nutritional requirements, and appropriate and diligent skin care, it is quite possible that a further investigation will not be pursued. On the other hand, if a patient has a trigger such as weight loss during the last MDS period, yet no documentation is present that addresses the situation or circumstances, the surveyor will likely be prompted to further investigate other similar situations.

Avoiding Fraud

Because the MDS serves various purposes within an organization, it is vital that the information contained within it is accurate. The primary purpose of the MDS is to provide a basis for reimbursement. With any method of billing comes the risk of inaccuracy, which may result in accusations of purposeful fraudulence. To avoid these allegations of fraud, it is imperative that the MDS coordinator remains aware of the patient's true status, as well as the documentation occurring about that patient's care at all times. The MDS team members must actively communicate with patients and/or staff members continuously and do so at a level that makes him or her trustworthy. Otherwise staff members may feel that the MDS team members have ulterior motives for looking for deficiencies in documentation. In addition, if the team members do not have established relationships with patients, it may be extremely difficulty to obtain necessary information from them pertaining to the MDS.

Documentation is a fundamental source of reference for the MDS. All supporting documentation for the MDS should be available and easily accessible. Any daily documentation tool, such as an ADL worksheet, must be filled out completely to avoid fraudulent claims. Changes in the patient's overall status, as well as onset and resolution of isolated clinical conditions, should be addressed in the permanent record. Because therapy services provide a significant source of reimbursement, it is vital that the therapy logs are consistent with days and minutes recorded on the MDS.

The MDS team members should perform routine and consistent chart audits to ensure proper documentation and consequential billing. It may be within the MDS coordinator's role to provide inservices to the staff regarding proper documentation techniques. In addition to correct documentation within the patient's record, it is essential that this record corresponds to the patient's care plan and that this care plan addresses the needs that are evident within the record. When possible, the patient and/or family should be involved in the care planning process.

Conclusion

The MDS is a multipurpose tool used primarily by long-term care facilities. It provides a concise overview of a patient at any given point in time. The MDS and its associated documentation can be used not only for reimbursement purposes, but also for review of patient care. The first priority of health care providers should be the proper and effective care of the patient. If this care is appropriately provided, the patient benefits. If this care is appropriately documented and used, the organization will have the added advantage of reaping the rewards that accompany the principle of putting the patient first.

References

American Health Care Association. (1999, June). *The muse study.* Washington, DC: AHCA.

Baker, J. J., & Baker, R. W. (2000). *Health care finance: Basic tools for nonfinancial managers.* Gaithersburg, MD: Aspen.

Dodson, V. (2001a, November). RUG tree. Presented at the annual regional meeting of the National Healthcare Corporation, Murfreesboro, TN.

Dodson, V. (2001b, November). Sample of MDS. Presented at the annual regional meeting of the National Healthcare Corporation, Murfreesboro, TN.

Fisher, C. (1998a, March). Linking payment and quality. *Provider,* 16–23.

Fisher, C. (1998b, August). Subacute providers seek safe landing under PPS. *Provider,* 28–40.

Harris, C. J. (1998, July). RUGS: A new bridge to payment. *Provider,* 27–31.

Hawryluk, M. (1998a, June). Details improve view of consolidated billing. *Provider,* 23–24.

Hawryluk, M. (1998b, June). Medicare audit finds $20 billion in improper claims. *Provider,* 10.

Hawryluk, M. (1998c, June). PPS, consolidated billing rule out. *Provider,* 9.

Hoffman, R. (1999, May). Growing pains on the front line: Implementing PPS. *Provider,* 24–30.

Klitch, B. A., & Mowris, S. V. (1999). The RUG-III & MDS connection: Interdisciplinary handbook. Des Moines, IA: Briggs Corporation.

Lovvorn, B. (Ed.). (1998). *Resident assessment instrument user guide: MDS version.* Albertsville, AL: W.H. Heaton.

Shephard, R. (2001, October). MDS documentation guide. Presented at the meeting of the American Association of Nurse Assessment Coordinators, Pittsburgh, PA.

Skilled nursing facility prospective payment system. (n.d.). Retrieved November 4, 2001 from http://www.hcfa.gov/medicare/snfppsuprate.htm.

Wagner, L. (1999, February). Managing medications under PPS. *Provider,* 24–35.

Williams, K. (2003, May). Improving MDS skills and performance. Presentation of Cross Country seminar, Nashville, TN.

Resources

CMS (formerly HCFA)
www.cms.gov

Office of Inspector General (OIG)
Department of Health and Human Services
www.dhhs.gov/progorg/oig

Briggs Corporation
www.BriggsCorp.com
1-800-247-2343

American Association of Nurse Assessment Coordinators
www.aanac.org
303-758-7647

Appendix

Minimum Data Set (MDS)–Version 2.0

Numeric Identifier_____

MINIMUM DATA SET (MDS) — *VERSION 2.0*
FOR NURSING HOME RESIDENT ASSESSMENT AND CARE SCREENING

BASIC ASSESSMENT TRACKING FORM

SECTION AA. IDENTIFICATION INFORMATION

1.	RESIDENT NAME⊕				
		a. (First)	b. (Middle Initial)	c. (Last)	d. (Jr/Sr)
2.	GENDER⊕	1. Male	2. Female		
3.	BIRTHDATE⊕	Month — Day — Year			
4.	RACE/⊕ ETHNICITY	1. American Indian/Alaskan Native 2. Asian/Pacific Islander 3. Black, not of Hispanic origin	4. Hispanic 5. White, not of Hispanic origin		
5.	SOCIAL SECURITY⊕ AND MEDICARE NUMBERS⊕ [C in 1st box if non med. no.]	a. Social Security Number __ __ __ — __ __ — __ __ __ __ b. Medicare number (or comparable railroad insurance number)			
6.	FACILITY PROVIDER NO.⊕	a. State No. b. Federal No.			
7.	MEDICAID NO. ["+" if pending, "N" if not a Medicaid recipient] ⊕				

8. | REASONS FOR ASSESS-MENT | [Note—Other codes do not apply to this form]

a. Primary reason for assessment
1. Admission assessment (required by day 14)
2. Annual assessment
3. Significant change in status assessment
4. Significant correction of prior full assessment
5. Quarterly review assessment
10. Significant correction of prior quarterly assessment
0. *NONE OF ABOVE*

b. *Codes for assessments required for Medicare PPS or the State*
1. *Medicare 5 day assessment*
2. *Medicare 30 day assessment*
3. *Medicare 60 day assessment*
4. *Medicare 90 day assessment*
5. *Medicare readmission/return assessment*
6. *Other state required assessment*
7. *Medicare 14 day assessment*
8. *Other Medicare required assessment*

9. | Signatures of Persons who Completed a Portion of the Accompanying Assessment or Tracking Form

I certify that the accompanying information accurately reflects resident assessment or tracking information for this resident and that I collected or coordinated collection of this information on the dates specified. To the best of my knowledge, this information was collected in accordance with applicable Medicare and Medicaid requirements. I understand that this information is used as a basis for ensuring that residents receive appropriate and quality care, and as a basis for payment from federal funds. I further understand that payment of such federal funds and continued participation in the government-funded health care programs is conditioned on the accuracy and truthfulness of this information, and that I may be personally subject to or may subject my organization to substantial criminal, civil, and/or administrative penalties for submitting false information. I also certify that I am authorized to submit this information by this facility on its behalf.

Signature and Title	Sections	Date
a.		
b.		
c.		
d.		
e.		
f.		
g.		
h.		
i.		
j.		
k.		
l.		

GENERAL INSTRUCTIONS

Complete this information for submission with all full and quarterly assessments (Admission, Annual, Significant Change, State or Medicare required assessments, or Quarterly Reviews, etc.)

⊕ = Key items for computerized resident tracking

☐ = When box blank, must enter number or letter   [a.] = When letter in box, check if condition applies

MDS 2.0 September, 2000

MDS MEDICARE PPS ASSESSMENT FORM
(VERSION JULY 2002)

Numeric Identifier _____

AB5.	RESIDEN-TIAL HISTORY 5 YEARS PRIOR TO ENTRY	*(Check all settings resident lived in during 5 years prior to date of entry.)*
		a. Prior stay at this nursing home
		b. Stay in other nursing home
		c. Other residential facility—board and care home, assisted living, group home
		d. MH/psychiatric setting
		e. MR/DD setting
		f. NONE OF ABOVE

A1.	RESIDENT NAME				
		a. (First)	b. (Middle Initial)	c. (Last)	d. (Jr/Sr)

A2.	ROOM NUMBER	

A3.	ASSESS-MENT REFERENCE DATE	a. Last day of MDS observation period
		Month — Day — Year

A4a	DATE OF REENTRY	Date of reentry from most recent temporary discharge to a hospital in last 90 days (or since last assessment or admission if less than 90 days)
		Month — Day — Year

A5.	MARITAL STATUS	1. Never married 3. Widowed 5. Divorced 2. Married 4. Separated

A6.	MEDICAL RECORD NO.	

A10.	ADVANCED DIRECTIVES	*(For those items with supporting documentation in the medical record, check all that apply)*
		b. Do not resuscitate ☐ c. Do not hospitalize ☐

B1.	COMATOSE	*(Persistent vegetative state/no discernible consciousness)* 0. No 1. Yes *(If Yes, skip to Section G)*

B2.	MEMORY	*(Recall of what was learned or known)*
		a. Short-term memory OK—seems/appears to recall after 5 minutes 0. Memory OK 1. Memory problem
		b. Long-term memory OK—seems/appears to recall long past 0. Memory OK 1. Memory problem

B3.	MEMORY/RECALL ABILITY	*(Check all that resident was normally able to recall during last 7 days)*
		a. Current season
		b. Location of own room
		c. Staff names/faces
		d. That he/she is in a nursing home
		e. NONE OF ABOVE are recalled

B4.	COGNITIVE SKILLS FOR DAILY DECISION-MAKING	*(Made decisions regarding tasks of daily life)*
		0. INDEPENDENT—decisions consistent/reasonable
		1. MODIFIED INDEPENDENCE—some difficulty in new situations only
		2. MODERATELY IMPAIRED—decisions poor; cues/supervision required
		3. SEVERELY IMPAIRED—never/rarely made decisions

B5.	INDICATORS OF DELIRIUM—PERIODIC DISORDERED THINKING/AWARENESS	*(Code for behavior in the last 7 days.)* [Note: Accurate assessment requires conversations with staff and family who have direct knowledge of resident's behavior over this time]. 0. Behavior not present 1. Behavior present, not of recent onset 2. Behavior present, over last 7 days appears different from resident's usual functioning (e.g., new onset or worsening)
		a. EASILY DISTRACTED—(e.g., difficulty paying attention; gets sidetracked)
		b. PERIODS OF ALTERED PERCEPTION OR AWARENESS OF SURROUNDINGS—(e.g., moves lips or talks to someone not present; believes he/she is somewhere else; confuses night and day)
		c. EPISODES OF DISORGANIZED SPEECH—(e.g., speech is incoherent, nonsensical, irrelevant, or rambling from subject to subject; loses train of thought)
		d. PERIODS OF RESTLESSNESS—(e.g., fidgeting or picking at skin, clothing, napkins, etc; frequent position changes; repetitive physical movements or calling out)
		e. PERIODS OF LETHARGY—(e.g., sluggishness; staring into space; difficult to arouse; little body movement)
		f. MENTAL FUNCTION VARIES OVER THE COURSE OF THE DAY—(e.g., sometimes better, sometimes worse; behaviors sometimes present, sometimes not)

C4.	MAKING SELF UNDER-STOOD	*(Expressing information content—however able)*
		0. UNDERSTOOD
		1. USUALLY UNDERSTOOD—difficulty finding words or finishing thoughts
		2. SOMETIMES UNDERSTOOD—ability is limited to making concrete requests
		3. RARELY/NEVER UNDERSTOOD

C6.	ABILITY TO UNDER-STAND OTHERS	*(Understanding verbal information content—however able)*
		0. UNDERSTANDS
		1. USUALLY UNDERSTANDS—may miss some part/intent of message
		2. SOMETIMES UNDERSTANDS—responds adequately to simple, direct communication
		3. RARELY/NEVER UNDERSTANDS

D1.	VISION	*(Ability to see in adequate light and with glasses if used)*
		0. ADEQUATE—sees fine detail, including regular print in newspapers/books
		1. IMPAIRED—sees large print, but not regular print in newspapers/books
		2. MODERATELY IMPAIRED—limited vision; not able to see newspaper headlines, but can identify objects
		3. HIGHLY IMPAIRED—object identification in question, but eyes appear to follow objects
		4. SEVERELY IMPAIRED—no vision or sees only light, colors, or shapes; eyes do not appear to follow objects

E1.	INDICATORS OF DEPRES-SION, ANXIETY, SAD MOOD	*(Code for indicators observed in last 30 days, irrespective of the assumed cause)* 0. Indicator not exhibited in last 30 days 1. Indicator of this type exhibited up to five days a week 2. Indicator of this type exhibited daily or almost daily (6, 7 days a week)

VERBAL EXPRESSIONS OF DISTRESS

a. Resident made negative statements—e.g., "Nothing matters; Would rather be dead; What's the use; Regrets having lived so long; Let me die"

b. Repetitive questions—e.g., "Where do I go; What do I do?"

c. Repetitive verbalizations—e.g., calling out for help, ("God help me")

d. Persistent anger with self or others—e.g., easily annoyed, anger at placement in nursing home; anger at care received

e. Self deprecation—e.g., "I am nothing; I am of no use to anyone"

f. Expressions of what appear to be unrealistic fears—e.g., fear of being abandoned, left alone, being with others

g. Recurrent statements that something terrible is about to happen—e.g., believes he or she is about to die, have a heart attack

h. Repetitive health complaints—e.g., persistently seeks medical attention, obsessive concern with body functions

i. Repetitive anxious complaints/concerns (non-health related) e.g., persistently seeks attention/reassurance regarding schedules, meals, laundry, clothing, relationship issues

SLEEP-CYCLE ISSUES

j. Unpleasant mood in morning

k. Insomnia/change in usual sleep pattern

SAD, APATHETIC, ANXIOUS APPEARANCE

l. Sad, pained, worried facial expressions—e.g., furrowed brows

m. Crying, tearfulness

n. Repetitive physical movements—e.g., pacing, hand wringing, restlessness, fidgeting, picking

LOSS OF INTEREST

o. Withdrawal from activities of interest—e.g., no interest in long standing activities or being with family/friends

p. Reduced social interaction

E2.	MOOD PERSIS-TENCE	One or more indicators of depressed, sad or anxious mood were not easily altered by attempts to "cheer up", console, or reassure the resident over last 7 days
		0. No mood indicators 1. Indicators present, easily altered 2. Indicators present, not easily altered

Resident Identifier _____   Numeric Identifier _____

E4.	BEHAVIORAL SYMPTOMS	(A) *Behavioral symptom frequency in last 7 days* 0. Behavior not exhibited in last 7 days 1. Behavior of this type occurred 1 to 3 days in last 7 days 2. Behavior of this type occurred 4 to 6 days, but less than daily 3. Behavior of this type occurred daily (B) *Behavioral symptom alterability in last 7 days* 0. Behavior not present OR behavior was easily altered 1. Behavior was not easily altered		(A)	(B)
		a. WANDERING (moved with no rational purpose, seemingly oblivious to needs or safety)			
		b. VERBALLY ABUSIVE BEHAVIORAL SYMPTOMS (others were threatened, screamed at, cursed at)			
		c. PHYSICALLY ABUSIVE BEHAVIORAL SYMPTOMS (others were hit, shoved, scratched, sexually abused)			
		d. SOCIALLY INAPPROPRIATE/DISRUPTIVE BEHAVIORAL SYMPTOMS (made disruptive sounds, noisiness, screaming, self-abusive acts, sexual behavior or disrobing in public, smeared/threw food/feces, hoarding, rummaged through others' belongings)			
		e. RESISTS CARE (resisted taking medications/injections, ADL assistance, or eating)			

G1.	(A) ADL SELF-PERFORMANCE—*(Code for resident's PERFORMANCE OVER ALL SHIFTS during last 7 days—Not including setup)*
	0. *INDEPENDENT*—No help or oversight —OR— Help/oversight provided only 1 or 2 times during last 7 days
	1. *SUPERVISION*—Oversight, encouragement or cueing provided 3 or more times during last 7 days —OR— Supervision (3 or more times) plus physical assistance provided only 1 or 2 times during last 7 days
	2. *LIMITED ASSISTANCE*—Resident highly involved in activity; received physical help in guided maneuvering of limbs or other nonweight bearing assistance 3 or more times —OR—More help provided only 1 or 2 times during last 7 days
	3. *EXTENSIVE ASSISTANCE*—While resident performed part of activity, over last 7-day period, help of following type(s) provided 3 or more times: — Weight-bearing support — Full staff performance during part (but not all) of last 7 days
	4. *TOTAL DEPENDENCE*—Full staff performance of activity during entire 7 days
	8. *ACTIVITY DID NOT OCCUR* during entire 7 days

	(B) ADL SUPPORT PROVIDED—*(Code for MOST SUPPORT PROVIDED OVER ALL SHIFTS during last 7 days; code regardless of resident's self-performance classification)*		(A)	(B)
	0. No setup or physical help from staff 1. Setup help only 2. One person physical assist 3. Two+ persons physical assist 8. ADL activity itself did not occur during entire 7 days		SELF-PERF	SUPPORT
a.	BED MOBILITY	How resident moves to and from lying position, turns side to side, and positions body while in bed			
b.	TRANSFER	How resident moves between surfaces—to/from: bed, chair, wheelchair, standing position (EXCLUDE to/from bath/toilet)			
c.	WALK IN ROOM	How resident walks between locations in his/her room			
d.	WALK IN CORRIDOR	How resident walks in corridor on unit			
e.	LOCOMOTION ON UNIT	How resident moves between locations in his/her room and adjacent corridor on same floor. If in wheelchair, self-sufficiency once in chair			
f.	LOCOMOTION OFF UNIT	How resident moves to and returns from off unit locations (e.g., areas set aside for dining, activities, or treatments). If facility has **only one floor,** how resident moves to and from distant areas on the floor. If in wheelchair, self-sufficiency once in chair			
g.	DRESSING	How resident puts on, fastens, and takes off all items of **clothing,** including donning/removing prosthesis			
h.	EATING	How resident eats and drinks (regardless of skill). Includes intake of nourishment by other means (e.g., tube feeding, total parenteral nutrition)			
i.	TOILET USE	How resident uses the toilet room (or commode, bedpan, urinal); transfer on/off toilet, cleanses, changes pad, manages ostomy or catheter, adjusts clothes			
j.	PERSONAL HYGIENE	How resident maintains personal hygiene, including combing hair, brushing teeth, shaving, applying makeup, washing/drying face, hands, and perineum (EXCLUDE baths and showers)			

G2.	BATHING	How resident takes full-body bath/shower, sponge bath, and transfers in/out of tub/shower (EXCLUDE washing of back and hair.) **Code for most dependent in self-performance.**	(A)
		(A) BATHING SELF PERFORMANCE codes appear below 0. Independent—No help provided 1. Supervision—Oversight help only 2. Physical help limited to transfer only 3. Physical help in part of bathing activity 4. Total dependence 8. Activity itself did not occur during entire 7 days	

G3.	TEST FOR BALANCE (see training manual)	*(Code for ability during test in the last 7 days)* 0. Maintained position as required in test 1. Unsteady, but able to rebalance self without physical support 2. Partial physical support during test; or stands (sits) but does not follow directions for test 3. Not able to attempt test without physical help	
		a. Balance while standing	
		b. Balance while sitting—position, trunk control	

G4.	FUNCTIONAL LIMITATION IN RANGE OF MOTION	*(Code for limitations during last 7 days that interfered with daily functions or placed residents at risk of injury)*		
		(A) *RANGE OF MOTION* 0. No limitation 1. Limitation on one side 2. Limitation on both sides	(B) *VOLUNTARY MOVEMENT* 0. No loss 1. Partial loss 2. Full loss	(A) (B)
		a. Neck		
		b. Arm—Including shoulder or elbow		
		c. Hand—Including wrist or fingers		
		d. Leg—Including hip or knee		
		e. Foot—Including ankle or toes		
		f. Other limitation or loss		

G5.	MODES OF LOCOMOTION	*(Check if applied during last 7 days)*
		b. Wheeled self ☐

G6.	MODES OF TRANSFER	*(Check all that apply during last 7 days)*
		a. Bedfast all or most of time ☐
		b. Bed rails used for bed mobility or transfer ☐

G7.	TASK SEGMENTATION	Some or all of ADL activities were broken into subtasks during **last 7 days** so that resident could perform them 0. No 1. Yes

H1.	CONTINENCE SELF-CONTROL CATEGORIES *(Code for resident's PERFORMANCE OVER ALL SHIFTS)*
	0. *CONTINENT*—Complete control [includes use of indwelling urinary catheter or ostomy device that does not leak urine or stool]
	1. *USUALLY CONTINENT*—BLADDER, incontinent episodes once a week or less; BOWEL, less than weekly
	2. *OCCASIONALLY INCONTINENT*—BLADDER, 2 or more times a week but not daily; BOWEL, once a week
	3. *FREQUENTLY INCONTINENT*—BLADDER, tended to be incontinent daily, but some control present (e.g., on day shift); BOWEL, 2-3 times a week
	4. *INCONTINENT*—Had inadequate control BLADDER, multiple daily episodes; BOWEL, all (or almost all) of the time

a.	BOWEL CONTINENCE	Control of bowel movement, with appliance or bowel continence programs, if employed	
b.	BLADDER CONTINENCE	Control of urinary bladder function (if dribbles, volume insufficient to soak through underpants), with appliances (e.g., foley) or continence programs, if employed	

H2.	BOWEL ELIMINATION PATTERN	c. Diarrhea	
		d. Fecal impaction	

H3.	APPLIANCES AND PROGRAMS	a. Any scheduled toileting plan		d. Indwelling catheter	
		b. Bladder retraining program		i. Ostomy present	
		c. External (condom) catheter			

For Section I : check only those diseases that have a **relationship** to current ADL status, cognitive status, mood and behavior status, medical treatments, nursing monitoring, or risk of death. (Do not list inactive diagnoses.)

I1.	DISEASES	a. Diabetes melitus		v. Hemiplegia/Hemiparesis	
		d. Arteriosclerotic heart disease (ASHD)		w. Multiple sclerosis	
				x. Paraplegia	
		f. Congestive heart failure		z. Quadriplegia	
		j. Peripheral vascular disease		ee. Depression	
		m. Hip fracture		ff. Manic depressive (bipolar disease)	
		r. Aphasia		gg. Schizophrenia	
		s. Cerebral palsy		hh. Asthma	
		t. Cerebrovascular accident (stroke)		ii. Emphysema/COPD	

I2.	INFECTIONS	*(If none apply, CHECK the NONE OF ABOVE box)*			
		a. Antibiotic resistant infection (e.g. **Methicillin resistant staph**)		g. Septicemia	
		b. Clostridium difficile (c. diff.)		h. Sexually transmitted diseases	
		c. Conjunctivitis		i. Tuberculosis	
		d. HIV infection		j. Urinary tract infection **in last 30 days**	
		e. Pneumonia		k. Viral hepatitis	
		f. Respiratory infection		l. Wound infection	
				m. NONE OF ABOVE	

Resident Identifier _____   Numeric Identifier _____

I3.	OTHER CURRENT DIAGNOSES AND ICD-9 CODES	a. ⎸ ⎸ ⎸ • ⎸ ⎸ b. ⎸ ⎸ ⎸ • ⎸ ⎸

J1.	PROBLEM CONDITIONS	*(Check all problems present in last 7 days unless other time frame is indicated)*

INDICATORS OF FLUID STATUS

a. Weight gain or loss of 3 or more pounds within a 7-day period

b. Inability to lie flat due to shortness of breath

c. Dehydrated; output exceeds input

d. Insufficient fluid; did **NOT** consume all/almost all liquids provided during **last 3 days**

OTHER

e. Delusions

g. Edema

h. Fever

i. Hallucinations

j. Internal bleeding

k. Recurrent lung aspirations in **last 90 days**

l. Shortness of breath

n. Unsteady gait

o. Vomiting

J2.	PAIN SYMPTOMS	*(Code the highest level of pain present in the last 7 days)*

a. **FREQUENCY** with which resident complains or shows evidence of pain

0. No pain *(skip to J4)*
1. Pain less than daily
2. Pain daily

b. **INTENSITY** of pain

1. Mild pain
2. Moderate pain
3. Times when pain is horrible or excruciating

J4.	ACCIDENTS	*(Check all that apply)*

a. Fell in **past 30 days**

b. Fell in **past 31-180 days**

c. Hip fracture in **last 180 days**

d. Other fracture in **last 180 days**

e. *NONE OF ABOVE*

J5.	STABILITY OF CONDITIONS	a. Conditions/diseases make resident's cognitive, ADL, mood or behavior patterns unstable—(fluctuating, precarious, or deteriorating) b. Resident experiencing an acute episode or a flare-up of a recurrent or chronic problem c. End-stage disease, 6 or fewer months to live d. *NONE OF ABOVE*

K1.	ORAL PROBLEMS	a. Chewing problem b. Swallowing problem

K2.	HEIGHT AND WEIGHT	Record (a.) **height in inches** and (b.) **weight in pounds**. Base weight on most recent measure in **last 30 days**; measure weight consistently in accord with standard facility practice—e.g., in a.m. after voiding, before meal, with shoes off, and in nightclothes a. HT (in.) ⎸ ⎸ ⎸ b. WT (lb.) ⎸ ⎸ ⎸

K3.	WEIGHT CHANGE	a. **Weight loss**—5 % or more in **last 30 days**; or 10 % or more in **last 180 days** 0. No 1. Yes b. **Weight gain**—5 % or more in **last 30 days**; or 10 % or more in **last 180 days** 0. No 1. Yes

K5.	NUTRITIONAL APPROACHES	*(Check all that apply in last 7 days)* a. Parenteral/IV b. Feeding tube h. On a planned weight change program

K6.	PARENTERAL OR ENTERAL INTAKE	*(Skip to Section M if neither 5a nor 5b is checked)* a. Code the proportion of **total calories** the resident received through parenteral or tube feedings in the **last 7 days** 0. None 3. 51% to 75% 1. 1% to 25% 4. 76% to 100% 2. 26% to 50% b. Code the average **fluid intake** per day by IV or tube in **last 7 days** 0. None 3. 1001 to 1500 cc/day 1. 1 to 500 cc/day 4. 1501 to 2000 cc/day 2. 501 to 1000 cc/day 5. 2001 or more cc/day

M1.	ULCERS (Due to any cause)	*(Record the number of ulcers at each ulcer stage—regardless of cause. If none present at a stage, record "0" (zero). Code all that apply during last 7 days. Code 9 = 9 or more.) [Requires full body exam.]* **Number at Stage**

a. Stage 1. A persistent area of skin redness (without a break in the skin) that does not disappear when pressure is relieved.

b. Stage 2. A partial thickness loss of skin layers that presents clinically as an abrasion, blister, or shallow crater.

c. Stage 3. A full thickness of skin is lost, exposing the subcutaneous tissues - presents as a deep crater with or without undermining adjacent tissue.

d. Stage 4. A full thickness of skin and subcutaneous tissue is lost, exposing muscle or bone.

M2.	TYPE OF ULCER	*(For each type of ulcer, code for the highest stage in the last 7 days using scale in item M1—i.e., 0=none; stages 1, 2, 3, 4)*

a. Pressure ulcer—any lesion caused by pressure resulting in damage of underlying tissue

b. Stasis ulcer—open lesion caused by poor circulation in the lower extremities

M3.	HISTORY OF RESOLVED ULCERS	Resident had an ulcer that was resolved or cured **in LAST 90 DAYS** 0. No 1. Yes

M4.	OTHER SKIN PROBLEMS OR LESIONS PRESENT (*Check all that apply during last 7 days*)	a. Abrasions, bruises b. Burns (second or third degree) c. Open lesions other than ulcers, rashes, cuts (e.g., cancer lesions) d. Rashes—e.g., intertrigo, eczema, drug rash, heat rash, herpes zoster e. Skin desensitized to pain or pressure f. Skin tears or cuts (other than surgery) g. Surgical wounds h. *NONE OF ABOVE*

M5.	SKIN TREATMENTS (*Check all that apply during last 7 days*)	a. Pressure relieving device(s) for chair b. Pressure relieving device(s) for bed c. Turning/repositioning program d. Nutrition or hydration intervention to manage skin problems e. Ulcer care f. Surgical wound care g. Application of dressings (with or without topical medications) other than to feet h. Application of ointments/medications (other than to feet) i. Other preventative or protective skin care (other than to feet) j. *NONE OF ABOVE*

M6.	FOOT PROBLEMS AND CARE (*Check all that apply during last 7 days*)	a. Resident has one or more foot problems—e.g., corns, calluses, bunions, hammer toes, overlapping toes, pain, structural problems b. Infection of the foot—e.g., cellulitis, purulent drainage c. Open lesions on the foot d. Nails/calluses trimmed during **last 90 days** e. Received preventative or protective foot care (e.g., used special shoes, inserts, pads, toe separators) f. Application of dressings (with or without topical medications) g. *NONE OF ABOVE*

N1.	TIME AWAKE	*(Check appropriate time periods over last 7 days)* Resident awake all or most of time (i.e., naps no more than one hour per time period) in the: a. Morning c. Evening b. Afternoon d. *NONE OF ABOVE*

(If resident is comatose, skip to Section O)

N2.	AVERAGE TIME INVOLVED IN ACTIVITIES	*(When awake and not receiving treatments or ADL care)* 0. Most—more than 2/3 of time 2. Little—less than 1/3 of time 1. Some—from 1/3 to 2/3 of time 3. None

O1.	NUMBER OF MEDICATIONS	*(Record the number of different medications used in the last 7 days; enter "0" if none used)*

O3.	INJECTIONS	*(Record the number of DAYS injections of any type received during the last 7 days; enter "0" if none used)*

O4.	DAYS RECEIVED THE FOLLOWING MEDICATION	*(Record the number of DAYS during last 7 days; enter "0" if not used. Note—enter "1" for long-acting meds used less than weekly)* a. Antipsychotic d. Hypnotic b. Antianxiety e. Diuretic c. Antidepressant

P1.	SPECIAL TREATMENTS, PROCEDURES, AND PROGRAMS	a. SPECIAL CARE—*Check treatments or programs received during the last 14 days*

TREATMENTS

a. Chemotherapy
b. Dialysis
c. IV medication
d. Intake/output
e. Monitoring acute medical condition
f. Ostomy care
g. Oxygen therapy
h. Radiation
i. Suctioning
j. Tracheostomy care
k. Transfusions
l. Ventilator or respirator

PROGRAMS

m. Alcohol/drug treatment program
n. Alzheimer's/dementia special care unit
o. Hospice care
p. Pediatric unit
q. Respite care
r. Training in skills required to return to the community (e.g., taking medications, house work, shopping, transportation, ADLs)
s. *NONE OF THE ABOVE*

Resident Identifier _____   Numeric Identifier _____

P1.	SPECIAL TREAT-MENTS, PROCE-DURES, AND PROGRAMS	b. **THERAPIES** - *Record the number of days and total minutes each of the following therapies was administered (for at least 15 minutes a day) in the last 7 calendar days (Enter 0 if none or less than 15 min. daily)* [Note — count only post admission therapies] (A) = # of days administered for **15 minutes or more** (B) = total # of minutes provided in **last 7 days**		
			DAYS (A)	MIN (B)
		a. Speech - language pathology and audiology services		
		b. Occupational therapy		
		c. Physical therapy		
		d. Respiratory therapy		
		e. Psychological therapy (by any licensed mental health professional)		

P3.	NURSING REHABILITA-TION/ RESTOR-ATIVE CARE	*Record the NUMBER OF DAYS each of the following rehabilitation or restorative techniques or practices was **provided to the residents for more than or equal to 15 minutes per day in the last 7 days** (ENTER 0 if none or less than 15 min. daily.)*		
		a. Range of motion (passive)		f. Walking
		b. Range of motion (active)		g. Dressing or grooming
		c. Splint or brace assistance		h. Eating or swallowing
		TRAINING AND SKILL PRACTICE IN:		i. Amputation/prosthesis care
		d. Bed mobility		j. Communication
		e. Transfer		k. Other

P4.	DEVICES AND RESTRAINTS	Use the following codes for *last 7 days:* 0. Not used 1. Used less than daily 2. Used daily	
		Bed rails	
		a. —Full bed rails on all open sides of bed	
		b. —Other types of side rails used (e.g., half rail, one side)	
		c. Trunk restraint	
		d. Limb restraint	
		e. Chair prevents rising	

P7.	PHYSICIAN VISITS	In the **LAST 14 DAYS** (or since admission if less than 14 days in facility) how many days has the physician (or authorized assistant or practitioner) examined the resident? *(Enter 0 if none)*	

P8.	PHYSICIAN ORDERS	In the **LAST 14 DAYS** (or since admission if less than 14 days in facility) how many days has the physician (or authorized assistant or practitioner) changed the resident's orders? *Do not include order renewals without change. (Enter 0 if none)*	
Q1.	DISCHARGE POTENTIAL	a. Resident expresses/indicates preference to return to the community 0. No 1. Yes	
		c. Stay projected to be of a short duration—discharge projected **within 90 days** (do not include expected discharge due to death) 0. No 2. Within 31-90 days 1. Within 30 days 3. Discharge status uncertain	
Q2.	OVERALL CHANGE IN CARE NEEDS	Resident's overall level of self sufficiency has changed significantly as compared to status of **90 days ago** (or since last assessment if less than 90 days) 0. No change 1. Improved—receives fewer supports, needs less restrictive level of care 2. Deteriorated—receives more support	

R2.	SIGNATURE OF PERSON COORDINATING THE ASSESSMENT:
a. Signature of RN Assessment Coordinator (sign on above line)	
b. Date RN Assessment Coordinator signed as complete	Month Day Year

T1.	SPECIAL TREATMENTS AND PROCE-DURES	*Skip unless this is a Medicare 5 day or Medicare readmission/return assessment*	
		b. **ORDERED THERAPIES**—*Has physician ordered any of the following therapies to begin in FIRST 14 days of stay—physical therapy, occupational therapy, or speech pathology service?* 0. No 1. Yes	
		c. Through day15, provide an estimate of the number of days when at least 1 therapy service can be expected to have been delivered.	
		d. Through day15, provide an estimate of the number of therapy minutes (across the therapies) that can be expected to be delivered.	

T3.	CASE MIX GROUP	Medicare					State				

OMB 0938-0739 expiration date 12/31/2002

PART III

Home Care Issues

Home health care has been an accepted set of services delivered to individuals in their homes since modern medicine was developed. Home health care services are often provided after an individual has received care in an inpatient facility, such as a hospital or rehabilitation center. Unfortunately, the current prospective reimbursement mechanism does not provide sufficient funds to provide continuous care for people with chronic medical problems. Chapter 8 will introduce you to types of services provided, who pays for this care, and who qualifies for home care. You will also learn about the comprehensive data collection tool, the Outcome and Assessment Information Set (OASIS), that is required in order to receive Medicare and Medicaid certification and reimbursement.

Chapter 9 takes the nurse administrator thought the various skills needed to successfully manage the staffing and budgeting process in home care. This chapter defines home health care agency types, discusses payer issues such as payer types, charges and reimbursements, contractual allowances, and what services are covered. Expenses are defined and outlined, along with staffing requirements. Then the nurse administrator can compare revenue with expenses to make sure the agency is staying within a viable range. This is extremely important under prospective payment.

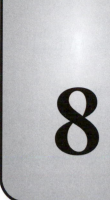

8

Introduction to Home Health Care

Gail Gerding, PhD, RN

and Karen Cober, MSN, RN, CCRN

Introduction

Home health care is an accepted set of services delivered to individuals in their homes since modern medicine was developed. Home health agencies developed in the 1880s and have continued to be a vital part of health care delivery. Home health care services are often provided after an individual has received care in an inpatient facility, such as a hospital or rehabilitation center. Clients who used early agencies could afford to pay for services out-of-pocket (National Association of Home Care, 2001). Medicare has covered home health care services since its inception in 1965, providing the opportunity for tremendous growth in this industry. When first implemented, Medicare covered most people over 65 years of age. In 1973, legislation was adopted to extend coverage to the disabled and to those with end stage renal disease, regardless of age. In 1966, 19.1 million people were enrolled in Medicare, and by 2004, 42 million had been enrolled (CMS, 2005).

According to the National Association of Home Care (NAHC), Medicare is the largest single payer of home health care services. Since 1989, fifty percent of home health care visits have been to Medicare beneficiaries, and sixty percent of these visits have been reimbursed by Medicare (National Association of Home Care, 2001). Given these statistics, Medicare may, in fact, drive the home health care market. Therefore, any change in reimbursement imposed by Medicare has repercussions on all home health care agencies.

History and Growth of an Industry

The number of enrollees who had used home health care in 1974 was 4 million. Within 20 years that number had increased to 32 million enrollees. Medicare defines a home health care visit as any visit providing skilled care: skilled nursing, physical therapy, speech therapy, and occupational therapy (CMS). Supportive services, CNA care, and social work are incidental to skilled services. Nursing and therapy are 'qualifying services.' Physician's orders for one or more of these disciplines qualifies the Medicare patient for home health care. Once the patient is qualified, non-qualifying support services may be added with a physician's order. Support services in this context are those not critical to the patient's health but are important to patient well-being; for example, personal care and social work services. Support services cannot be provided to the Medicare beneficiary unless there is a need for, and delivery of, a qualifying service. For example, a stroke patient requires physical therapy. This qualifying service allows the patient to receive personal care from a CNA. The average number of Medicare home health visits per beneficiary steadily increased from 21 in 1974, to 27 in 1989, to 76 in 1996 (Cooper and Gustafson, 1996; Meyer, 1997; and Vladeck and Miller, 1994). The largest change was in the number of supportive service visits. However, by 1999, after the Balanced Budget Act of 1997, the average number of visits per beneficiary had decreased to 41.7 (National Association of Home Care, 2001). The most recent statistics indicate in most states the average number of visits per beneficiary per PPS episode is 18–20.

Medicare reimbursements for home health care *increased* from $25 million in 1967 to approximately $17.8 *billion* in 1997 (Cohen and Tumlinson, 1997; Jitramontree, 2000; Meyer, 1997; and Scalzi et al., 1994). By 2002, because of the Balanced Budget Act of 1997, Medicare reimbursements to home health agencies had *decreased* to $12.2 billion (www.cms.hhs.gov/default.asp?). Up until this time home health care had been the fastest growing component of Medicare expenditures. This increase in expenditures could be credited not only to an increased number of patients served, but also to the number of visits per patient and the distribution of these visits.

The distribution of visits rose from only 4 percent of persons receiving 100 visits or more in 1988, to 25 percent of persons receiving over 100 visits by 1994, and by 1997 10 percent of beneficiaries received 200 or more visits (www.cms.hhs.gov/default.asp?). The average cost of visits per patient across all agencies rose from an average of $17 per visit in 1974, to an average of $83 per visit by 1994, to $98 per visit by 1999 (Bishop and Skwara, 1993; Centers for Medicare and Medicaid Services Chart Book, 1999; Hays and Willborn, 1996). By 1998, the cost per visit across agencies by service type demonstrated wide variation from a low of $55 for a home health aide in a government agency to $67 in a proprietary agency, and $134 for a medical social worker in a government agency to $153 in a proprietary agency (Centers for Medicare and Medicaid Services Chart Book, 1999).

To decrease the escalating costs of home care, and to extend the solvency of the Medicare trust fund, major changes in home care reimbursement were implemented. The Balanced Budget Act of 1997 mandated that by October 1, 1999, a prospective payment system for home health care agencies be in place. To aid in the transition from retrospective payment to prospective payment, the Interim Payment System for home health agencies was implemented. Home health care agencies were targeted for $16.2 billion in reduced costs. These reductions imposed significant fiscal challenges to reduce costs for certified home health care agencies (National Association of Home Care, 1997).

The Interim Payment System reduced the per-visit-limit from 112 percent of the costs of a freestanding agency to 105 percent. Also, home health agency costs were subjected to an aggregate per-beneficiary cost limitation. This per-beneficiary cost limitation was based upon a 12-month cost reporting period from the agency, ending in fiscal year 1994. For those agencies that did not have a 12-month cost report from fiscal year 1994, the per-beneficiary limitation was based upon the national median of the per-beneficiary limits for home health agencies. Home health agencies were paid the lesser of actual cost, the per-visit limits, or the per-beneficiary limits (Forster, 1998; and National Association for Home Care, 1997).

The Interim Payment System retained a cost-based reimbursement foundation with changes in how home health care agencies would be compensated. Home health care agencies would be paid the lowest of: 1) actual allowable costs; 2) the per-visit cost limits; or 3) agency-specific aggregate per-beneficiary annual limit. The cost limits were based on 1994 data and reduced the costs in two ways. Costs were calculated on 105 percent of the median per visit costs of freestanding agencies rather than the 112 percent of the mean. Additionally, home health care agencies could not take into account the market basket increase that occurred during the July 1, 1994 to June 30, 1997 freeze on cost limits. Thus costs were based upon three-year-old prices that did not allow for inflation (National Association of Home Care, 1997).

The aggregate per beneficiary limit was introduced by the Interim Payment System to prevent further increases in *utilization per patient*. This limit allowed higher cost patients and lower cost patients to be balanced because visits were not restricted on individuals, but focused on the agency visits per the aggregate. These provisions were expected to reduce costs by 14–22 percent, and to prepare agencies for the coming prospective payment system mandated by the Balanced Budget Act of 1997 (National Association of Home Care, 1997).

Consumer Price Index or CPI—Perhaps the best known price index, the CPI measures the price of a "market basket of goods and services for an urban family of four."

Market Basket—a colloquial term, derived from the definition of the CPI, market basket indicates the change in prices for a set of goods and/or services. Price indices, or market baskets, are measured for consumer prices, wholesale prices, and specific industries such as health care.

From: Marquette, R. (2006) Chapter 11 in *Health Care Financial Management for Nurse Managers: Merging the Heart with the Dollar,* Sudbury, MA: Jones & Bartlett, p. 372.

Home health agencies faced enormous challenges as the Medicare Prospective Payment System (PPS) reimbursement revisions altered the method of payment for home care. Medicare home care moved from a retrospective cost-based, per-visit reimbursement to a 60-day episode of care, which included most supplies.

The PPS payment method parallels Medicare's shift in hospital payments to slow the growth of expenditures in 1983 to diagnosis related groups (DRGs). Hospitals responded to the Prospective Payment System with shortened lengths of stay, more efficient methods of delivering hospital services, better use of outpatient services, and more specific coding techniques for DRGs. Medicare anticipated most of these changes, which resulted in substantially reduced hospital costs and delivery system changes (Goldfarb and Coffey, 1992; Russell and Manning, 1989). A similar response was expected from home health care agencies to decrease the growth of Medicare expenditures for home health care services.

In order for home health care agencies to remain economically solvent during the transition from a retrospective fee-per-visit payment system to a prospective episodic reimbursement, adjustments to reduce costs have had to be made. Agencies had to become more efficient and effective. Length of stay and number of visits decreased, staff increased productivity while concentrating on teaching patients self care and ensuring good outcomes. Accurate coding and specific documentation of the patient's assessment via the OASIS (the Outcome and Assessment Information Set) became essential. Ultimately agencies developed ways to integrate clinical and financial information to analyze episodes, utilization, and cost of providing care (Jitramontree, 2000; Stoker, 2000; and St. Pierre and Dombi, 2000). PPS resulted in consolidation in the industry and closure of one-third of the home health agencies in the country.

Even with the decreases in certified home health care agencies, eligible beneficiaries need access to home health care. Given the economic climate of reduced costs and utilization, agencies may decide to accept clients that are a better fit with the services the agency delivers. What services are provided, and how effectively agencies can deliver these services, now play a major role in how the agency maintains a strong revenue flow.

Qualifying for Home Health Care

To qualify for the home health care benefit covered by Medicare, several criteria must be met: 1) the beneficiary must be home-bound; 2) in need of skilled intermittent care (no more than 35 hours per week); and 3) under the care of a physician with an established written plan of care that is periodically reviewed by a physician (www.cms.hhs.gov/default.asp?). Only a Medicare-certified home health care agency can provide services to Medicare beneficiaries. These services are provided as long as they are considered medically reasonable and necessary for treatment of the disorder.

Although the criteria for home health care has remained the same over the years, legislative changes in the delivery and dissemination of services have been amended. When first implemented, only nonprofit agencies were allowed to be certified for Medicare home health care visits. Originally, to qualify for home health services, at least three days of prior hospitalization was required. The beneficiary had to pay a $60 deductible. The number of visits allowed was limited according to medical diagnosis. (Visit limits are still common in state Medicaid home care programs.) In 1980 the Omnibus Reconciliation Act (OBRA) removed these limitations. The existing limits on the number of allowable home health visits was removed, as were the existing three-day-prior-hospitalization requirement and the $60 deductible. In order to encourage expanded use of home care, proprietary (for-profit) agencies were allowed to become Medicare-certified health care providers (Benjamin, 1993).

By 1982 two legislative developments had great impact on home health care agencies. The Tax Equity and Fiscal Responsibility Act (TEFRA) authorized Medicare reimbursement for hospice care for the terminally ill. The second development, which had a more profound impact on home health care, was the implementation of the Medicare prospective payment system for hospitals. The prospective payment system (DRGs) created a discharge incentive for hospitals and physicians. No longer reimbursed for lengthy hospital stays, patients were discharged "quicker and sicker." Post-acute care came to the forefront of public attention, and home health care visits, along with home health care agencies, began to expand.

As the number of agencies expanded, problems with inconsistent determinations in coverage increased because of narrow interpretations by Medicare intermediaries regarding "part time or intermittent" care. These narrow interpretations resulted in denial of care for eligible beneficiaries. A lawsuit was filed against Health Care Financing Administration (HCFA), now the Center for Medicare and Medicaid Services (CMS), in 1987 by a coalition of U.S. Congress members, consumer groups, and the National Association for Home Care (NAHC), *(Duggan vs. Bowen, 1988)*. As a result of this lawsuit, a revision of the *Medicare Home Health Agency Manual (HIM-11)* was developed and implemented in 1989. These revisions clarified coverage criteria and reduced inconsistencies in determinations of coverage (National Association of Home Care, 2000; and Vladeck and Miller, 1994).

In addition to legislation, the DRG/Prospective Payment System in hospitals required earlier discharges, thus stimulating the need for post-acute services in the home. The focus of care began to change to rehabilitating the patient to previous levels of functioning, and preventing further hospitalizations. For these reasons, as well as for profit motives, the home health care industry grew.

Types of Services Provided in Home Care

Home health care agencies deliver services in the home that range from skilled nursing directed at specific surgical procedures or disease process management to education regarding medications, treatments, and health promotion. Wound care, infusion therapy, intramuscular injections of medication for chronic conditions such as pernicious anemia and osteoporosis, and catheter changes are chronic care needs. Skilled services include therapy disciplines: Physical Therapy and Speech Therapy. While Occupational Therapy (OT) cannot stand alone as a skillable service, OT is very important to the rehabilitation and independence of the patient and has become a very necessary home care service.

Support services—personal care (home health aides) and social work—have become less frequently used than they were under the cost reimbursement model. Many home health agencies have supported and lobbied for Home- and Community-Based Services. These state-funded or state/federally-funded programs provide personal care, housekeeping, respite, and social services, often needed by the elderly or disabled patient in order to remain in the home. The availability of Home and Community Based Services varies from state to state and can be a valuable resource to the patient in need of home care services, particularly when there is no Medicare skillable service needed.

Who Pays For Home Health?

The cost of home care services is primarily dictated by Medicare reimbursement, although a home health agency may have numerous contacts with other third party payers (insurance companies), and some agencies specialize in self-pay (private duty) services. Home care costs a fraction of a day in the hospital, and significantly less than a day in a Skilled Nursing Facility (SNF). The Consumer Price Index (CPI) publishes these statistics each year, and NAHC (National Association for Home Care) reports the data in "Basic Statistics About Home Care" updated annually. For example, in 2000 the charges for an average hospital day were $3,753; SNF $421; and a home health visit cost $100.

Average cost for home care services vary depending upon the type of agency supplying the service. Average skilled nursing costs range from $102 for a government agency to $115 for a proprietary agency. Home health aide charges range from $56 for a government agency to $68 in a proprietary agency. (See Exhibit 8-1 for further examples.)

Exhibit 8-1   Skilled Services Range of Costs By Agency Ownership in 2001

	Average cost by visit type: All agencies	Average cost by visit type: Non-profit	Average cost by visit type: Government	Average cost by visit type: Proprietary
Skilled Nursing	$112	$111	$102	$115
Physical Therapy	$117	$115	$106	$106
Occupational Therapy	$119	$117	$110	$110
Speech Therapy	$119	$117	$109	$109
Medical Social Services	$148	$149	$144	$144
Home Health Aide	$66	$65	$56	$56

Data from: Health Care Financing Review, 2001, Vol 23.

As previously noted, Medicare has been the largest payer source for home health care agencies. Using data from the Ohio Department of Health from 1996 and 1998, a representation of the changes in distribution of visits and patients by payer source can be approximated. See Exhibits 8-2 and 8-3. In 1989, Medicare accounted for 59.19 percent of visits reimbursed, with Medicaid accounting for 24.89 percent. Over the next seven years the distribution of Medicare reimbursed visits increased as Medicaid reimbursed visits decreased. By 1996 the distribution

Exhibit 8-2   Distribution of Visits By Payer Source

Year	Medicare	Medicaid/ Medicaid Waiver	All Other Insurance and Private Pay	Other Subsidized
1989	59.19%	24.89%	13.60%	2.32%
1990	68.13%	19.25%	10.33%	2.29%
1991	69.23%	18.87%	8.98%	2.90%
1992	73.44%	16.16%	8.42%	1.98%
1993	74.60%	14.93%	6.97%	3.50%
1994	79.12%	12.08%	7.34%	1.46%
1995	80.33%	10.45%	7.02%	2.20%
1996	80.83%	9.37%	5.85%	3.96%
1997	76.03%	12.32%	7.82%	3.84%
1998	70.80%	12.08%	10.53%	6.59%

Data from: Ohio Department of Health, 1996 and 1998.

Exhibit 8-3 Distribution of Patients By Payer Source

	Payer category			
Year	Medicare	Medicaid/ Medicaid Waiver	All Other Insurance and Private Pay	Other Subsidized
1989	64.81%	14.86%	17.39%	2.94%
1990	70.43%	11.68%	14.68%	3.21%
1991	69.71%	12.35%	13.59%	4.33%
1992	73.44%	10.91%	12.79%	2.86%
1993	68.67%	10.57%	12.04%	8.73%
1994	78.28%	8.64%	11.28%	1.80%
1995	74.76%	9.55%	12.66%	3.02%
1996	74.70%	8.79%	12.44%	4.07%
1997	70.06%	9.17%	16.61%	4.16%
1998	64.56%	8.92%	21.51%	4.95%

Data from: Ohio Department of Health, 1996 and 1998.

of visits by source of reimbursement peaked with Medicare at 80.83 percent and Medicaid at 9.37 percent. The next two years saw a decline in visits by Medicare reimbursements and an increase in visits by Medicaid, other insurance, and private pay (Ohio Department of Health, 1996 and 1998). A similar trend can be noted in the distribution of patients by source of reimbursement (Exhibit 8-3) with Medicaid patients remaining more stable from 1996 to 1998 and insurance and private pay patients increasing by approximately 9 percent (Ohio Department Health, 1996 & 1998). The reason for this change in distribution is unclear.

Given the changes in distribution of patients by source of reimbursement, it seems logical to conclude that who pays for services influences what services are delivered and ultimately used.

Types of Home Care Agencies

The number of home health care agencies has increased over the last two decades. In 1975 there were 2,254 Medicare certified agencies. Between the years 1980 and 1995 the number of agencies more than doubled from 2,858 to 7,827, and peaked at over 10,000 agencies in 1997. By 2001, after the implementation of the PPS, the number of Medicare certified home health agencies decreased to 7,152. According to the National Association of Home Care, this 31.5 percent decline since 1997 can be attributed to reimbursement changes imposed by the Balanced Budget Act of 1997 and 2000. In 1980 proprietary and hospital-based agencies comprised 6.4 percent and 12.3 percent of all home health care agencies respectively. By the early 1990s, largely as a result of the Omnibus Reconciliation Act, home health care agencies grew to 17.6 percent voluntary, 23.4 percent government; 42.1 percent proprietary, and 17 percent private non-profit (Scalzi, Zinn, Guilfoyle, and Perdue, 1994). By 1996, a total of 8,434 home health care agencies delivered services to the home-bound population in this country. Of these agencies, 50.2 percent were proprietary, 33.7 percent nonprofit (voluntary and private), and 16.1 percent were governmental (Centers for Medicare and Medicaid Services website, 1999). These agencies delivered over $4 billion worth of Medicare health care services to Medicare beneficiaries.

Agencies are characterized as proprietary, non-profit, and governmental. See Exhibit 8-4. These categories, or types of agencies, often indicate the structure and purpose of the agency (Ohio Department of Health, 1996). Note that:

- Visiting Nurse Associations (VNA), health departments, and some hospital-based agencies can be characterized as *voluntary non-profit*. Voluntary non-profit agencies focus their efforts on clients with Medicare, Medicaid, and insurance but often deliver services to clients with no visible means of support.

- *Private non-profit agencies* are similar to voluntary non-profit agencies, and may receive financial support from specific charities such as the United Way.

- *Governmental agencies* provide diverse services that meet the needs of the community above and beyond the home health issues/needs. These agencies are supported through public funding in addition to Medicare, Medicaid, and private payers. They tend to focus their efforts on indigent populations as well as those community members with few resources.

- *Proprietary agencies* are for-profit, and focus their efforts on those clients with third party insurance and/or those able to pay out-of-pocket.

Exhibit 8-4   **Percent of Agency Type and Percent of Agency Ownership**

2001 Type Of Agency	%	2001 Agency Ownership	%
Visiting Nurse Assoc.	5.7	Non-Profit	35.4
Official	11.9	Governmental	15.5
Combination	0.5	Proprietary	49.0
Hospital-Based	29.6		
SNF-Based	2.0		
Proprietary	40.0		
Private Non-Profit	10.0		

Data from: www.cms.hhs.gov/researchers/pubs/03cmsstats.pdf (p. 19).

- *Private agencies* can be a mix of any of these agency types (Ohio Department of Health, 1996).

- Ownership of *skilled-nursing-facility-based (SNF) home health agencies* can be any of the above structures, depending on the organization of the parent institution.

Characteristics of Home Care Users

Home health care users tend to be concentrated in urban areas (Kenney, 1993; Kenney and Dubay, 1992; and Hammond, 1985). Studies show this may be related to number of agencies per Medicare enrollee (Benjamin, 1986; Cohen and Tumlinson, 1997). Because of geographies and sparse populations, home health agencies are more concentrated in urban areas. Because of this imbalance, little research has been focused on home health care provided for rural elderly (Esposito, 1994).

Geography and sparse populations often determine the development of viable home health care agencies. Rural areas often dictate long distances between homes, therefore increasing time on the road and thus decreasing revenues. In addition, there are more visits per patient in rural areas. In 1997 the average number of visits for rural home health users was 81 versus 69 for urban elders. This may suggest that home health care substitutes for fewer community resources in rural areas (Centers for Medicare and Medicaid Services, 1999).

The new Prospective Payment System (PPS) reimburses agencies per episode of care. PPS is designed to provide incentives to decrease services while increasing efficiency (Herbert, 2000; St. Pierre and Dombi, 2000). According to Herbert (2000) research indicates that smaller rural agencies will find PPS challenging because of their case mix and the increase in cost necessary to adapt to PPS. If rural home health agencies substitute for community resources, and therefore provide more visits per beneficiary, it is logical they will have difficulty with PPS. Thus, Congress provided a small additional reimbursement to rural agencies (10 percent, later 5 percent per PPS episode) to help with the burden on rural agencies.

Home health care users tend to be a very heterogeneous population. Even so, studies have attempted to predict use of home health care by patient characteristics. Most studies validate that being greater than 75 years old, female, having a low income, having limited formal education, and living alone, constitute the home health care user (Branch, Goldberg, Cheh, and Williams, 1993; Frederiks, te Wierik, van Rossum, Visser, Volovics, and Sturmans, 1992; Kempen, and Suurmeijer, 1991; and Mauser and Miller, 1994). Variables correlating with the increased use of home health care include: age, gender, nursing diagnoses, medical diagnoses, bed disability days, number of RN visits, number of home health aide visits, length of stay during home health care, cognitive status, ADLs, and IADLs (Adams and Kramer, 1996; Branch, Goldberg, Cheh, and Williams, 1993; Hays, 1992; Fredman, Droge, and Rabin, 1992; Hays and Willborn, 1996; Marek, 1996; Williams, Phillips, Torner, and Irvine, 1990).

Diagnosis

Medical diagnoses have been examined for a correlation with home health care use. Williams et al. (1990) found that primary medical diagnosis was a poor predictor of home health care use and that more specific patient characteristics may be more predictive. Marek (1996) used medical diagnosis and nursing diagnoses as independent variables to determine hours of nursing care and number of nursing visits. Correlations were small and it appears need variables continue to be the most predictive, with functional status and age the strongest predictor of home health care use; as we might anticipate, higher acuity, or need, influences the number of visits and overall use.

Reason For Discharge

As a companion variable to diagnosis, reason for discharge is used to classify patients as they are discharged from the agencies. Multiple reasons for discharge were documented prior to PPS; only one reason for discharge is now submitted. If patients are stable at discharge, they are less likely to be readmitted during the same 60-day episode of care. This is important to the agency in terms of reimbursement and resource utilization.

Case Mix

Kempen and Suurmeijer (1991) found that as functional status measured by ADLs and IADLs decreased, home health care visits increased. They also found social networks correlated with home health care use. The closer the networks, the less home health care was used. Fredman, Droge, and Rabin (1992) found that home health care users were more limited in all ADLs and IADLs. Specific limiting ADLs were bathing, dressing, and going outside. Specific limiting IADLs were shopping and heavy housework. These studies suggested that supportive services are linked with skilled post-acute care. However, due to the predictive ability of ADLs and IADLs, supportive services seem to be the more needed service.

The distribution of visits has dramatically changed. In 1988, only four percent of beneficiaries received 100 visits or more. By 1991 this percentage had tripled (Bishop and Skwara, 1993). In 1994, persons with 100 visits or more accounted for more than a quarter of the total charges. This group of beneficiaries tends to be frailer and uses a larger mix of supportive and skilled services, thus consuming a large proportion of resources. The mix of clients served, those with many needs versus those with fewer needs, becomes an important indicator of the financial viability of an agency.

Why the Change in Home Health Reimbursement?

Costs per visit have increased from an average of $17 per visit in 1974 to an average of $83 per visit in 1994. Rapid growth in Medicare home care expenditures provided the impetus for major changes in the reimbursement policies sanctioned by CMS. As noted, home health care moved from a retrospective payment system to a prospective payment system. CMS projected that changing to PPS would alleviate the rapid cost growth of Medicare home care, and make Medicare expenditures more controllable and predictable (Jitramontree, 2000).

The Balanced Budget Act of 1997 mandated that CMS develop a system to replace the costly retrospective payment system. The Interim Payment System was implemented in October of 1997, with new reimbursement methods implemented in January of 1998. This payment system was intended to decrease spending and utilization while preparing agencies for the coming Prospective Payment System.

The Prospective Payment System Proposed Rule was published in the *Federal Register* (Vol. 64, No. 208) on October 28, 1999. The final Rule was published in July of 2000. CMS implemented the Prospective Payment System (PPS) on October 1, 2000. The PPS reimburses agencies for episodes of care instead of for individual visits. Along with other major changes in reimbursement patterns, CMS expected to slow the rate of expenditures while supporting delivery care to all beneficiaries. PPS changed the way home care is delivered.

OASIS and the Prospective Payment System

In 1995 the Outcome and Assessment Information Set (OASIS) was developed by the Center for Health Services Research at the University of Colorado in Denver. As part of a Medicare Demonstration Project the Center, in conjunction with 50 home health agencies in the project, developed and tested the outcomes based interventions and data collection tool.

The goal of the OASIS was to produce a comprehensive data collection tool that could be used to measure patient outcomes, plan care, and assess patient changes during care. This assessment data collection system became a requirement of CMS in 1999 as a condition of participation for home health care agency certification nationwide (St. Pierre and Dombi, 2000 and Sperling, 1997). The wording of the OASIS questions may not be changed. The OASIS questions, frequently referred to as "MOO" questions because of their numbering (MO 190, MO 220, etc.), do not provide a complete patient assessment; CMS requires these questions as part of an integrated patient assessment documented for Medicare and Medicaid patients (www.cms.hhs.gov/default.asp?).

(A good source on OASIS is: OASIS: "Final Rule. Medicare and Medicaid Guide," Issue No. 1120 No. 1115, July 12, 2000. It is availabe from Department of Health and Human Services, Attention: HCFA (CMS) 1059-P, P.O. Box 8010, Baltimore, MD. To download the OASIS forms, go to http://www.cms.hhs.gov/basis/all.pdf.)

Prior to the Balanced Budget Act of 1997, home health care visits were paid/covered under a retrospective reimbursement system. In essence, the more care provided to the patient, the more the agency was reimbursed. While most agencies were ethical and honest, there were a few agencies that took advantage of this system, acted fraudulently, and paid a high price in fines and jail time for their dishonesty. While these fraudulent claims were few, and the home care industry was a relatively small contributor to fraudulent activities compared to other sectors of health care, home health was prominent in the changes required by the Balanced Budget Act of 1997 (BBA). Many 'clean' agencies were negatively affected by these legislative efforts to improve the health care system. Thirty percent of the agencies in the country closed and many beneficiaries lost service. In 2005, the industry is stabilizing and adjusting to a completely new structure for providing home care as outlined in the BBA.

Hospitals were the first to experience a PPS system. Since the advent of DRGs, CMS has developed and implemented PPS systems in rehabilitation hospitals, Skilled Nursing Facilities, and Home Health agencies.

OASIS is the foundation of the home care prospective payment system (PPS). No longer cost reimbursed, home care's reimbursement is directly tied to the OASIS assessment. The assessment projects the level of care required—functional, clinical, and service needs—and assigns a reimbursement amount to that care. This reimbursement includes supplies, supervisory activities, and essentially all home health care services provided to the patient during the 60 day episode.

The PPS and OASIS regulations and requirements are too numerous to examine in this context. Assessments or updates are required at prescribed times and for prescribed reasons including admission, changes in the patient's condition, transfer to another facility, discharge, etc. Each assessment has a time frame for completion and for transmission of the data. A subset of the OASIS is used to calculate the Home Health Resource Group (HHRG) value, which reflects the level of care the patient requires and results in the amount of reimbursement the agency will receive for this care. OASIS content changes frequently as does the reimbursement for a Medicare 60-day episode of care. The data collected is used by CMS to monitor patient outcomes and guide the survey process.

Home Health Coding

In the past coding and billing was a necessary and relatively simple process. For example, a physician gave the patient a flu shot and sent the bill to the insurance company. He might simply write "injection" and the charge. The introduction of Medicare in 1965, the development of DRGs in the 1980s, the growth of the health care industry, and the increase in health care fraud and abuse all created the need for tighter control of billing processes. Billing forms, codes, and procedures became extremely complex. A new job description, that of "clinical coding specialist," became a necessity and certification specific to coding was developed. Many organizations now certify coders, among them the American Health Information Management Association (AHMA).

Physician's offices generally bill for services using a Form 1500. The billing process requires International Classification of Diseases, 9th Revision (ICD-9-CM) code(s) to designate the patient's diagnosis. A Common Procedural Terminology (CPT) code or HCFA Current Procedural Coding System (HCPCS) Code(s) designate specific procedures. ICD-9 Codes may have three, four, or five digits depending on the degree of specificity required. Coding is further explained in Chapter 10, Nurse Practitioner Reimbursement in Primary Care.

The home health industry uses the UB (Uniform Billing) 92 billing form, requiring even greater detail. ICD-9 codes are used and additional codes are required for other fields/sections of the billing form. Revenue codes, for example 551 for a skilled nursing visit, are just one of the many additional codes required on the UB 92. PPS has stimulated a greater understanding of coding in home care and, for the first time, coding classes specific to home health coders are available.

Coding is the way home care agencies identify the services provided to the patient, and coding is the process whereby third party payors determine reimbursement. The volume of information available on the UB 92 (and other billing documents) is collected and used in a variety of ways. Payors, in particular the government, gather demographic and disease-related information, compile these statistics and use the information in research, reimbursement decisions, and a multitude of other ways. Accurate coding is absolutely essential, and one safe guard against allegations of fraud or abuse.

Summary

Home health care agencies supply services that are broad and diverse. Medicare has covered home health care services since its inception in 1965 and funded tremendous growth in this industry. As of 2003, 4.1 percent of all Medicare expenditures are distributed to home health care agencies—more than ten billion dollars. To decrease the tremendous growth of home care costs in the 1980s and 1990s, the Prospective Payment System was implemented (CMS 2003). With its history of flexibility, innovation, and commitment to quality care at home, agencies have continued to furnish the consumer with much needed services.

Given the continued economic desire to reduce costs and utilization, home health care administrators need to deliver quality care to those clients who need it, and develop strategies to streamline care and to increase productivity. Home care service is more focused on specific needs, and provides more acute care. The need for service to patients with chronic, debilitating disorders must not be overlooked simply based on financial constraints. Reimbursement strategies that allow for delivery of care to those clients with more long-term needs, especially those clients who can still manage much of their care themselves with little assistance, must be developed. As our population ages, more creative service-delivery strategies need to be developed to meet the demands of home care and a more chronically debilitated clientele.

References

Adams, C.E. and Kramer, S. (1996). Home health resource utilization: Health maintenance organization versus fee-for-service subscribers. *Journal of Nursing Administration, 26*(2), 20–27.

Benjamin, A.E. (1986). Determinants of state variations in home health utilization and expenditures under Medicare. *Medical Care, 24*(6), 535–547.

Benjamin, A.E. (1993). A historical perspective on home care policy. *The Milbank Quarterly, 71*(1), 129–166.

Bishop, C. and Skwara, K.C. (1993). Recent growth of Medicare home health. *Health Affairs, 12*(3), 95–110.

Branch, L.G., Goldberg, H.B., Cheh, V.A. and Williams, J. (1993). Medicare home health: A description of total episodes of care. *Health Care Financing Review, 14*(4), 59–74.

Centers for Medicare and Medicaid Services. Health Care Finance Administration. (1999). A profile of Medicare home health: Chart book. Retrieved from www.hcfa.gov/stats/cbookhha.pdf.

Centers for Medicare & Medicaid Services. (2005). Medicare a brief summary. Retrieved February 5, 2005 from: http://www.cms.hhs.gov/publications/overview-medicare-medicaid/default3.asp.

Cohen, M., and Tumlinson, A. (1997). Understanding the state variation in Medicare home health care: The impact of Medicaid program characteristics, state policy, and provider attributes. *Medical Care, 35*(6), 618–633.

Cooper, B., and Gustafson, T. (Eds.) (1996). *Healthcare Financing Review: Medicare and Medicaid Statistical Supplement, 1996.* Baltimore: U.S. Department of Health and Human Services.

Esposito, L. (1994). Home health case management: Rural caregiving. *Home Healthcare Nurse, 12*(3), 38–43.

Forster, T.M. (1998). Home care, the Balanced Budget Act of 1997, and IPS. *Caring,* February, 8–13.

Frederiks, C., te Wierik, M., van Rossum, H., Visser, A., Volovics, A., and Sturmans, F. (1992). Why do elderly people seek professional home care? Methodologies compared. *Journal of Community Health, 17*(3), 131–141.

Fredman, L., Droge, J., and Rabin, D. (1992). Functional limitations among home health care users in the national health interview survey supplement on aging. *The Gerontologist, 32*(5), 641–646.

Goldfarb, M.G. and Coffey, R. (1992). Change in the Medicare case-mix index in the 1980s and the effect of the prospective payment system. *Health Services Research, 27*(3), 385–415.

Hammond, J. (1985). Analysis of county-level data concerning the use of Medicare home health benefits. *Public Health Reports, 100*(1), 48–55.

Hays, B. (1992). Nursing care requirements and resource consumption in home health care. *Nursing Research, 41*(3), 138–143.

Hays, B., and Willborn, E. (1996). Characteristics of clients who receive home health aide service. *Public Health Nursing, 13*(1), 58–64.

Herbert, W. (2000). PPS—How will it impact your agency and your practice? *Home Healthcare Nurse, 18*(2), 94–97.

Jitramontree, N. (2000). The impact of Medicare reimbursement changes on home healthcare: A nursing perspective. *Home Healthcare Nurse, 18*(2), 116–122.

Kempen, G., and Suurmeijer, P. (1991). Professional home care for the elderly: An application of the Andersen-Newman model in the Netherlands. *Social Science Medicine, 33*(9), 1081–1089.

Kenney, G. (1993). Is access to home health care a problem in rural areas? *American Journal of Public Health, 83*(3), 412–414.

Kenney, G. and Dubay, L. (1992). Explaining area variation in the use of Medicare home health services. *Medical Care, 30*(1), 43–57.

Marek, K. (1996). Nursing diagnoses and home care nursing utilization. *Public Health Nursing, 13*(3), 195–200.

Mauser, E. and Miller, N. (1994). A profile of home health users in 1992. *Health Care Financing Review, 16*(1), 17–33.

Meyer, H. (1997). Home (care) improvement. *Hospitals & Health Networks, April 20,* 40–42.

National Association of Home Care. (1997). Transition to PPS: The Interim Payment System for Medicare home health services. National Association of Home Care Research Department: Washington, DC.

National Association of Home Care. (2000). Basic statistics about home care. Retrieved February 5, 2005 from http://www.nahc.org/Consumer/hcstats.html.

National Association of Home Care. (2001). Basic statistics about home care. Retrieved February 5, 2005 from http://www.nahc.org/Consumer/hcstats.html.

OASIS: "Final Rule. Medicare and Medicaid Guide" Issue No. 1120. No. 1115. July 12, 2000. Department of Health and Human Services, Attention: HCFA (CMS) 1059-P, P.O. Box 8010, Baltimore, MD 21244-8010.

Ohio Department of Health. (1996). Ohio Certified Home Health Agencies Annual Registration Report—1996. Columbus: Ohio Department of Health.

Ohio Department of Health. (1998). Ohio Certified Home Health Agencies Annual Registration Report—1998. Columbus: Ohio Department of Health.

Russell, L.B. and Manning, C.L. (1989). The effect of prospective payment on Medicare expenditures. *The New England Journal of Medicine, 320*(7), 439–444.

Scalzi, C.C., Zinn, J.S., Guilfoyle, M.J., and Perdue, S.T. (1994). Medicare-certified home health services: National and regional supply in the 1980s. *American Journal of Public Health, 84*(10), 1646–1648.

Sperling, R. (1997). Frequently asked questions about OASIS: Answers from a rural agency participant. *Home Healthcare Nurse, 15*(5), 340–342.

Stoker, J. (2000). Unresolved Medicare reimbursement issues. *Home Healthcare Nurse, 18*(5), 296.

St. Pierre, M. and Dombi, W.A. (2000). Home health PPS: New payment system, new hope. *Caring,* January, 6–11.

U.S. Department of Health and Human Services. http://www.hcfa.gov.

Vladeck, B.C. and Miller, N.A. (1994). The Medicare home health initiative. *Health Care Financing Review, 16*(1), 7–16.

Waid, M.O. (1998). Brief summaries of Medicare and Medicaid. Retrieved from http://www.hcfa.gov/banner.map.

Williams, B.C., Phillips, E.K., Torner, J.C. and Irvine, A.A. (1990). Predicting utilization of home health resources: Important data from routinely collected information. *Medical Care, 28*(5), 379–391.

9

Putting It All Together: Managing Resources in a Home Health Agency

Karen Cober, MSN, RN, CCRN

Introduction

Previous chapters in this book provide management and financial information applicable to a variety of health care delivery models. This chapter applies these concepts to managing a home health care agency. The general budgeting principles discussed may be used to develop a budget for a new business line in a small home care agency, as well as to develop the budget for a multi-million dollar, multi-state home health conglomerate. A variety of financial terms are used and defined in text boxes throughout this chapter. Graphs, charts, and examples are included to illustrate significant concepts.

Staffing is the single largest expense in home care, indeed in most health care delivery systems. To provide a more complete guide to budgeting, staffing is examined in some detail, and various staff reimbursement models as well as productivity are discussed. In addition tips for successful home care financial management are provided for your consideration.

Budgeting and staffing decisions are among the greatest challenges in health care management. A multitude of variables influence these decisions and one's emotions can too easily become involved in the process. The successful health care manager strives to be *fair but firm*. Team members rely on the stability of the agency for their livelihood. Decisions made at budgeting time can improve the agency's financial status, or can place the agency in financial jeopardy. In most organizations, budgeting experts and mentors with years of experience are available to assist the new manager with the budgeting process. Take advantage of these resources and do not neglect to make yourself available to help others after you have honed your budgeting skills.

Barriers to Budgeting Success

The greatest barrier to budgeting is a health care professional's *knowledge deficit* related to financial matters. Financial expertise has been neither an expectation of nursing programs nor a goal for most health care professionals. Nurses and therapists have not been educated in basic principles of finance and accounting. This knowledge deficit becomes a major barrier when the successful staff nurse is promoted to a management position. Just how deficient one's financial education is becomes all too clear when the home health care agency manager meets with the agency's accountant or the hospital finance team to 'present the budget'! Accountants tend to be very analytical, and health care providers (frequently nurses) are generally nurturing and patient-care centered. These two professional groups speak different languages and frequently process information differently. Nurse managers, and those aspiring to be managers, may benefit from a general accounting course or continuing education classes designed to enhance the nurse's understanding of financial principles and to improve effective communication with the organization's financial experts. A general understanding of finance assists the nurse manager to successfully plan program development, evaluate the viability of a product line, and advocate effectively for the financial needs of the agency and team members.

Product Line and Service Line— A group of similar products or services. Responsibility for these services may be assigned to one manager as in a strategic service unit management model.

After overcoming the barrier of knowledge deficit in the area of financial terms and tools, the nurse manager may encounter another barrier: Lack of staff buy-in.

*Buy-In—*Acceptance of and commitment to a concept or task.

In most successful business operations, team members (staff) feel connected to the agency/operation. If a business is to succeed, and make no mistake health care *is* a business, the team members must "buy-in" to budget constraints and accept necessary changes. Team members' suggestions for improvement and their participation in decision making are critical to agency success, clinical success, and especially financial success.

A barrier to success exists when care staff resist involvement in, and understanding of, financial issues, and resist change and/or participation in anything other than direct patient care. Staff may view financial principles as conflicting with the care provider's philosophy of health care. "I just want to take care of my patients." and "Money should not be a consideration in healthcare decisions." are frequent comments from nurses and therapists. How can the manager overcome these barriers?

- **Develop understandable reports and share financial data with all team members.** While there will be specific proprietary or strategic information one can not discuss, generally the more team members know and understand about financial decisions and changes in the agency, the more likely change will be adopted and decisions supported. Not knowing *why* changes occur is a major roadblock to understanding. When one has no knowledge, one is likely to "fill in the knowledge gap," leading to rumors and poor morale. The successful manager is as open as possible with financial information, and includes team members in the management and budgeting process to the greatest extent possible. This approach adds to the development of potential managers from among the team. In the book *Good to Great*, Collins identifies developing the next generation of leaders as a primary responsibility of a great leader. The leader charged with managing and budgeting for a home health agency must develop his/her financial and management skills and then seek to develop those skills in promising members of their team (Collins, 2001).

Proprietary (Information)— A profit-oriented organization type. May refer to information about revenue or strategic plans that could affect revenue.

Team Building—A long-term process that uses a variety of strategies to develop a diverse group of individuals into a team with common goals. The team is supportive of each other and the whole and functions effectively to problem solve and improve processes.

- **Maintain an open dialog with the team.** An open-door policy with easy access to the manager can be a challenge for the busy manager but provides team security, promotes team building, and reduces staff turnover. The successful manager answers questions, including financial questions, as openly and honestly as possible. More importantly, the manager *listens* to team members. It is amazing what can be learned by listening to those one leads.

- **Focus on quality.** Develop a culture where doing *the right thing is the most important thing*. By sharing the team's commitment to quality care the manager can assist the staff to understand that fiscal responsibility and delivery of quality patient care are **not** mutually exclusive.

  Additionally, emphasizing ethical practices offers a degree of safety in the highly regulated world

Turnover—A term used to indicate resignations and terminations within an organization. Usually reported as a percent of total staff as: "The agency averages a turnover rate of 21 percent per year."

of home health. A reputation as a "clean" provider (one that enforces Medicare regulations) can be a recruitment tool and a marketing plus.

- **Understand every team member impacts the quality of care *and* the agency's financial viability.** The leader may want to accomplish many goals. For example, he/she may want to provide raises for staff, or pay for travel to seminars. However, the manager's responsibility is to ensure financial stability for all team members by insuring financial liability for the agency. Consider the truism "No Margin, No Mission." Expect some resistance despite the best efforts. However, consistent openness builds trust and decreases resistance. Build an agency where *every* position and each individual is important and vital to the agency's success.

Agency Types

Many factors influence budget development, including the type of agency, also discussed in Chapter 8. Following is a summary of agency types.

The For-Profit Agency

The *for-profit* agency exists to serve and expects to make money. To this end, the for-profit agency is very conservative with resources. For example, the agency may limit the types of patients admitted and/or determine specific types of patients not accepted for admission because of the resources they require. These determinations will be documented in the agency's *admission criteria*. Limiting admissions is within the rights of the agency, as long as the admission criteria are applied consistently.

> *Case Weight*—A measure of the amount of care or a value assigned to the resources a patient requires.

> *HHRG*—Home Health Resource Groups. Eighty-eight classifications of the Prospective Payment System (PPS) based on the patient's clinical, service, and functional needs.

How does the type of patient admitted influence budgeting? The complexity of the patient and the resources required to care for the patient are documented on the federally mandated OASIS admission assessment and generate a *case weight*. Case weight is similar to acuity ratings in the acute care setting. In Medicare language, the case weight is designated by one of 88 HHRGs.

The reimbursement system for the Medicare home care patient converts the HHRG to a Health Insurance Prospective Payment System (HIPPS) Code and determines the reimbursement for the patient's episode of care. At times the reimbursement for a patient will not cover the expense of care delivery.

One of the primary Conditions of Participation for the Medicare Home Care Program is that the agency must have the resources to care for the patients admitted. The manager must not jeopardize the agency's Medicare Certification by accepting patients who require more resources than the agency can provide. Patients unsafe at home, and those unable to provide a safe environment for agency staff, are inappropriate for admission to home care. Some questions to consider are:

- Will the agency accept a limited number of resource-intensive wound care patients requiring extensive dressing supplies and multiple visits?

- What about the patient requiring nursing, personal care, and physical and speech therapy?

- What about the patient who is technically within the agency's service area but lives 75 miles from the office?

After determining the financial and human resources available in the agency, management may need to restrict the admission criteria. The for-profit agency is likely to adopt a very conservative response to these situations.

The Not-for-Profit Agency

The *not-for-profit* agency's admission criteria may be more expansive. This agency may choose to accept all types of patients without regard to the patient's complexity or ability to pay for services. This agency must also be sure it can provide the resources necessary to adequately care for the patient. However, profit is not a primary emphasis. Nevertheless, not-for-profit does not mean "for loss," and the not-for-profit company/agency must make money in order to survive.

Not-for-Profit—Financial structure and philosophy primarily designed to serve or provide a service rather than make a profit.

Equipment must be replaced, new services developed, and the cost of doing business, including salaries, continues to increase. However the primary purpose of the not-for-profit agency is service, not profit.

NOTE: *Non-Profit* is yet another financial structure. Usually reserved for fraternal organizations or benevolent associations, non-profit status requires all revenues be used or given away with an ultimate zero bottom line.

Agency Case Mix and Size

Case mix and *size* of the agency are considerations. Size is a factor because a large number of paying patients is necessary to compensate financially for both those patients who have no insurance and no ability to pay for the services needed, and to offset the expense of patients requiring vast amounts of resources. Case mix

Case Mix—A measure of the acquity of patients the agency serves, based on different diagnosis, or HHRGs.

is important because no agency has the financial resources to care for only expensive, high-use patients. Ideally a variety of patient types (i.e., those requiring few visits and supplies, as well as a limited number of extremely complex patients), provide a manageable case mix. See Exhibit 9-1.

Is the Agency Freestanding or Hospital-Based?

A *freestanding agency* is not part of a hospital or health care institution and is frequently owned by an individual or group of investors. The freestanding agency typically spends significant amounts of money on marketing, employee bonuses, and administrative salaries. While not always the case, the freestanding agency is more likely to be a for-profit entity. The freestanding agency may benefit from less bureaucracy and have the ability to make decisions and changes more quickly.

Exhibit 9-1   An Example of an Agency Case Mix

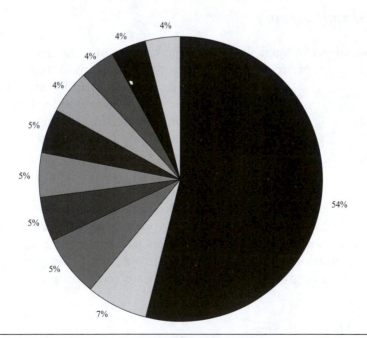

The majority of patients in this example have a diagnosis of 'abnormality of gait.' This indicates a condition requiring physical therapy—a very lucrative discipline in the PPS era. Other major diagnoses are diabetes and coronary artery disease/CHF/cardiac arrhythmias. Pneumonia and COPD, followed by CVA, and osteoarthrosis, and breast cancer complete the top 10 in this example. This is a typical mix for Medicare certified agencies.

It is possible that 50% of these patients are actually wound care patients. The abnormality of gait may be caused by recent total hip or knee replacement. Home health coding refers to the underlying cause of the problem with modifiers (V codes) explaining surgical status.

The *hospital-based agency* is owned by a hospital and meets the CMS criteria for "hospital based" status. These criteria require a governance relationship between the hospital, the agency, and shared services. (See CMS website for criteria.) The manager of a *hospital-based* agency may have a very real challenge to avoid being managed like any other hospital unit. Both the agency and the hospital benefit when hospital administration recognizes home health management needs are different from those of other hospital units or departments. To be successful a home care agency requires as much flexibility as possible in the areas of salary structure, location of the office and branches, advertising, and so forth. Home care decisions must be made quickly as the home care climate changes and the business evolves; the manager of a hospital-based agency can expect higher costs of care delivery. One issue is that *management allocations* are from the hospital or hospital system.

> *Management Allocations*—A portion of corporate costs of administrative and general services assigned to the agency or department.

Other increased costs that hospital-based agencies may experience include:

- Richer Benefit Packages for team members with associated higher costs. Benefit packages for hospital-based home health agencies typically cost the organization 18–23 percent of the team member's base salary.

- Complex and Expensive Information Systems. Specific computer requirements and standards may be necessary to permit interface between the hospital system, and the hospital-based home care agency.

- If the agency is housed in the hospital, furnishings must meet higher standards (fire retardancy, for example) are more expensive.

Conversely, hospital-based agencies may benefit from reduced costs of insurance and supplies, better buying contracts, access to cash, and the security of the hospital structure, along with greater access to managed care contracts.

New or Established?

Is the agency *established* with many years of operation and budget history? Historic data removes many of the uncertainties associated with budgeting. The manager can research the statistics, trends, and budget exceptions of the agency's recent past and develop a reasonable budget projection for the coming year.

A new company, or *"start-up"* agency, presents special challenges. This budget is a blank sheet of paper with no specific data history to guide the budgeting process. There are industry resources providing guidelines, average expenditures, projected staffing needs, and so forth. The National Association of Home Care (NAHC), and other industry organizations listed in this chapter's references, have developed a wide variety of educational materials. Nevertheless the new agency's anticipated revenues and expenses are educated guesses. During this first year of operation a start-up agency's volumes (number of patients/admission) and expenses may double or triple. The budget will require revision—sometimes dramatic and frequent revisions.

> *Line of Credit*—A preapproved amount of money that may be borrowed/accessed as needed.

In the new agency, revenue may be difficult to predict, and collection of revenues may be delayed. Management can expect a significant gap between the initiation of operations with the associated expense, and the collection of the first cash. It takes time to bill and collect claims, and a 60–90 day lag-time is to be expected. During this time the cost of staff and supplies, rent and utilities, insurance and telephones goes on. Significant capital resources and/or a line of credit with a lending institution is necessary.

> *Productivity*—A measure of the amount of work performed by an employee or group in a given time frame. For example, an RN makes six home health visits one day, and five, six, seven, and six the remainder of the week. The employee's average productivity is six per day.

How quickly will the agency grow? How many staff will be needed? The budget can be constructed with a corollary such as, "for every sustained increase of 50 admissions X amount of revenue will be generated and the agency will add X number staff."

Expenses such as rent and computer costs can be projected following a reasonable evaluation. Other projections are more difficult. For example, productivity for each discipline, the ratio of discipline use (e.g., ratio of CNA visits to skilled nursing visits) and revenue per patient are dependent on an unlimited

> *Tip*: Build as much flexibility into the budget as possible. Be conservative in estimating revenue and slightly liberal when estimating expenses.

number of variables. Time and experience are required to determine accurate budget projections.

Niche versus One-Stop-Shop

Health care organizations generally follow one of two basic philosophies regarding care delivery. One is that the public prefers to have all services available from one organization—the *one-stop-shop* concept. In the case of home health agencies, this can mean access to pediatric nurse specialists, disease management programs, wound care expertise, occupational, physical, and speech therapists, psychiatric home care, and so forth, at one agency. Beyond skilled care in the home, many organizations deliver durable medical equipment (DME) and infusion products (IV therapy). Hospice is another home-based service that may be offered. The one-stop-shop intends to provide every home-based service to the physician or case manager ordering home care for a patient. The "one call does it all" concept is very appealing to busy physicians and case managers.

The manager/administrator of a comprehensive home care agency must have a working knowledge of the various regulations impacting each discipline and the numerous financial reimbursement requirements. There is expense associated with each discipline—for example, multiple licenses, a wider variety of necessary publications, and multiple accreditation surveys and fees. Printing expenses must be considered as each discipline requires numerous forms and documents specific to their service line. It can be difficult to maintain proficiency and appropriately manage multiple service lines. One must keep up with multiple regulations, be prepared for multiple licensure and accreditation surveys, keep up with the latest clinical information in all areas, and recruit and train staff for each diverse area of service.

The *niche agency* is designed to specialize in one (or a very few) services, for example, admission and care of the pediatric patient. The advantage of a niche agency is the ability to develop expertise in one specific area while limiting expenses to those associated with delivering one type of care. Marketing is a major factor in the success of a niche agency and marketing expenses may be a larger-than-average portion of budgeted expenses. Obtaining managed care contracts may be a challenge for the niche agency. This model generally works best in large metropolitan areas where the population is diverse enough to support a specialty agency. A niche service limits the number of patients applicable for the service, and requires the referrer to make multiple calls if other services are required for the patient.

> *Niche*—A small and specialized service designed to fill a specific need or serve a specific market segment.

Budget Types

The organization or agency constructs the budget within the framework of the company's *mission*. The mission, stated or unstated, will determine the agency type and a variety of budget-related decisions. Regardless, most organizations recognize three basic budget types:

- Capital,
- Cash, and
- Operating.

The *capital* budget covers purchases of equipment and major items having a long usable lifespan. Organizations define major items and usable lifespan according to their business philosophy, such as, "purchases over $1,000 with a useful life of two or more years."

Home health agencies have fewer capital needs than a hospital, or than most other health care organizations. Common home health agency capital expenditures may include: tele-monitoring equipment, computer systems, and copiers. Start-up agencies will have additional capital expenses such as furniture. Items, such as a videocamera and portable ultrasound units, may be capital expenditures depending on the organization's definition.

One of the stresses in any business, and particularly for the owner/operator of a home health agency, is the cash budget, or *cash flow*. Employees must be paid, supply companies send their bills each month, equipment breaks and must be repaired, and health insurance and social security taxes must be paid. These bills are as regular as the sunrise, even though reimbursement from Medicare and other insurance companies is not! It is not unusual for claims payment to require 90 days or more. There may be unexpected recoupment of monies already paid to the agency when denials or other factors require repayment of funds already deposited (and spent?). The agency has paid the staff to deliver the care, paid for the supplies, and covered the other expenses of keeping the agency functional, and now must wait three months for a check in the mail. Significant planning and management of cash is required for an entity to remain open.

Expected and unexpected payment delays require the home health agency to have adequate cash, or a line of credit at a bank, to cover operating expenses during payment delays. The days of service outstanding (DSO), or accounts receivable (AR), are measurements of cash flow. Cash requirements for day-to-day operations, and efficiency in billing and collecting for services provided, drive the cash budget.

When one discusses "the budget," one is generally referring to the *operating budget*. This budget is the financial map and guide for the agency's day-to-day operations. Based on the agency's fiscal year (a 12-month time frame not necessarily following the calendar year), the operating budget includes expected revenues and expenses for those 12 months. See Exhibit 9-2.

Exhibit 9-2   Sample Agency Budget

Categories	Previous Year's Actual	Current Year Projected	Coming Year's Projection
Revenues:			
Outpatient Revenue	$110,000	$108,000	$112,000
Expenses:			
Salaries	$65,000	$69,000	$72,000
Other Expenses	$34,000	$41,000	$40,000

In this example the revenues for the current year *decreased* from the previous year. The projections for the coming year show an increase over both the current year and the previous year. The projected increased revenue indicates the agency expects greater volume in the coming year. This projected increase in volume and revenue may be due to a new program, a new physician in the area, or other significant changes anticipated by the agency management.

The Budgeting Process

Developing and distributing a budget from upper management without input from those who must make the budget work is a common management error—one roadblock previously discussed. A budget document is a powerful tool only when the entire team (all employees) buys-in to the process. Buy-in is achieved by involving the team in budget development. The effective leader seeks input from employee groups in the agency. Multiple sources of information improve the quality of the budget document and provide the foundation for staff buy-in.

What approaches are effective and practical for gathering data?

- *Staff meetings* may include discussing budget issues such as productivity and input on how to decrease mileage expense. This discussion is particularly successful when the staff has been informed of the financial status of the agency on an ongoing basis. The knowledgeable staff can consider then the challenge "we must cut expenses by 2 percent this budget year" and offer specific suggestions for achieving this goal.

- Ask the team/staff to choose a representative from each employment group (physical therapy, CNAs, nurses, and so forth). *The representative participates* with leadership in budget planning sessions and reports back to his/her group.

- *Questionnaires* are good data gathering tools. Examples of budget-related questions include: "How would you recognize and reward exceptional performance in our organization?" and "How many miles do you drive, on average, each day?" To ensure participation distribute the questionnaire at a staff meeting—i.e., to a captive audience—or provide a small incentive for completing and turning in the survey (for example, a candy bar or company pen).

The Leadership Team gathers budget information from every source available: historical data, monthly budget reports, staff input, hospital/organization goals and objectives for the coming year, professional organization membership, publication projections, complaint forms, patient satisfaction surveys, performance improvement projects, and so on. Compile the data in a usable form, identify key leaders to assist in the process, and get to work.

One necessary calculation for budget preparation is *annualizing of statistics*. The budget is prepared several months before the beginning of the fiscal year. The manager works with statistics of the partial year to project revenues and expenses for the coming year. To reach an average of the expenses and revenues for the current year, year to date statistics are annualized, using the budget given in Exhibit 9-3.

Revenue

MSA or Non-MSA—Metropolitan Area or Non-Metropolitan Service Area. Designations of urban and rural status used for example in Medicare reimbursement.

We have been discussing budget information. Now let's examine revenue, followed by expense. Revenue is influenced by numerous variables. The volume of patients, number of episodes of care for each patient, length of stay, average case weight, payor type, and contractual agreements are just some of these. Is the agency in a Metropolitan Service Area (MSA) or a non-MSA?

Exhibit 9-3   Budget Using Annualized Statistics

Example

You prepare the budget for the coming fiscal year in January. The fiscal year begins July. You have six (6) months of actual data for the *current* year (July through January). To annualize, divide the total year-to-date (expenses or revenues) by the 6 months the total represents. This gives you an *average* for each of the six months. Now to annualize this average, multiply by 12 (months).

The result is the projected revenue (or expense) for the current year.

Annualization may be based on days rather than months for greater specificity.

1. If we know that January year-to-date (YTD) revenue is $63,000 (July fiscal year = 7 months data).
2. $63,000 ÷ by 7 (months) = $9,000 (Average Monthly Revenue).
3. $9,000 × 12 (months) = $108,000.
4. The projected revenue for this year is $108,000.

Formula

Total Revenue/Expense YTD (Number of Months YTD =
Average Revenue/Expense Per Month
Multiply the average by 12 = Projected Annual Costs/Revenue.

One also needs to consider the federal wage index rating in your region. This index changes and is available on government websites (http://www.hcfa.gov) and in manuals.

Finally, one must consider payer information. Is the agency primarily serving Medicare patients? Is managed care a strong influence in the area? Does the agency participate in Medicaid? Does the agency provide home and community-based services? Does the agency target self-pay or private duty patients? Are there specific disease management programs in place with alternate sources of funding? Each of these factors impacts revenue.

Payor Type

It is important to be able to identify each *payor type* along with the volume for each type projected. Payor types include private insurance, Medicare, Medicaid, or out-of-pocket expense. See an example in Exhibit 9-4.

PPS—Prospective Payment System. Medicare's method of reimbursement based on specific criteria and, in home health, a 60-day time frame. A fixed reimbursement for care provided to a classification of patients.

Medicare reimburses on a prospective payment system (PPS) model, using a 60-day episode of care. The episodic reimbursement includes routine supplies as well as visit expenses.

Private insurance companies generally reimburse on a per visit basis, less than two hours of care. If the care requirements exceed this time frame generally there are additional negotiated charges OR an alternate form of care may be more appropriate (nursing home, etc.). Private insurance companies may or may not reimburse separately for supplies. Services covered vary widely, as does reimbursement. Each patient's insurance coverage will need to be verified and pre-authorized.

Per Diem—Literally "per day" reimbursement based on a day's total care. In a hospice a flat fee for each day of care, including all services provided to the patient (medication, equipment, nursing, etc.).

A hospice is commonly reimbursed on a per diem (literally "per day") basis. The manager will need to know what the per diem covers for a specific patient population. Have DME (Durable Medical Equipment) or certain drugs been *carved out* of the contract?

Some services are reimbursed on an hourly basis. Most frequently these include private duty, and home- and community-based services. *Home- and*

Exhibit 9-4 Average Payor Mix: For-Profit Agency

Private Insurance	23.5%
Out-of-Pocket/Private	24.4%
Medicare	28.4% (Single largest payor)
Medicaid	18.5%
Other Public	5.2%

> Carve-Out—Designation of a service or patient type to be excluded from a contract or financial reimbursement agreement. A group to be treated differently.

community-based services is a general term that refers to the various Medicaid Waiver programs and to state funded support services delivered in the home setting. Personal care, respite, and homemaker services are the types of care delivered through these programs. These services are designed to provide the elderly with support, allowing clients to stay in their home or extend the period of independence, postponing nursing home placement.

When developing the revenue portion of the operating budget, the manager must know what volume (amount) of care is delivered to patients in each payor category (see Exhibit 9-5.) Given the volumes, the amount of revenue for each type can be predicted and the total revenue projected. (See Exhibit 9-6.)

Charges and Reimbursement

One concept must be clearly understood by all those involved in budgeting and care delivery: There is little or no relationship between *charges* (what amount is charged for services given) and *reimbursement* (what is billed or received from the payor).

The agency determines *charges* based on the cost of delivering the care, the Medicare reimbursement limits, and other factors. These charges will be the same for a service regardless of payor type.

> *Tip*: A Medicare participating agency may not charge any payor less than they charge Medicare for the same service.

Exhibit 9-5   Example of Payor Type in Revenue Budget

The manager projects admissions/volumes as follows:

Medicare Episodes:	110 per month × 12 months = 1,320 episodes annually.
	Average reimbursement per episode: $2,100 (based on average case weight).
	Projected Medicare revenue for fiscal year: $2,772,000.
Private Insurance Visits:	70 admissions per month.
	Average # Visits/Admissions = 3.
	Total Visits = 210/month.
Revenue:	$70/Visit × 210 visits/month = $14,700 per month × 12 months.
Total Revenue:	$176,400 per year.
Projected Annual Revenue:	$2,772,000 + $176,400 = $2,948,400.

Exhibit 9-6   Common Revenue Categories in Home Care

Gross Revenue

Outpatient Revenue (visits):

Skilled Nursing

LPNs

Aides

Physical Therapy

Occupational Therapy

Speech Therapy

Social Work

Medical/Surgical Supplies

Other Revenue

Revenue Total:

Contractual Adjustment

Contractual Adjustment

Charity

Other Adjustments

Total Contractual Adjustment:

Total Net Revenue

After the charges are determined, the agency begins contract negotiations with insurance companies to determine acceptable reimbursement for the services. The difference between the amount charged and the contracted reimbursement is called the *contractual allowance.*

> Contractual Allowance = Amount Charged − Negotiated Reimbursement

The contractual allowance can easily be fifty percent of the total charges. When considering the revenue portion of the budget one must be certain to take into account all deductions from revenue, including contractual allowances.

Confusing? It can be. Let us look at an example. A cost analysis determines the actual cost of delivering a skilled nursing visit to a home health patient is $101.00. This includes nursing time and benefits, supplies, mileage reimbursement, and indirect expenses. The agency decides to charge $125.00 for the skilled nursing visit. Medicare will pay the federally mandated reimbursement per episode (based on the

HHRG—Home Health Resource Groups—value) regardless of the number of visits made to the patient during the 60-day episode (excluding LUPAs). LUPA refers to Low Utilization Payment Adjustment, the decrease in reimbursement implemented by Medicare when a patient had fewer than five visits during the 60-day episode. LUPAs and outliers are the exceptions to the HHRG reimbursement. Outliers refer to patients who incur unusually high costs during the home care episode. For these patients, CMS (Medicare) provides an additional reimbursement in excess of the usual HHRG payment. If the average reimbursement for the agency is $2,000.00, the agency will want the average number of visits per episode to be less than 20. Most States average from 18–20 visits per episode.

One insurance company may contract to reimburse the agency $75.00 per visit. Another insurance company's contract may pay "charges minus 20 percent" (a discount-off-charges model) or $100.00 per visit. So one would multiply the charge, $125, by 80 percent to determine what will actually be reimbursed ($125 × 0.80 = $100).

To summarize, the manager projecting the budget must take into account all of these variables when determining the amount of projected revenue for the budget year.

How Many? How Sick? Who Pays?

In addition to contractual allowances other deductions from revenue may influence the budget. *Charity* care, *bad debt*, and *denials* are all very common and must be considered in the budgeting process. *Charity* and *bad debt* are self-explanatory.

Denials are more complicated. Medicare uses various edits, or computer programs, to screen and monitor home health claims. The Medicare Fiscal Intermediary (FI) may screen by an "edit" placed in the computer system to look at all of a certain type of claim, (e.g., CHF patient with physical therapy). Alternately, Medicare may target a provider they wish to scrutinize more closely because of claims history. This is called Focused Medical Review (FMR). These edits may result in requests for more information, or Additional Development Requests (ADRs). This is Medicare's attempt to gather more information about the patient's care to determine if the care was medically necessary, provided in the amount appropriate for the patient, and delivered to a patient who qualified for the services.

A majority of the agencies in this country fail to respond to ADRs. *Failure to respond results in an immediate denial with a resulting recoupment of monies paid and loss of revenue for the episode of care.*

> **Tip**: *Always* respond to an ADR. The window of opportunity for response is short (30 days). Answer all ADRs in a timely manner.

After providing additional information to the FI (Medicare Fiscal Intermediary), payment may be made to the agency, or the agency may receive a denial. Medicare has a prescribed process for appealing a denial. Again many agencies fail to take this additional step, and again, time is limited. The vast majority of appeals are settled in the favor of the care provider, and appeals should be vigorously pursued by the agency.

Private insurance companies have appeals processes specific to their companies. These will be enumerated in the contract. The manager should be aware of the appeal process and use these processes whenever a claim is denied.

> *Tip*: An agency should have a 100-percent appeal philosophy, BUT if a technical error has occurred—for example, someone failed to pre-authorize the visits—the appeal is frivolous. Do not squander the agency's credibility on a losing cause.

Expenses

There are a multitude of expenses associated with a home health agency. These expenses, or line items, in the budget are generally grouped into two categories: *direct* and *indirect* expenses.[1]

Direct expenses are those expenses directly associated with the delivery of care. Salaries are generally the greatest percentage of direct expenses, often 50 percent or more of the total expense budget. Mileage reimbursement and supplies are other direct expenses.

Indirect expenses may include benefits, utilities, rent, and other overhead expenses not directly associated with patient care but that are necessary for the operation of the agency. When constructing a budget and when calculating the cost of delivering a service, both direct and indirect expenses must be considered. Benefits, for example, may cost the agency 20 percent of salaries—a very significant expense and one you do not want to overlook in your calculations.

If the agency is hospital-based, or part of a large corporate entity, *management allocations* are a reality. Management allocations are fees paid for corporate or support services provided to the agency by the corporate body or hospital. Human Resources is one service often centrally located in the corporate offices or hospital and designed to service all parts of the organization. Information Systems, Employee Health, and Maintenance/Engineering are other examples of services that may be included in management allocations. Administrators and support staff of the corporate body must be paid, and these expenses are apportioned or allocated to the agencies or departments in the organization as part of the management allocation.

---

[1]For more information on budget terms, see Chapters 10 and 11 in Dunham-Taylor and Pinczuk (2006) *Health Care Financial Management for Nurse Managers: Merging the Heart with the Dollar*. Sudbury, MA: Jones & Bartlett.

Costing Out a Service

Cost accounting is a fairly complex and precise accounting concept. The nurse manager is unlikely to master this level of accounting without additional education. However, learning to cost out a service is fairly simple. The manager uses this process when considering a new service, determining if an existing service is profitable, drilling down in statistics that are unclear, and other situations.

For example, you discover a benchmark that states the cost of a skilled nursing visit averages $46.00 direct expense and $55.00 indirect expense in agencies similar to yours. You want to know how your costs compare to this benchmark. If the results are positive (you deliver services for less than this average) you may want to share this information with your accountant or hospital finance department. How do you determine your costs for a skilled nursing visit?

Direct Costs

Salary: RN salary per hour times average visit time: $20.00 x 1.33 (hrs.) = $26.60

Benefits: 20% times salary cost: $26.60 x 20% = $5.32
Mileage: Average 15 miles per visit x current reimbursement. 15 x 0.36 = $5.40

Supplies: Est. $1.00
(A routine visit without wound care requires gloves, thermometer cover, soap, towels, etc. Calculate costs based on your average.)

Total Direct Costs: $38.32

Indirect Costs

This is where calculations become more difficult. Supervision and management costs must be budgeted. These individuals must be available to support the team member making the visit. Management schedules visits, reviews documentation, and performs a multitude of other functions absolutely necessary to the nurse in the field.

The receptionist answering the phone, file and payroll clerks, the team member who reviews certifications and audits charts, the supply clerk, etc., all contribute to and add to the cost of the visit.

Performance Improvement Coordinators, agency educators, and computer technologists, and so forth contribute less directly but also must be considered in the indirect cost of this visit.

How do we determine these costs? A cost accountant might examine the amount of time spent by each support person and assign a cost to the activity. Most managers know there are numerous individuals who have an impact on the cost of this visit and it is extremely difficult to calculate these costs with a degree of certainty. The simplest way to account for these costs is to:

> **ADD ALL SUPPORT STAFF COSTS (SALARY AND BENEFITS).**
> **DIVIDE BY THE TOTAL NUMBER OF VISITS.**

This provides a rough estimate of the cost of indirect support personnel per visit. Now let's apply this to an example.

Example

$33.00	The cost of support staff divided by number of visits. (Support staff includes supervisors, managers, administrators at a higher cost per hour than RNs.)
$18.00	Combine rent, utilities, insurances, etc., and divide by the number of visits.
$10.00	If hospital-based there will be additional expense in the form of a hospital allocation.
	Miscellaneous additional expenses might include overtime, contract labor, depreciation, or incentive pay
$61.00	**Total Indirect Expense**

Determine Cost of a Skilled Nursing Visit

To determine the cost of a skilled nursing visit, one would add the direct and indirect costs.

What is the Cost of a Skilled Nursing Visit?

$38.32	Direct Cost
$61.00	Indirect Cost
$99.32	**Total, or Cost of a Skilled Nursing Visit**

Now you can compare your cost of $99.32 for a skilled nursing visit to the benchmark of $101.00, and you have something to share with the finance department and your team. This is the kind of information needed to plan, and it should be shared. ***Give your team a pat on the back!***

To determine the viability of the service the next step is to compare this cost with the reimbursement you receive for the visit. At this step consider the percent of charity care and bad debt in the calculation.

Staffing and Salary Expense

Direct Expense: FTEs

In staff budgets, there is a difference between the number of employees and Full-Time Equivalents or FTEs. An agency may employee 200 individuals and budget for 120 FTEs. How is this computed? An FTE is a calculation of paid hours. For example, two part-time employees may, together, work 2080 hours (40 hours/week times 52 weeks) and be considered one FTE. Several PRN employees may work variable hours and equal less than one FTE.

> *FTE*—Full-time equivalent. 2,080 hours of worked time. 40 hours per week x 52 weeks.

Overtime hours increase the number of FTEs but not the number of people employed. Each overtime hour worked is calculated as 1.5 hours (or more). Depending on the organization's pay system, premium pay, shift differential, and call pay may also increase cost. Include in staffing calculations projected time off[2]—vacation (80 hours), holiday (48 hours), and sick time. Will a substitute be required during these periods? 128 hours of paid time off is equal to 0.06 FTE. When budgeting a critical full-time position with these benefits, one would budget 1.06 FTEs. Many organizations use an "average salary per FTE" calculation as one parameter of the budget. The average salary considers all of the adjustments to pay at all pay levels, and results in a calculated average salary expense per worked hour.

Staffing Models

When determining the staffing model for the agency a manager considers the need for flexibility, the value of several available PRN staff, job sharing, and other innovative approaches to staffing. Then, the manager balances the benefits of these resources with the cost incurred by each individual employed. For example, malpractice or liability insurance, worker's compensation insurance,

---

[2]This is called nonproductive time. Much greater detail on budget terms and calculations is presented in Dunham-Taylor and Pinczuk (2006). *Health Care Financial Management for Nurse Managers: Merging the Heart with the Dollar.*

and the cost of some other benefits such as FICA are based on the number of individuals employed.

The manager may consider a policy that encourages flexibility in the staffing plan while controlling costs for unproductive PRN staff. One approach is to develop a policy for PRN staff with limiting criteria. For example, "PRN employees who have not worked during the past quarter (three months) will be terminated from the employment role," or "PRN employees must work a minimum of one weekend each quarter to maintain their employment status."

Does the agency staff 24/7, or is the agency primarily an 8:00–5:00 entity? Is the agency a Monday through Friday provider? How many patients are seen twice a day requiring a 3–11 shift? What about daily visits and the need for several weekend staff? Is the agency paying differentials for evenings or weekends? Are Baylor positions budgeted (working only weekends for premium pay)? All these factors must be considered when choosing staffing models and determining staffing costs.

With the expanding shortage of nurses, therapists, pharmacists, and other health care professionals, contract staff and 'travelers' are used more often. (These individuals may not be available in all areas of the country, and experienced home health contract staff are not commonly available.) This method of staffing is extremely expensive. The manager will need to make additional calculations to determine if contract staff is a viable option for the agency. If the agency is Joint Commission of Accreditation of Healthcare Organizations (JCAHO) or Community Health Accreditation Program, Inc. (CHAP) accredited, contract staff must meet the specific requirements of the accrediting agency. Check the accreditation standards for this information. Include the requirements for the contract document in your review.

Staff Reimbursement Models

Staff reimbursement models vary as much as third party payor reimbursement methods, and greatly influence the cost of employing the home health staff. Productivity may also be influenced by agency pay policies, and salary levels influence agency recruitment and retention.

The most common reimbursement structure in home health is *hourly* reimbursement. A per-hour pay structure may be used for all agency personnel, or for specific segments of the team. For example, office-based support staff are commonly reimbursed on an hourly basis. When reimbursing hourly, the manager includes overtime in the calculation of total salary expense. This structure is simple and well accepted. The wage and hour laws are clear and defined. Productivity may be an issue, and may require monitoring by management. Overtime has a habit of 'creeping' up. Process review and vigilance can maintain overtime for the organization below two percent.

Reimbursement by *salary* is another common model for staff reimbursement. A salaried individual may be exempt or non-exempt. The *exempt* team member is paid for the specified job description and group of duties, rather than a specified number of hours. There is no reimbursement for overtime. A full-time salaried, exempt individual may work 35 hours one week and 50 hours the next week, and the salary collected by the individual remains based on the pre-arranged rate with no variation for the number of hours worked. Exemption of a salaried employee requires specific criteria—for example, supervision of other team members. Check specific state and federal wage and hour laws, or discuss these issues with the Human Resources Department or labor law attorney for specific guidelines. An employee may be salaried and non-exempt. In this model there is a pre-determined salary for an individual, usually a non-supervisory team member. However, when applicable, overtime is paid.

Some agencies pay *per visit*. Health care professionals performing a unique service or working on a contract basis may be reimbursed on a per visit basis. To avoid violating wage and hour laws, this method of pay is generally reserved for professionals providing complex care and working autonomously. Registered nurses and licensed therapists may qualify depending on their job duties, level of autonomy, and supervisory responsibilities.

The per-visit pay policy should define exactly what is included in the per-visit reimbursement. Does the visit include travel time, time spent documenting and calling the physician, direct care, case conferences, and attendance at staff meetings? How many meetings are required and included in the per visit reimbursement? This salary model can be more complicated because a visit is not necessarily a physical visit. Will a three-hour admission visit and the associated paperwork count as a routine one-hour visit, or two visits, or some permutation of these? How will a high tech visit requiring monitoring of a six-hour intravenous infusion be paid? These are determinations agency management must make before embarking on this method of reimbursement.

> *Tip*: When this model is used, the agency cannot mix per-visit reimbursement with hourly reimbursement in the same pay period. It is possible to develop a salary-based model with a per-visit bonus rewarding specific levels of productivity.

Since the implementation of Medicare PPS, *per-visit pay* has become very popular with home health agencies. The system generally has a very positive effect on productivity and recruitment. The challenge is that staff must be monitored *very* closely to ensure quality of care does not suffer as staff attempt to do more visits than is reasonable in a day. Another negative is the tendency of team members to become task-oriented, and concentrate on the visit rather than care management.

Productivity and FTEs

Productivity levels of staff can be determined. Exhibit 9-7 shows how to determine the productivity level of a home health RN.

The average visit takes 1 hour and 20 minutes (1.33 hours).

An 8-hour day ÷ 1.33 hours = ***Average Productivity***, or ***6 visits/day***

The industry is examining a *per-episode* salary model. At this time the literature has not documented successful use of this structure. Many challenges must be overcome before per-episode reimbursement becomes a workable reimbursement system. Continuity of caregivers is one challenge to making this model feasible. However, with Medicare episodic reimbursement and an emphasis on outcomes, a per-episode pay model could be very attractive.

Another critical staffing consideration is the *ratio of office* or *support staff to direct care givers*. Direct care givers produce revenue. Support staff cost the agency money. The support is absolutely critical to the operation of the agency, and this segment of the staff can grow quickly. New supervisors and managers have a tendency to hire more people in an attempt to solve problems. Adding an FTE (particularly a support FTE) may be necessary, but should be considered a last resort. Before hiring, the manager should examine processes, re-engineer paper flow, and examine all aspects of the in-house workload. Benchmarks exist for agencies in various governance systems and these ratios are good tools for the manager, particularly when defending the budget to owners or administrators.

Recruitment and *retention* are staffing issues often overlooked. Estimates on the cost of recruiting and training a new team member vary widely—$18,000 to $50,000 dollars or more per new hire (depending on the position filled). Money spent recognizing and providing incentives for retention of team members may be far less costly. When defending a budget request for these additional monies, gather the statistics specific to your area and organization, and be prepared to explain the request in purely financial terms.

Exhibit 9-7   Productivity Calculations for Home Health RN

Visit Time (Hands-on care)	30–50 Minutes	Average 45 Minutes	45 Minutes
Documentation Time	10–20 Minutes	Average 15 Minutes	15 Minutes
Travel Time	20 Minutes		20 Minutes
Total			**1 hour and 20 minutes**

Mileage is a huge direct expense in home health, and one not generally a factor in other health care delivery models. It is not unusual for employees in a medium-size agency to drive one and a half million miles a year. At the current federal mileage reimbursement rate, this is an expense of over $500,000 annually. Agencies are not required to reimburse for mileage. The individual employee can document work-related mileage and deduct this expense on their income tax return. Direct reimbursement for mileage is an expectation of home health care employees and may be a recruitment tool.

Supplies are also a large direct expense, especially for the agency providing wound care. Generally, supplies are bundled into the Medicare or insurance reimbursement. This means the full cost of the supplies is borne by the agency. For example:

Mr. B. requires several hundred 4 × 4's and ABD dressings, tape, saline, and other supplies twice a day. The cost of these supplies is $20.00 per visit, $40.00 per day, and $1,200.00 per month. The patient has an existing colostomy unrelated to the agency's plan of care, and Medicare requires the agency to provide the ostomy supplies, an additional $120.00 per month. Supply costs for this patient during the 60-day episode exceed $2,650.00. Add staffing costs of two visits per day or $10,800.00, and the cost of care exceeds $13,450.00. The maximum Medicare reimbursement per episode is 2.81 times the average episodic payment or approximately $6,000.00. This is an example of the impact of case mix on the budgeting process. One hopes the agency admits several patients with low supply costs to offset the expense of the more resource intensive patients.

History is a helpful indicator of supply costs. Consider the historical average supply cost per patient and add an inflation factor when budgeting for the coming year. Consider any exceptional factor—for example, a new surgeon with a desire for a specific and expensive wound treatment, or a precipitous increase in the cost of a commonly used supply. If the agency has added a new service and has no history of costs, consider requesting benchmarking data from the National Association of Home Care (NAHC), do a literature search, and/or talk to others in the industry so your estimate is as accurate as possible.

The popularity of technology, such as point-of-service documentation, has increased tremendously in home care. Point-of-service care delivery refers to the computerized technology in the patient's home. Data is entered into the computer device by the nurse/therapist at the time the care is delivered. The data then populates the required fields in the Plan of Treatment (485) or creates the visit record used by the agency. The 485 is the common name given to the home health Plan of Treatment. The home health plan of treatment documents the patient's demographics, medications, equipment in use, and the physician's order for care including duration and frequency of visits. The 485 provides the official guidelines for the patient's care. The 485 may be augmented by supplemental orders throughout the patient's 60-day episode. This technology has both decreased the paper burden and added its own expenses to home care. Adopting this technology requires long-range planning for replacement of hardware, upgrades to software, computer technology support, and extensive training of care staff.

Indirect Expense

Depending on the agency structure and the budget format, employee benefits may be a direct or indirect expense. Utilities, billing and collection costs, recruitment, and insurances are examples of indirect expenses.

A note about benefits: Benefits are a significant and growing expense for all industries. In health care a benefit package may easily cost the agency an additional 20 percent of the employee's base salary. When recruiting and interviewing, be sure to include benefits in the total reimbursement package presented to the prospective employee. When calculating costs of delivering care, include benefit costs in the total.

Home health is very documentation, and therefore paper, intensive. The OASIS initial comprehensive assessment may well be 25 pages in length. If the agency does not use point-of-service computer technology, these forms must be printed. Nurses and therapists feel most secure when they have copies of several chart forms in their hand, and copying is a significant expense in most agencies. Folders, chart binders, pens, paperclips, etc., are other examples of necessary office supplies.

Other indirect expenses include: telephones, fax expenses, education programs, orientation, and repairs to equipment. Other common expenses that may be overlooked include: licenses, subscriptions, dues, and accreditation expenses (CHAP, JCAHO). Marketing activities and expenses are frequently excluded from the hospital-based agency budget. In my opinion, this is one of the most serious errors an agency can make. Because the home care community is extremely competitive, and educating the community, working with potential referral sources to insure their understanding of the agency's services, and problem solving with physician's offices, are marketing efforts critical to the success of a home care agency, these activities should always be included in the budget.

A sample expense budget follows in Exhibit 9-8.

Exhibit 9-7   Sample Expense Budget Items

Expense		Other	
	Productive Salary		**Leases & Rentals Office**
	Non-Productive Salary		**Leases–Storage**
	Contract Staff		**Travel, Meetings**
	Employee Benefits		
	• Payroll Taxes–FICA		**Mileage**
	• Administrative Fees		• Nursing
	• Employee Appreciation		• Phys. Therapy
	• Tuition Reimbursement		• Occ. Therapy
	• Education Loan Forgiveness		• Social Work
	Professional Fees		**License & Permits**
	• Consulting		**Postage**
	• Medical Dir. Fees		**Courier**
	• Physician Fees		**Repairs**
	Supplies		**Repairs–Equipment**
	• General & Adm. Supplies		**Maintenance Contracts**
	• Printing		**Marketing**
	• Medical Supplies–Chargeable		• Creative
	• Medical Supplies–Non-Chargeable		• Productive
	• Medical Supplies–Rented		• Other
	• Non-Medical Supplies		**Infectious Waste**
	• Drugs & Pharmaceuticals		**Disposal**
	• Food		
	• Non-Capital Equipment		**Insurance**
	• Books/Manuals		
	• Miscellaneous Supplies		**Other Expenses**
	Utilities		
	• Telephone–Local		
	• Telephone–Long Distance		
	• Cellular Telephones & Pagers		
	• Utilities & Electricity		
	• Gas & Oil		
	• Water & Sewer		
	• Trash Collection		

Defending Your Budget

After spending hours gathering information, discussing the numbers with your staff, projecting revenues, and documenting expected costs, you put it all together in the format requested by the organization. The difference between the revenue and the expense is your bottom line or *gross margin*. This total may be a positive number—a *profit margin*—or a negative number—a *deficit*. Deficits are generally placed in parentheses ( ). The hospital finance department, agency owner, or investors don't like to see any ( )! Even if the bottom line on your projected budget promises a profit, you may be asked several questions about individual revenue projections or expense items. *Be prepared*. Have a reasonable explanation for each of the projections. Explain what changes you plan to correct the deficit, or what exceptional situation is beyond your control that is causing you to project these numbers. When requesting additional staffing, be prepared to demonstrate the additional revenue expected to be generated by the additional staff, or to indicate the regulation requiring the additional staffing expense.

How does an agency change the gross margin? It can be done in one of two ways:

1. To increase the revenue.
2. To decrease the expenses.

If the agency's financial situation requires a change in the bottom line the manager should decide which of these approaches will be implemented and how. Will a new service be added, or marketing expanded to increase revenue? Will services be restructured, staff positions eliminated, or other steps taken to reduce costs?

In the past there was little statistical information related to home health agencies. Home health agencies were often privately owned, and proprietary statistics were 'secret.' Independent financial audits were infrequent. With the introduction of OASIS, and the health care industry's emphasis on costs and outcomes, there is now a wide variety of cost and quality benchmarking data available for home health agencies. Sources of statistics and benchmarks include National Association of Health Care (NAHC), state hospital organizations, and publications such as *The Remington Report* and "home health line." Statistics exist for average supply cost per visit and there are salary surveys for home care positions. Unfortunately many of the best sources of home health information require a commitment of finances. For example "home health line" (customer@decisionhealth.com) is a very popular newsletter for the industry and the current subscription price is $457.00 per year.

> *Benchmarks*—A goal to be reached. A standard. Common benchmarks exist for productivity and average cost of a visit. Medicare publishes clinical benchmarks. (See Exhibit 9-9.)

Exhibit 9-9 is a reproduction of the type of graph provided by CMS to home health agencies for benchmarking purposes. Over 40 parameters are measured and the reports are accessible through the Internet. The reference bar refers to the national agency average for the time period monitored. OASIS data is compiled from assessments performed by the agency and transmitted to the government,

Exhibit 9-9   Improvement in Ambulation/Locomotion

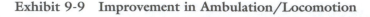

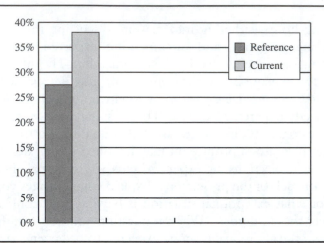

then the national average is computed. The report provides individual agencies with their outcome for the time period, allowing comparison with the average. In the actual report, a third bar provides the agency's previous quarter's results, and therefore provides a means of tracking improvement (or decline) in outcomes. These results are reviewed by surveyors before they make licensure and certification visits to the agency. The surveyors use the outcomes to target areas where the agency may have a problem or opportunity for improvement.

Come to the budget meeting armed with this data. These are valuable tools when defending your budget.

Present an action plan. For example, if bad debt is extensive, explain the steps taken to reduce the debt and the improvement you anticipate in the coming year. If charity care is projected at an all-time high, explain how the agency saves the hospital money by accepting charity patients and freeing up hospital beds for other patients. Back this up with statistics. Presenting the budget to the Administration is the agency manager's opportunity to promote the agency. Present the good things accomplished during the past year. Request changes in the projected budget designed to enhance the agency's services and/or reward the staff.

Budget Variances:
Evaluating the Budget Throughout the Year

The hospital or agency accountant provides a report on the budget for management on a regular basis, usually monthly. These reports are often called *variance reports*. The variance report documents *actual* revenues and expenses for the month compared to those projected at the time the budget was developed, and clearly documents variances from what was projected in the budget. As the year progresses the variance report will include year-to-date as well as monthly results. Following is an example of a variance report.

Exhibit 9-10   Nurse's Heaven Home Care and Hospice Statement of Revenue and Expenses

	MONTH OF MARCH					NINE MONTHS YEAR TO DATE				
	Actual	Budget	Bud Var	Prior Yr	PY Var	Actual	Budget	Bud Var	Prior Yr	PY Var
Patient Revenue										
Inpatient Revenue	0	0	0.0%	0	0.0%	0	0	0.0%	0	0.0%
Outpatient Revenue	1,483,820	1,612,282	-8.0%	1,581,501	-6.2%	13,651,461	14,510,538	-5.9%	14,483,087	-5.7%
Total Gross Patient Revenue	1,483,820	1,612,282	-8.0%	1,581,501	-6.2%	13,651,461	14,510,538	-5.9%	14,483,087	-5.7%
Deductions from Revenue										
Contractual Adjustments	497,924	608,586	18.2%	650,977	23.5%	4,624,531	5,477,274	15.6%	5,492,832	15.8%
Bad Debt	(58)	0	100.0%	7,166	100.0%	(1,024)	0	100.0%	42,852	102.4%
Charity	0	2,083	100.0%	29,902	100.0%	19,864	18,747	-6.0%	46,647	57.4%
Total Deductions	497,866	610,669	18.5%	688,044	27.6%	4,643,371	5,496,021	15.5%	5,582,331	16.8%
Net Patient Service Revenue	985,954	1,001,613	-1.6%	893,458	10.4%	9,008,090	9,014,517	-0.1%	8,900,757	1.2%
Other Operating Revenue	2,612	4,849	-46.1%	9,111	-71.3%	30,589	43,641	-29.9%	30,427	0.5%
Total Operating Revenue	988,565	1,006,462	-1.8%	902,569	9.5%	9,038,678	9,058,158	-0.2%	8,931,183	1.2%
Operating Expense										
Salaries	472,419	464,369	-1.7%	477,556	1.1%	4,072,794	4,173,623	2.4%	4,037,880	-0.9%
Contract Labor	3,346	1,242	-169.4%	1,648	-103.0%	17,832	11,142	-60.0%	23,831	25.2%
Employee Benefits	220,264	108,585	-102.8%	90,184	-144.2%	964,649	977,265	1.3%	798,995	-20.7%
Fees	229,867	202,332	-13.6%	200,164	-14.8%	1,734,137	1,826,388	5.1%	1,726,664	-0.4%
Supplies	61,273	50,011	-22.5%	51,726	-18.5%	466,263	450,099	-3.6%	399,612	-16.7%
Utilities	6,308	7,787	19.0%	2,517	-150.6%	46,493	70,083	33.7%	27,611	-68.4%
Other Expense	63,780	71,496	10.8%	41,800	-52.6%	559,361	643,464	13.1%	360,787	-55.0%
Depreciation	6,229	9,003	30.8%	3,333	-86.9%	64,928	81,027	19.9%	25,986	-149.9%
Amortization	0	0	0.0%	0	0.0%	0	0	0.0%	0	0.0%
Interest & Taxes	0	0	0.0%	0	0.0%	0	0	0.0%	0	0.0%
Management Fees	30,848	30,848	0.0%	19,705	-56.5%	254,224	254,224	0.0%	196,787	-29.2%
Total Operating Expense	1,094,333	945,673	-15.7%	888,633	-23.1%	8,180,680	8,487,315	3.6%	7,598,152	-7.7%
Net Operating Income	(105,767)	60,789	-274.0%	13,936	-859.0%	857,998	570,843	50.3%	1,333,032	-35.6%
Investment Income	37	28	31.9%	49	-24.3%	2,130	252	745.2%	371	474.6%
Realized Gain on Investments	0	0	0.0%	0	0.0%	0	0	0.0%	0	0.0%
Gain / (Loss) from Affiliates	0	0	0.0%	0	0.0%	0	0	0.0%	0	0.0%
Gain / (Loss) on Disposal	(207,835)	0	100.0%	0	100.0%	(207,835)	0	100.0%	0	100.0%
Minority Interest	0	0	0.0%	0	0.0%	0	0	0.0%	0	0.0%
Incentive Pay	0	0	0.0%	0	0.0%	0	0	0.0%	0	0.0%
Other Non Operating Income	0	0	0.0%	0	0.0%	0	0	0.0%	0	0.0%
Total Revenue Over Expense Before CFVIRS	(313,565)	60,817	-615.6%	13,985	-2342.2%	652,293	571,095	14.2%	1,333,402	-51.1%
Change in Fair Value of Interest Rate Swaps	0	0	0.0%	0	0.0%	0	0	0.0%	0	0.0%
Total Excess Revenue Over Expense	(313,565)	60,817	-615.6%	13,985	-2342.2%	652,293	571,095	14.2%	1,333,402	-51.1%
Net Unrealized Gain / (Loss) on Investments	0	0	0.0%	0	0.0%	0	0	0.0%	0	0.0%
Total Increase in Unrestricted Net Assets	(313,565)	60,817	-615.6%	13,985	-2342.2%	652,293	571,095	14.2%	1,333,402	-51.1%
EBITDA Before CFVIRS	(307,336)	69,820	-540.2%	17,318	-1874.7%	717,221	652,122	10.0%	1,359,388	-47.2%
EBITDA	(307,336)	69,820	-540.2%	17,318	-1874.7%	717,221	652,122	10.0%	1,359,388	-47.2%

Source: National Association of Home Care (www.nahc.org)

In this example, the left side of the variance report refers to the previous month. Revenues are below budget, with a greater than expected decrease in contractual adjustments. This results in a slightly positive Total Operating Revenue to budgeted projections. Expenses indicate salaries were less than budgeted; this is what we would expect with a decrease in revenues (volume). If revenues were up, then we expect the cost of delivering that care (salaries, mileage, etc.) to also increase. The manager places more emphasis on relationships between line items and trends rather than to specific monthly numbers. In this example, the bottom line: earnings before interest, taxes, depreciation and amortization (EBITDA) is *very* positive for the month and for the year-to-date.

The right side of this table provides year-to-date statistics. This is where the trends become more evident. Numerous issues may affect statistics for one month and the statistics may be insignificant; however, several months of statistics make a trend. In this example, revenues have consistently been below budget for the year, however, other expense has been controlled and the agency is actually exceeding budgeted EBITDA. This is a trend we want to see!

Variance reports are usable management tools. It is important to consider questions like: Are revenues down? Is the decrease related to volume or bills not being sent in a timely fashion? Are expenses up? Is the cause an increase in overtime or an unexpected expense? It is helpful to share these reports with key supervisors in the agency, and to share at least an aggregate with the entire staff. When the budget review is positive, an opportunity arises to give a collective pat-on-the-back to the team. If the picture is less rosy, processes can be changed and direction given to bring things back in line.

Conclusion: Future Challenges

The number of home health agencies grew dramatically during the 1980s and early 1990s. The Balanced Budget Act of 1997 dramatically changed home care reimbursement and caused an equally dramatic decline in the number of home care agencies. See Exhibit 9-11.

The number of agencies has stabilized. Acquisition and growth are once again increasing in the industry. Most likely, we can expect further consolidation with larger for-profit home care organizations. It will become more and more difficult for small agencies to survive, whether independent or hospital-based. For financial stability, to offset the increasing expense and volume of high acuity patients and charity patients, a large volume of patients will be needed.

Regulations and competition are likely to increase. Good management and delivery of quality care will continue to be primary to success.

Technology will continue to increase. Disease management will become a primary focus as CMS moves toward prevention and outcomes reimbursement.

Home care has always been a challenging area of health care and those challenges will continue. Home care has also been a caring, innovative, productive segment of health care. This too will continue. Best wishes as you manage your agency.

Exhibit 9-10   Number of Home Health Agencies in the United States

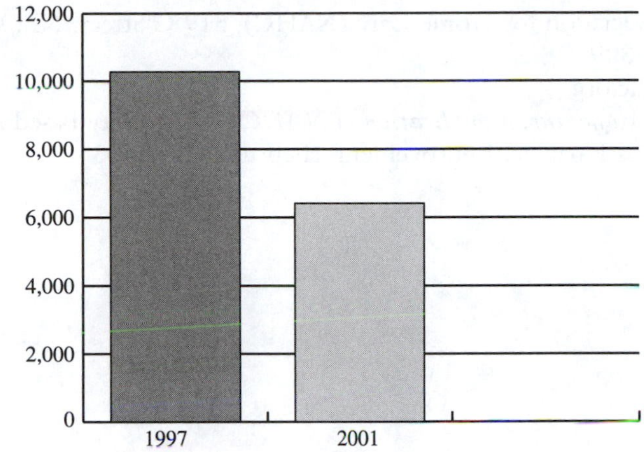

Source: National Association of Home Care (www.nahc.org).

References

Collins, J. (2001). *Good to Great.* New York: HarperCollins.

National Association For Health Care. Retrieved from NAHC.org/consumer/hcstats.html.

Rooney, H. & Long, C. (January/February 2003). Key Performance Measures. *The Remington Report*, 4–20.

Helpful References and Websites

American Health Care Association: www.AHCA.org

Baker, J., & Baker, R. (2000). *Health Care Finance.* Gaithersburg, MD: Aspen.

Centers for Medicare and Medicaid Services (CMS): www.CMS.hhs.gov/default.asp?
(The CMS website has numerous links for statistics, regulations, industry updates and other information.) Their address is:
Centers for Medicare and Medicaid Services
7500 Security Boulevard,
Baltimore, MD 21244-1850

Health Care Advisory Board, Washington, DC (chenga@advisory.com)
The Advisory Board provides research and reports among other services to members including industry projections and trends. The focus of the Board is acute care hospitals and the statistical information can be very helpful to the home care manager. Advisory.Com, Finance Watch of the Financial Leadership Council.

Home Health Care Nurse. J.B. Lippincott Co., 12107 Ins. Way, Hagerstown, MD 21740

"Home Health Line" (customer@decisionhealth.com) Current subscription price: $457/year.

National Association for Home Care (NAHC), 519 C Street, NE, Washington, DC 20002-5809
www.nahc.org
Caring Magazine, a publication of NAHC. Productivity-based Annual Budget Hardwires Financial Improvement. (February 27, 2003)

PART IV

Ambulatory Care Issues

Chapter 10 covers the reimbursement process in ambulatory settings—community health centers, rural health centers, or private practice settings—where the advanced nurse practitioner is either employed or self-employed. This chapter describes the different clinic types, administrative operations, and the types of contracts that affect their environment, as well as the important issues that should be addressed before signing the contract as a provider of health care services. Information is provided regarding how to determine allowable costs for billing as well as policies and procedures that must be in place for compliance with federal and state regulations. The types of insurance providers such as MCOs, PSOs, and PPOs and basic billing procedures for coding and identifying levels of services are also discussed. There are also helpful definitions of terminology used in the billing setting for diagnosis coding.

Chapter 11, written by an administrator in ambulatory care, discusses managing ambulatory care resources—both staff and equipment/supplies—and the importance of increasing the revenue flow to the organization. This is critical now with prospective payment in effect. The author discusses, and gives examples, of the capital and operating budgets as well as an explanation of being able to determine the contribution margin using volume projections based on reimbursement rates. Lastly, she uses this information to determine charges and cost out services. She points out the importance of both quality and patient satisfaction as they will have a direct impact on the budget.

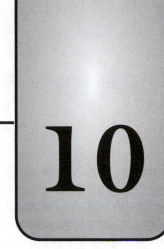

10

Nurse Practitioner Reimbursement in Primary Care

Carol Lee Logan

Introduction

Reimbursement is like a puzzle, constantly changing with different sized pieces that have to be fitted together. There are several "tools" available to help one to more effectively fit these pieces together. This chapter addresses the reimbursement process in ambulatory settings—private practice settings, rural health clinics, or community health centers—where the advanced nurse practitioner is either employed or is self-employed.

Primary Care Settings

Private Practice Offices/Contracted Services

Nurse practitioners are primarily employed in private practice, nursing homes, school-based health centers, or industrial settings; or are under contract to provide primary, specialized or occupational health care. Depending on the employment status, advanced nurse practitioners may be contracted to provide independent direct services, or to provide services as a physician extender. Note: State rules regarding the scope of practice vary from state to state. An employment contract is a written agreement defining the scope of services to be performed, as well as the responsibilities and expectations of the contract employee. This comprehensive agreement should protect both the employee and the employer, and indicate how the compensation is to be calculated. This rate could be hourly, a straight salary, a percentage of net receipts, or a base salary with an incentive bonus such as a percentage of a preset goal. Other issues one might include are: the benefit package, leave for continuing education, vacation and sick leave, malpractice expense, and other specifics about the work environment (Buppert, 1999).

The contract should also consider the type of reimbursement for providing these services. Reimbursement differs greatly depending on the employment status of the nurse practitioner. These complications are covered later in this chapter, under the section titled "*Who Reimburses Advanced Nurse Practitioners?*"

Rural Health Clinic

Another primary care practice setting is the Rural Health Clinic. The Rural Health Clinics Act (P.L. 95-210) was passed by Congress in 1977 and implemented in 1978. The goal of this Act is twofold. First, it encourages the use of midlevel practitioners by providing Medicare and Medicaid reimbursement for their services, even in the absence of a full-time physician. Second, it creates a cost-based reimbursement mechanism to generate additional revenue to eligible rural practices. This Act provides a reimbursement option for primary care practices located in rural areas with an underserved designation (Travers, Ellis, and Dartt, 1995). There are two types of rural health clinics identified in this Act— independent and provider-based. An independent rural health clinic is a free-standing practice that is not part of a hospital, skilled nursing facility, or home health agency. The provider-based rural health clinic is an integral part of a health care organization, housed within a hospital, skilled nursing facility, or home health agency.

A rural health clinic must be located in a rural area with a federal designation as medically underserved. This designation includes the following categories:

a medically underserved population, a health profession shortage area, a health profession shortage population, or a high migrant impact area. The governor of the state can designate an area as having a shortage of personal health services, which is then certified by the Secretary of the Department of Health and Human Services.

Federally Qualified Health Center

A third primary care practice setting is the federally qualified health center program, which was enacted under the Omnibus Budget Reconciliation Act (OBRA) in 1989, and expanded under OBRA in 1990. This program was started to provide medical services for Medicare and Medicaid beneficiaries at a reasonable cost. This covers migrant health needs as well as homeless health care (included in the Public Health Services Act: Section 329, Migrant Health Center; Section 330, Community Health Center; and Section 340, Health Care for the Homeless), and Tribal Indian Health Centers, which are automatically eligible for federally qualified health center status.

A federally qualified health center can either be located in a medically underserved area, or serve a medically underserved population. There are no requirements for midlevel staffing in a federally qualified health center. A practice not receiving federal funding may obtain federally qualified health center status from the Center for Medicare and Medicaid and is referred to as a look-alike.

Rural Health Clinic versus Federally Qualified Health Center

Both rural health clinics and federally qualified health center programs share a common theme. The preservation and expansion of needed primary care health services in underserved areas is a primary goal. Associated with the primary goal is the legitimate recovery of reasonable costs medical services provided to Medicare and Medicaid beneficiaries. The cost-based reimbursement is basically the same for a federally qualified rural health center and a federally qualified health center. There are, however, some differences in the eligibility criteria (location, federal designation, corporate structure, board of directors, staffing requirements, scope of services, and the type of provider) and reimbursement. For more information, see the website at: http://cms.hhs.gov/pubforms.

When making the choice between the two programs, the financial effect is a key factor. Rates are determined yearly by Medicare based on the center's cost report. Reimbursement is based on allowable costs that result from providing covered medical services. Allowable costs include direct costs for providing patient care, such as salaries and supplies, and an allocated portion of overhead for administrative and facility expenses. As shown in Exhibit 10-1, this example facility's total costs are $700,000.

Exhibit 10-1   Allowable Costs Resulting from Providing Covered Medical Services

Direct Costs	Provider salaries	$440,000
	Other professional salaries	$120,000
	Medical supplies	$ 15,000
Overhead	Administrative salaries	$ 70,000
	Office supplies	$ 10,000
	Rent and utilities	$ 45,000
TOTAL		$700,000

If the practice provides non-covered services, such as inpatient services, these costs are excluded from the all-inclusive reimbursement rate. Inpatient services are billed on a fee-for-service basis rather than a cost-based formula. In this case, there is a complicated formula on the cost report to determine the allowable overhead. Exhibit 10-2 presents the most commonly used allocation method.

The steps involved in allocating overhead are as follows:

1. Determine the allowable and non-allowable direct service costs and the practice overhead costs, as show in the *direct costs* line on the table.

2. Calculate the percentages of allowable and non-allowable direct costs to total costs less overhead costs, as shown in the *percent of direct costs* line.

3. Multiply the overhead cost times each direct cost percentage, as calculated in Step 2, to arrive at the overhead allocation amount, as shown in the *overhead allocation* line.

4. Add the allocation of overhead, which was calculated in Step 3, to the direct service cost, as shown in the *total* line (Travers, Ellis, and Dartt).

The allowable costs ($560,000) are then divided by the number of rural health center/ federally qualified health center visits (8,000). Thus, the all-inclusive reimbursement rate equals $70.00 per visit, as shown in Exhibit 10-3.

Exhibit 10-2   Determining Allowable Costs

	Total Costs	Overhead	Non-Allowable	Allowable
Direct Costs	$700,000	$100,000	$120,000	$480,000
% of Direct Costs			20% *	80% **
Overhead Allocation		($100,000)	$ 20,000	$ 80,000
Total allowable				$560,000

* Twenty percent of the overhead is non-allowable (20% of $100,000)
** Eighty percent of the overhead is allowable (80% of $100,000)

Exhibit 10-3   **Determining the Reimbursement Rate**

$560,000 Allowable Costs ÷ 8,000 Visits = $70.00 Reimbursement Rate

However, there are caps on the reimbursement rate depending on the category; see Exhibit 10-4.

There are different caps on the reimbursement rate depending on the center's status. Medicare reimburses Rural Health Centers (RHC) and Federally Qualified Health Centers (FQHC) at the maximum rates, as shown in Exhibit 10-4.

Who Reimburses Advanced Nurse Practitioners?

Advanced nurse practitioners are reimbursed by a majority of third-party payers. The rules and regulations of reimbursement vary by payer. Third-party payers include Medicare, Medicaid, commercial indemnity insurers, managed care organizations, and negotiated contracts. (There is more information about providers and various insurance plans in Dunham-Taylor and Pinzcuk (2006) *Health Care Financial Management for Nurse Managers: Merging the Heart with the Dollar.*

Medicare

The Balanced Budget Act of 1997 (BBA) removed the limitations on nurse practitioners to bill Medicare directly for services provided regardless of the geographic area of practice. (Prior to 1997, nurse practitioners had to bill "incident to" a physician's professional service except in a federally qualified rural health center or community health center. The billing physician was required to have "direct supervision" of the non-physician practitioner providing the service, and the physician had to initiate the treatment.) There are three types of provider supervision:

Exhibit 10-4   **Medicare Maximum Reimbursement Rate**

Year	RHC	Urban FQHC	Rural FQHC
1999	$60.40	$93.77	$80.62
2000	$61.85	$96.02	$82.56
2001	$63.14	$98.03	$84.28
2002	$64.78	$100.57	$86.47
2003	$66.68	$103.58	$88.99
2004	$68.65	$106.58	$91.64

www.cms.hhs.gov/providers/fghc

Direct supervision (also referred to as collaboration) is interpreted as the billing physician being physically present in the same facility where the services are provided. The Centers for Medicare and Medicaid Services (CMS) "Incident to" definitions are available in the *Medicare Carriers Manual*, Section 2050.3. *Incident to* means auxiliary personnel are allowed to provide services under the supervision of a physician or practitioner who supervises them. When a nurse practitioner's services are billed under the physician's provider number, Medicare reimburses at 100 percent of the customary allowable charge. Billing under the nurse practitioner's provider number reduces the reimbursement to 85 percent of the customary allowable charge.

Personal Supervision—Provider is in the room and performs the services.

Direct Supervision—Provider is in the office suite when the services are performed by auxiliary personnel.

General Supervision—Provider can be reached via telephone/beeper but is not in the office.

There is a "three to one" rule that pertains to auxiliary personnel—nurse practitioners are excluded from this rule. Here, the supervising provider must initiate a treatment plan and delegate follow-up services to auxiliary personnel. The third visit must be provided by the supervising provider, or if the patient's condition changes, the supervising provider needs to see the patient at the appropriate time before the third visit.

Medicaid

Title XIX of the Social Security Act, establishing Medicaid, is a program that provides medical assistance, jointly funded by the state and the federal government, to qualified beneficiaries. Medicaid became law in 1965 to provide adequate medical care to eligible needy persons. It covers children, the blind and/or disabled, and those that need federally assisted income maintenance payments. Medicaid services (where the reimbursement dollars are provided by both state and federal monies) are defined by each state, so reimbursement guidelines may differ from state to state. The federal government has determined that each state must meet the following guidelines:

1. Establish its own eligibility standards;

2. Determine the type, amount, duration, and scope of services;

3. Set the rate of payment for services; and

4. Administer its own program.

In addition, the Code of Federal regulations, Title 42-Public Health, Chapter IV—Centers for Medicare and Medicaid Services Section § 438.12, states "Provider discrimination [is] prohibited." Under General Rules it further

MCO—Managed Care Organization

PIHP—Prepaid Inpatient Health Plan

PAHP—Prepaid Ambulatory Health Plan

states: "An MCO, PIHP, or PAHP may not discriminate for the participation, reimbursement, or indemnification of any provider who is acting within the scope of his or her license or certification under applicable State law, solely on the basis of that license or certification."

Commercial Indemnity Insurers

Indemnity insurers reimburse health care providers on a fee-for-service basis, meaning that fees are paid for specifically defined services as they are rendered. Each organization has its own policy regarding reimbursement of advanced nurse practitioner-provided services.

Managed Care Organizations

Managed Care Organization (MCO) is an umbrella term that includes health maintenance organizations (HMO), provider-sponsored organizations (PSO), or physician-hospital organizations (PHO). Advanced nurse practitioners can be included in many Managed Care Organization (MCO) provider panels. If a managed care organization reimburses advanced nurse practitioners, a pre-application is needed before care is given, and before the credentialing process begins. (The following section further defines Credentialing Requirements.) When an advanced Nurse Practitioner is a member of a provider panel, he/she is designated as a primary care provider (PCP). The primary care provider: 1) oversees the management of care and is responsible for providing primary care, referring care to a specialist when medically necessary; 2) maintains proper credentials; 3) is included in the managed care organization's directory listing; and 4) is reimbursed for providing care according to the provider schedule and contract (*Code of Federal Regulations*, Title 42—Public Health, Chapter IV—Centers for Medicare and Medicaid Services Section).

Business/Agency Contracts

A business or agency may contract individually with an advanced nurse practitioner, or with his/her employer, to provide preventive health care, occupational health, or employee assistance for their employees. Generally both the employer and employee benefit because "lost work" is reduced. A contract and/or agreement specifies the scope of services to be provided. The agency is then billed on an hourly, weekly, or monthly basis, or is billed per client served. An example of such a contract is one with a county jail that has state-mandated physicals of inmates. (See Appendix A.)

Credentialing Requirements

To bill and be reimbursed by Medicare, Medicaid, and managed care organizations, the provider must be credentialed with that agency/organization. This process ensures that only qualified practitioners are being paid as providers. Credentialing verifies that providers have the appropriate education and experience to render the provided services. The credentialing process includes: verifying degrees, licenses, and certifications; checking the references of the providers; and showing proof of having malpractice insurance (Appendix B). Credentialing rules and requirements vary by payer/agency. The basic requirements for nurse practitioners are state licensure, prescription writing rules and regulations, and board certification from either the American Academy of Nurse Practitioners, American Nurses Credentialing Center, National Certification Corporation, National Certification Board of Pediatric Nurse Practitioners and Nurses, Oncology Nursing Certification Corporation, or Critical Care Certification Corporation.

Effective January 1, 2003, nurse practitioners applying for a Medicare provider number must possess a master's degree from an accredited Nurse Practitioner program, as well as national certification and state licensure.

An Introduction to Third Party Reimbursement

At the beginning of this chapter, reimbursement was referred to as a puzzle. The pieces of the puzzle are:

- What medical services/procedure(s) were received?

  A code is required to describe the service/procedure (HCPCS).

- Why was the service(s) provided?

  A diagnosis code is required to describe the medical necessity for the service (ICD-9-CM).

- What fee will be charged for the service provided based on the complexity of the service provided?

  A fee schedule is developed for each CPT code used by the facility.

- Who is responsible for paying for the service provided?

  The person receiving the service, guarantor or contracting agency, and third-party payer(s) are responsible for payment.

To optimize reimbursement, the medical office must be in control of the billing process. This includes advising providers of changes in the coding process, conducting regular workshops, and performing chart audits to ensure that the providers are coding at the appropriate level. In addition, the billing staff must remain current on reimbursement issues, including primary versus secondary insurance carriers, and patients with multiple insurance plans. For example, a Medicare patient whose spouse carries a commercial plan that is primary to Medicare, or a child with coverage under both parents' commercial plans. (The rule here is the parent whose birthday is first in the fiscal year is the primary plan, while the other parent's plan is secondary.) Another frequent cause of confusion and improper reimbursement occurs when the patient presents with an injury. Often these services are not covered by the personal commercial plan, as the injury may be due to worker's compensation, automobile insurance, household insurance, or some other entity.

CPT—Current Procedural Terminology American Medical Association.

HCPCS—Health Care Financing Administration Common Procedure Coding System.

ICD-9-CM——International Classification of Diseases 9th Revision Clinic Modification. Revised by the World Health Organization. Annual updates published by Health Care Financing Administration, now Centers for Medicare and Medicaid Services (CMS).

Personnel must be trained to correctly document procedure(s) and diagnosis code(s) and remain current on insurance claim processing rules and regulations by each payer (Medicare, Medicaid, and commercial insurance carriers). It is important to make sure that:

- Policies and procedures support the billing, coding and collection process;

- Forms and documents are current, accurate, and conform to legal requirements;

- Current CPT, HCPCS and ICD-9-CM manuals are used for procedure and diagnosis coding;

- Providers and staff are trained in current coding and billing issues;

- Medical dictionaries and terminology reference books are available; and

- Effective strategies and systems are used that employ third-party-payer rules for maximum reimbursement with minimal effort. This includes:

  ○ Third-party usual, customary and reasonable (UCR) fee schedules; and

  ○ Third-party payer manuals and web site addresses are provided. For example, http://www.bcbst.com is the Web address for Blue Cross Blue Shield of Tennessee.

Basic Steps of Medical Billing

Exhibit 10-5 describes the steps involved in medical billing:

The collection and billing process begins when the patient makes an appointment to see a provider and ends when the patient's account balance is zero. There are several important steps involved for accurate coding and reimbursement. As stated before, for optimum reimbursement, the provider practice needs to be in control of the process.

1. Patient registration ensures that the demographic and insurance information is accurate and up-to-date. Can one reach the patient, if need be, after the appointment? Has the patient moved, changed telephone numbers, changed insurance plans?

2. A super-bill, or encounter form, is initiated with patient identification, date, account number, and prior balance. This form is then attached to the patient's medical record.

3. The provider performs the procedure(s) and/or services.

4. The procedure(s) and/or services are documented in the medical record.

5. The provider selects the proper procedure code(s) and appropriate diagnosis code to justify the level of service provided, as well as the medical necessity for the services.

Exhibit 10-5   Steps of Medical Billing

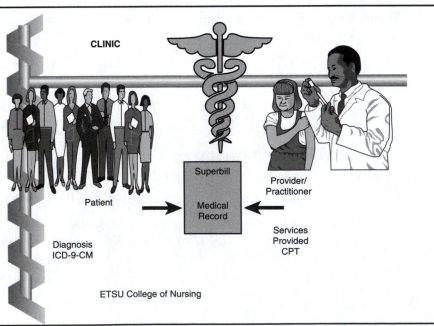

6. The patient is provided a copy of the super-bill indicating the amount due for each service entered, and the total amount due.

7. **If insurance is billed for the patient, go to Step # 9.**

8. The patient pays for the service; it is documented whether it was cash, check, money order, or credit card. The patient is informed that they must file their own claim with their insurance company.

9. The manual or computerized billing system is updated. (Some small private offices use a manual system rather than the more expensive computerized system.) The insurance claim form is prepared, either manually or electronically.

10. Super-bills are batched by date of service and filed for easy future reference.

11. Insurance claim copies are filed and kept for review and/or for refiling a claim.

12. When, or if, the insurance carrier payment is received, the explanation of benefits (EOB) on the insurance form is reviewed. If payment is satisfactory, the payment is posted.

13. The patient is billed for the balance due, if any, or the patient's secondary insurance carrier is billed with a copy of the explanation of benefits from the primary carrier attached.

14. If a secondary insurance carrier was billed in #13, the patient is billed for the balance.

15. Payment is received from the patient and posted to his/her account.

Note: Denied claims and collection efforts will be covered later.

Administrative Operations

Policies and Procedures

Policies and procedures must be in place for compliance with federal and state regulations that include: the Health Insurance Portability and Accountability Act (HIPAA), the Occupational Safety and Health Administration (OSHA), and third-party reimbursement rules and regulations.

Operational policies and procedures need to include clearly defined written instructions necessary for each step of the reimbursement management process.

Written policies are therefore needed, explaining how each of the medical office's documents and forms are completed and dispensed.

Policies need to include such things as:

- Does the medical office file insurance claims for all patients and all services?

- Does the medical office accept assignment all of the time? Does the medical office participate in Medicare; i.e., accept assignment for medical services?

- Does the practice participate in Medicaid/TennCare or other state funded programs?

- How does the medical office handle deductibles and coinsurance?

- Does the medical office file claims within the time periods specified by the third party payer?

Adapted from: Davis, J. (1996). *Reimbursement Manual for the Medical Office: A Comprehensive Guide to Coding, Billing and Fee Management* (3rd Ed). Los Angeles: Practice Management Information Corporation.

Assignment of Benefits—The subscriber authorizes the payer to send payment directly to the provider.

Medicare Assignment—When the client is covered under Medicare, the provider agrees to accept Medicare customary and allowable reimbursement and not bill the balance to the subscriber.

Usual Customary and Reasonable (UCR)

Usual—Provider's usual charge for a procedure.

Customary—Payer's customary fee for a procedure.

Reasonable—Payer's determination of a reasonable fee for a procedure.

The practice has to decide to accept assignment for claims filed to Medicare and third-party payers.

When the provider accepts the Medicare assignment, this means that the practice will accept the customary allowable charge from the third party payer as payment in full and will not bill the balance to the patient. The patient can only be billed for the co-pay and deductible. Co-pay is usually 80 percent of the customary and allowable charge. It is considered fraud to file a full charge to a third party and not collect co-pays and deductibles.

Some other billing terms are: usual, customary, and reasonable (UCR).

Here are some examples of possible patient billing:

- Provider A bills $100 for a procedure and accepts assignment. The Payer has set the customary fee at $120. This means that the customary fee is $20 more than Provider A charged ($120 − $100 = $20). Additionally, there is a co-insurance of 80 percent; the provider receives $80 (80 percent of $100 = $80 *or* $100 × 0.8 = $80). In this case, the Provider receives $80 and bills the patient 20 percent, or $20.

$100 Total billed by provider ($120 allowable customary fee that insurer has set).

    $120 customary fee

   -$100 billed amount

    $ 20

    The additional $20 cannot be billed by the provider.

− $ 80 Billed to insurer because there is 80 percent co-insurance ($100 x 0.8 = $80).

$ 20 Billed to patient ($100 × 0.2 = $20).

- Provider B bills $150 for a procedure and accepts assignment. The Payer has set the customary fee at $120. Provider B can therefore only charge $120 ($150 − $20 = $30). There is a co-insurance of 80 percent so the provider receives $96 ($120 × 0.8 = $96). In this case Provider B writes off $30, and bills the patient for 20 percent of $120, or $24.

$150 Provider bills $150.

− $120 Insurer sets this as the customary fee.

$ 30 Therefore, the provider can only bill $120 so provider either writes off $30 or will bill the patient for this.

$ 96 Billed to insurer because there is 80 percent co-insurance ($100 x 0.8 = $96).

+ $ 24 Billed to patient because of 20 percent co-insurance ($100 x 0.2 = $24).

$120 Total Provider Receives

- There are occasions when a payer will exceed the customary fee; such as in the following example. Provider C bills $150 for a procedure with documentation of unusual circumstance(s) and accepts assignment. The provider hopes the Payer will determine that $150 is a reasonable fee under the circumstance and will pay 80 percent of the $150 ($150 × 0.8 = $120). The patient would be billed 20 percent ($150 x 0.2 = $30).

$150 Billed by provider.

− $120 Billed to insurer because there is 80% co-insurance ($150 x 0.8 = $120).

$ 30 Billed to patient because there is 20% co-insurance ($15 x 0.2 = $30).

Forms and Documents

In addition to the forms required for the medical record, numerous forms are required to accurately code and bill third party payers. Fundamental and essential forms (shown more in Appendix C) include:

- Patient Registration Form

- Release of Medical Information to third-party payers

- Assignment of Benefits (May be included in the Patient Registration Form)

- Insurance Pre-authorization or Certification Form, if applicable

- Advanced Beneficiary Notice/Medicare Medical Necessity Form for providing non-covered Medicare medical services

- Consent to Treatment for surgeries or other invasive procedures. *Note: statutes vary from state to state* (Buppert, 1999, p. 238)

- Authorization to release medical records to another entity/facility

- Encounter Form/Superbill/form to capture services rendered and medical necessity, and

- HCFA 1500 Insurance Claim Form or UB92 Insurance Claim Form (discussed in Appendix D) (www.cms.hhs.gov).

The patient registration form includes demographic data, employer, name and address of the insurance carrier(s) (with member and group numbers), emergency contact, and so forth. The data contained on this form can affect the revenues of the center if the proper information is not obtained, and/or is not updated on a regular basis. ***Insurance coverage does not remain static as employers change employee insurance plans or insurance carriers, or as changes are made in coverage or plan expense.***

Authorization to release information, such as sharing the patient diagnosis and treatment with the patient's insurance carrier is required, and releases will be expanded under the Health Insurance Portability and Accountability Act (HIPAA) regulations. More detail regarding HIPAA can be found at the HIPAA website (http://www.cms.gov/hipaa/). This authorization may be part of the patient registration form or Superbill.

Some insurance carriers and managed care organizations require pre-authorization for a planned procedure, or referral to another health care provider. In this case, the provider will need to contact the insurance company before treating the patient.

The Superbill (also known as the encounter form, visit slip, fee ticket, or charge slip) is used to record the medical services provided, as well as to document the medical necessity for the service. This form might also include return visit criteria, release and assignment of benefits, and be used as a payment receipt.

The Medicare medical necessity form, also known as Advance Beneficiary Notice (ABN), is given to a Medicare beneficiary in advance of treatment if services to be provided may be denied by Medicare as a non-covered service. If an ABN has been obtained, the patient may be billed for non-covered services. This is most common for laboratory procedures and selected preventive procedures such as physical examinations. If there is no ABN, then the patient cannot be charged, and the charges have to be written off. It is illegal to bill the patient.

The insurance form is used to bill the patient's insurance carrier. The HCFA 1500 (shown in Appendix D) is the most common form used/required by third-party payers, including Medicare and Medicaid Part B carriers. Rural health clinics and federally qualified health centers use the UB 92 form to bill Medicare fiscal intermediaries under Part A.

> ### Helpful Definitions
>
> *Carrier (Medicare)*—Private contractor who administers claims for Part B Medicare (outpatient services).
>
> *Fiscal Intermediary*—Private contractor who administers claims for Part A Medicare (inpatient and rural health centers).

Fee Schedules

Managing fee schedules involves a great deal more than simply defining a charge associated with a particular service or procedure. Setting fees requires comprehensive knowledge about third party reimbursement by insurance carriers, including Medicare, Medicaid, and private insurance carrier billing rules and regulations. In the competitive market environment, it is important to understand that medical service fees are part of your marketing strategy. Fees should be reviewed and adjusted periodically. This does not necessarily mean an increase in fees charged, there may be a circumstance where a fee has to be reduced. Charging a fee that is less than an insurance carrier will pay benefits the insurance carrier, not the provider or his/her patient. It is important to continue to adjust for inflation and to cover cost increases. Traditional methods of adjusting fees include:

- Figure a percentage increase for all Current Procedural Terminology (CPT) codes

- Use the consumer price index as a tool to increase fees by an appropriate percentage

- Calculate increased operating costs

- Increase rates for selected procedure(s)

- Be aware of the community-accepted rate

- Know out-of-date rates, and

- Understand and adjust for relative values (Lucas, 2001).

A percentage increase is probably the most common method used because it is easy to calculate and implement. The danger in this method is that higher end fees may cause the practice to be noncompetitive, drive away patients, and further limit referrals to the practice.

Operating costs for the average medical practitioner have been increasing at the rate of about 9 percent per year. Increasing fees by 9 percent does not translate into increased revenues. Refer to the examples earlier in this chapter under Policies and Procedures. Rather than implement an across-the-board increase in fees, consider selective-fee raises by procedures and/or services. The key to this method is to pay attention to the volume of specific procedures and/or services you are reviewing. The evaluation and management fees may need to be adjusted without adjusting special procedures.

The acceptable fees for specific procedures or services should agree with what local community medical professionals charge and what the majority of the patients are willing to pay.

If the fee schedule has not been updated on a regular basis, it may be out of date and in serious need of "catching up." To avoid client shock, increase charges frequently by small amounts rather than one significant increase. Patients expect increases in health care costs; huge increases have a negative effect. The relative value system determines fees more scientifically and logical but is also more time-consuming. The Resource Based Relative Value Scale (RBRVS) is also the Medicare fee schedule and can be located on Medicare's website, http://www.cms.hhs.gov.

Procedure Coding with CPT and HCPCS

This section is a very important part of the reimbursement puzzle. One needs to know how to use the CPT and HCPCS manuals. Selecting the proper code has a *tremendous* impact on the financial aspects of a medical office. CPT is an acronym for Current Procedural Terminology and HCPCS is the acronym for HCFA (Health Care Finance Administration now Centers for Medicare & Medicaid Services) Common Procedure Coding System.

No universal medical services coding system existed prior to 1966. In some cases, each payer had their own coding system. For example, in Michigan in the seventies there were different procedure codes for Blue Cross/Blue Shield, Michigan Medicaid, and

Coding Terms

CPT—Current Procedural Terminology

HCPCS—HCFA Common Procedure Coding System

Medicare. Then the American Medical Association (AMA) developed the Current Procedural Terminology (CPT) codes. These procedure codes have been adopted by third-party payers. In 1970 the AMA expanded the procedure codes to consist of five digits and introduced modifiers.

The codes were supplemented in 1983 with a three-level system:

1. Level I contains the Current Procedural Terminology published and copyrighted by the American Medical Association (www.ama-assn.org)

2. Level II are national codes published by the Health Care Finance Administration (now Centers for Medicare and Medicaid Services) (www.cms.hhs.gov), and

3. Level III are *local codes* developed by local Medicare carriers—these are temporary codes used by different states. This is defined further in the chapter.

Key Points Regarding Current Procedural Terminology (CPT) and Health Care Financing Administration Common Procedure Coding System (HCPCS)

*   **Level I CPT** codes have five-digit numeric codes.

    (For instance, 59425 is used for ante-partum care only; four to six visits can be reported.)

    *   Describes procedures, services and supplies.

        (For example, CPT code 10060 describes incision and drainage of an abscess.)

    *   With few exceptions, third-party payers require CPT codes.

    *   Revised annually in December. Codes are added, changed or deleted each year.

    *   "Visit" codes were deleted in 1992 and replaced with Evaluation and Management codes (99201 through 99499).

        (99201 is reported when a new patient presents with a limited problem and needs an examination.) (American Medical Association *Physicians Current Procedural Terminology CPT '03*)

*   **Level II of the national HCPCS codes** are five-digit alphanumeric codes. The first digit is a letter to define the category and the second through fifth digits are numbers.

    (For instance, medical and surgical supplies start with the letter "A" followed by 4000–4999.)

- Includes two-digit modifiers at the National and Local levels which may be alphabetic or alphanumeric.

    (For example, the QB modifier states that services were provided in a rural Health Professions Shortage Area—HPSA.)

- Describes supplies, materials and services.

    (For example, J0290 is used when a 500 mg ampicillin sodium injection is given.)

- Revised annually in March. Again codes are added, changed or deleted.

- Follows a specific hierarchy of selection and use.

    (Commercial payers and Medicaid may want the CPT code 99070 to describe supplies; while Medicare wants the more specific Level II national HCPCS code—www.cms.hhs.gov.)

- **Level III local codes** take precedence over national Level II and national Level II takes precedence over CPT Level 1. There is some overlap of Level I, national Level II, and local Level III.

    Note: CPT and HCPCS coding can make a 25-percent difference (plus or minus) in your reimbursement. Choosing the wrong code for the particular payer will affect the rate of reimbursement. Accurate coding puts you in control of the reimbursement process (Davis, 1996).

Structure of CPT and HCPCS

The main body of the CPT manual is divided into six sections. Each section has subsections with subheadings. The six sections of CPT are:

- **Evaluation and Management**—99201 to 99499.

- **Anesthesiology**—00100 to 01999 and 99100 to 99140.

- **Surgery**—10040 to 69979.

- **Radiology**—70010 to 79999.

- **Pathology and Laboratory**—80002 to 89399.

- **Medicine**—90701 to 99199.

Specific "Guidelines" are presented at the beginning of each of the six sections. These Guidelines define items that are necessary to appropriately interpret and report the procedures and services contained in that section. These guidelines include:

Multiple procedures—Psychotherapy services in addition to a hospital visit.

Add-on Codes—Additional or supplemental procedures.

Separate procedures—Procedure/service that is unrelated to the primary procedure/service.

Current Procedural Terminology (CPT) Modifiers

A CPT modifier provides the means by which a provider can indicate that a service or procedure that has been performed has been altered by some specific circumstance, but not changed in its definition or code (AMA, 2003). Modifiers are appended after the CPT code. Examples may include:

- Mandated services—Modifier 32.

- A service or procedure has been increased or reduced—Modifier 52.

- Only part of a service was performed—Modifier 53.

- An additional service was performed on the same date of service—Modifier 25.

- Unusual procedural services—Modifier 22.

Ambulatory care providers mostly use the Evaluation and Management codes for "cognitive" services such as office/clinic visits, consultations, preventive examinations, and critical care services. A face-to-face contact between a patient and provider is considered a visit (encounter), and can occur in a variety of settings.

National Level II HCPCS

Level II of the HCPCS codes are used to bill for supplies, materials, injections, and other services provided by health care professionals. Level II codes start with a letter, and are followed by four numbers (A0000 through V0000). Primary care providers only use the codes from the medical and surgical supplies section, and drugs administered by means other than the oral method. These codes start with an A or J. For example, J0120 is used for injection of tetracycline, up to 250 mg.

There are no guidelines published with the Centers for Medicare and Medicaid Services version of Level II codes. Although HCPCS National Level II codes are uniform in description throughout the United States, the processing and reimbursement of these codes are not necessarily uniform. Some codes are reimbursed based on "carrier discretion." The Medicare bulletins published by the intermediaries and in the Medicare rules and regulations include this information. It is important, therefore, for providers and staff to keep current with the information provided in these "manuals."

National Level II Modifiers

Level II codes also use modifiers to further define a service. Examples include:

- Service was provided by a psychologist (Modifier AH), clinical social worker (Modifier AJ), or other nonphysician provider.

- Service was provided as part of a specific government program.

- Service was provided to a specific side of the body—L6010-F9 would be used when fitting a prosthetic device to the right hand, fifth digit.

- Social work visit, in the home, per diem—S9127-AJ.

Procedure Coding

As mentioned earlier, this first section of the Current Procedural Terminology (CPT) manual contains the Evaluation and Management (E&M) codes used by primary care providers. The descriptors for the different levels of E&M services have seven key components:

- History

- Examination

- Medical Decision-Making

- Counseling

- Coordination of Care

- Nature of Presenting Problem, and

- Time (*Documentation Guidelines for Evaluation and Management Services* (Nov 1997) jointly produced by the American Medicaid Association and HCFA (now CMS).

The first three components are the **key** components in determining the level of services provided.

History is divided into four types:

- Problem focused—chief complaint; brief history of present illness/problem.

  ○ Requires no Problem Pertinent Review of Systems and no Past, Family and/or Social History. *Example: Established minor patient with chronic secretory otitis media.*

- Expanded problem focused—chief complaint; brief history of present illness; problem-pertinent system review.

  ○ Requires one Problem Pertinent Review of Systems and no Past, Family and/or Social History. *Example: Established adult patient with chronic essential hypertension on multiple drug regimen presenting for a blood pressure check.*

- Detailed—chief complaint; extended history of present illness; problem pertinent system review extended to include a review of a limited number of additional systems; pertinent past, family and/or social history directly related to the patient's problems.

  ○ Requires Extended Review of Systems (2–9) and one Past, Family and/or Social History. *Example: Initial office visit for a seven-year-old patient with juvenile diabetes mellitus with past history of hospitalization times three.*

- Comprehensive—chief complaint; extended history of present illness; review of systems which is directly related to the problem(s) identified in the history of the present illness plus a review of all additional body systems; complete past, family, and social history (AMA, 2003).

  ○ Requires Complete Review of Systems (10 or more) and two Past, Family and/or Social History. *Example: Established patient with a three-month history of fatigue, weight loss, intermittent fever, and presenting with diffuse adenopathy and splenomegaly.*

Examination depends on clinical judgment and on the nature of the presenting illness/problem. There are four types:

- Problem focused—an examination of the affected body area or organ system.

  ○ *Example: Office visit for client presenting with severe rash and itching for 24 hours, positive history for contact with poison oak 48 hours prior to visit.*

- Expanded problem focused—an examination of the affected body area or organ system and other symptomatic or related organ system(s).

  ○ *Example: Office visit of a child with chronic secretory otitis media.*

- Detailed—an extended examination of the affected body area(s) and other symptomatic or related organ system(s).

  ○ *Example: Biannual follow-up of client with migraine variant having infrequent, intermittent, moderate to severe headaches with nausea and vomiting.*

- Comprehensive—A complete single system specialty examination or a complete multi-system examination.

  ○ *Example: Female with symptoms of rash, swellings, recurrent arthritic complaints, and diarrhea and lymphadenopathy. Client has had a 25-pound weight loss and was recently camping in the Amazon.*

Medical decision-making refers to the complexity of establishing a diagnosis and/or selecting a management option. This is measured by:

- The number of possible diagnoses and/or the number of management options considered

- The amount and/or complexity of medical records, diagnostic tests, and/or other information that must be obtained and analyzed, and

- The risk of significant complications, morbidity and/or mortality, as well as co-morbidities associated with the patient's presenting problem(s), the diagnostic procedure(s) and/or the possible management options.

Four types of medical decision making are defined in the CPT manual:

- **Straightforward**—Presenting problem: One self-limited or minor problem.

  ○ Minimal number of diagnoses or management options.

  ○ Minimal or no data reviewed.

  ○ Minimal risk of complications and/or morbidity or mortality.

- **Low Complexity**—Presenting problem: Two or more self-limited or minor problems; one stable chronic illness; acute uncomplicated illness or injury.

  ○ Limited number of diagnoses or management options.

  ○ Limited amount and/or complexity of data to be reviewed.

  ○ Low risk of complications and/or morbidity or mortality.

- **Moderate Complexity**—Presenting problem: One or more chronic illnesses with mild exacerbation or progression; two or more stable chronic illnesses; undiagnosed new problem.

  ○ Multiple diagnoses or management options.

  ○ Moderate amount and/or complexity of data to be reviewed.

  ○ Moderate risk of complications and/or morbidity or mortality.

- **High Complexity**—Presenting problem: One or more chronic illnesses with severe exacerbation; progression or side effects of treatment, acute/chronic illnesses or injuries that may post a threat to life or bodily function; an abrupt change in neurological status.

  ○ Extensive diagnoses or management options.

  ○ Extensive amount and/or complexity of data to be reviewed.

  ○ High risk of complications and/or morbidity or mortality.

The next three components: counseling, coordination of care, and the nature of the presenting problem, are considered **contributory** factors in the majority of encounters.

Counseling is a discussion with a patient and/or family concerning one or more of the following areas:

- Diagnostic results, impressions, and/or recommended diagnostic studies;

- Prognosis;

- Risks and benefits of management (treatment) options;

- Instructions for management (treatment) and/or follow-up;

- Importance of compliance with chosen management (treatment) options;

- Risk factor reduction; and

- Patient and family education (AMA, 2003).

The CPT does not define coordination of care. The only statement made is: "Coordination of care with other providers or agencies without a patient encounter on that day is reported using the case management codes" (Practice Management Information Corporation, 1996, p. 91). When counseling and/or coordination of care dominates (more than 50 percent) the face-to-face provider encounter, *time* is considered the key factor to qualify for a particular level of evaluation and management services. The extent of counseling and/or coordination of care must be documented in the medical record. *Example: A provider spends half an hour explaining diabetes nutrition and disease management, or the risks and benefits of different treatment options.*

Diagnosis Coding with ICD-9-CM

The Medicare Catastrophic Coverage Act of 1988 (P.L. 100-220) required diagnosis coding using the International Classification of Diseases, 9th Revision, Clinical Modification (ICD-9-CM) for all health care professionals submitting Medicare claims. To comply with the regulations, health care professionals must convert the reasons(s) for providing medical services into a diagnosis code. Changes made to Medicare are frequently followed by similar changes for Medicaid and private insurance carriers.

Key points include:

- ICD-9-CM codes are three to five numeric or alphanumeric codes
- They describe illnesses, injuries, signs and symptoms, and procedures
- ICD-9-CM codes, with few exceptions, are accepted or required by insurance carriers
- Most codes have a specific definition and some have more than one definition
- Correct diagnosis codes can make a difference in reimbursement as they define why the services were provided, and
- Proper use of diagnosis codes puts you in control of the reimbursement process.

The format of ICD-9-CM is published as a three volume set. The Tabular List (Volume 1) is a numeric listing of diagnosis codes and descriptions, and consists of 17 chapters that classify diseases and injuries, two sections with supplementary codes (V codes and E codes), and six appendices. Each chapter of the Tabular List (Volume 1) is structured into four components:

- Sections: groups of three-digit code numbers
- Categories—three-digit code numbers
- Subcategories—four-digit code numbers, and
- Fifth-Digit Sub-classifications—five-digit code numbers.

The Alphabetical Index (Volume 2) consists of an alphabetic list of terms and codes, two supplementary Sections following the alphabetic listing, plus three special tables found within the alphabetic listing and is structured as follows:

- Main Terms appear in **Boldface** type.
- Sub-terms are always indented two spaces to the right under the main terms.

- Carry-over lines are always indented more than two spaces from the level of the preceding line.

The supplementary sections following the Alphabetic Index are the Table of Drugs and Chemicals, and an index containing external causes of injuries and poisonings (E-Codes).

Volume 3 consists of procedures, used incorrectly by health care professionals unless they are in the hospital setting.

To effectively use the ICD-9-CM coding, it is important to follow nine steps. These are described in the following table.

Nine Steps for Accurate ICD-9-CM Coding

- Locate the main term within the diagnostic statement.

- Locate that main term in the Alphabetic Index (Volume 2).

- Refer to all notes under the main term.

- Examine any modifiers appearing in parentheses next to the main term.

- Take note of sub-terms indented beneath the main term.

- Follow any cross reference instructions such as "see" or "see also."

- Confirm the code selection in the Tabular List (Volume 1).

- Follow the instructional terms in Volume 1. Watch for exclusion terms, note and fifth-digit instructions.

- Assign the code number that you have determined to be correct (*ICD-9-CM Manual*).

A good example is Diabetes mellitus, which requires a fifth digit. The three digit code is 250. Diabetes with ketoacidosis is identified as 250.1. The fifth digit further defines whether it is Type 1 or Type 2, either controlled or uncontrolled. If it is a Type 2 non-insulin dependent, the code would be 250.10. The following diagram explains each number:

Additional codes may be required to describe any current coexisting conditions. Do not include codes for conditions that were previously treated and no longer exist. Diagnoses documented as probable, suspected, questionable, or rule out should not be coded as if the diagnosis is confirmed. The condition(s) should be coded by describing symptoms, signs, abnormal test results, or other reasons for the encounter. For example, the Client presented with a sore throat and lab tests are ordered to rule out strep throat. The diagnosis would be 462. On the follow-up visit, strep has been confirmed, so the diagnosis would be 034.0.

ICD-9-CM also provides codes to deal with visits other than a disease or injury, such as prenatal visit or a well physical. These codes are found in the V-code section and range from V01.0 through V82.9.

In the case of an injury, an additional E-code is required to describe the cause of the injury, poisoning, or other adverse effects. Any CPT code in the 80000 to 90000 range (Injury and Poisoning) triggers a denial if no E-code is assigned. Third-party payers need to know how the injury occurred to determine primary coverage for the medical services; such as Worker's Compensation, automobile accident, or homeowner's liability insurance.

Third-Party Reimbursement— Dealing with Insurance Carriers

Medicare

The Balanced Budget Act of 1997 allows nurse practitioners to have their own Medicare provider number and to bill directly for services. Nonphysicians, with their own provider number, are reimbursed by Medicare at 85 percent of the fee schedule amount. Carolyn Buppert's book, *Nurse Practitioner's Business Practice & Legal Guide*, proves an excellent reference on the definition of nurse practitioner qualifications state by state. Physician supervision varies from state to state.

The application form to participate in the Medicare program can be obtained from the Centers for Medicare and Medicaid Services (CMS, formerly the Health Care Finance Administration) website: http://www.cms.hhs.gov. The application forms changed effective January 1, 2002, and are available in electronic form. The individual application is 855I. Nurse practitioners must participate and accept assignment.

Medicaid

Section 4280 "Establishment and Use of Medicaid Unique Physician Identifier" Paragraph B states: "For planning purposes, States are advised that HCFA intends to require that States obtain the Medicare UPIN (Universal Physician Identification Number) on all physician billings submitted for Medicaid reimbursement." At the present time, some states already require Medicare participation in order to obtain a Medicaid provider number.

The Balanced Budget Act of 1997 made a number of changes in the federal law governing rural health clinics and federally qualified health centers, which allowed states to phase out the Medicaid cost-based reimbursement. This authority was enacted on October 1, 1999, but was repealed by President Clinton in December 2000. The Medicare, Medicaid, S-CHIP Benefit Improvement Protection Act (BIPA) repealed the 1115 state waivers and restored the requirement that state Medicaid programs pay Rural Health Clinics and federally qualified health centers 100 percent of their reasonable costs effective January 1, 2001. This was established by legislation known as the Safety Net Preservation Act and was called the New Prospective Payment System for Federally Qualified Health Centers and Rural Health Clinics (Section 702).

Commercial Third-Party Payers

Commercial carriers offer contracts to individuals and groups. The types of plans vary according to the contract with the individual and/or employer. Payments are made to the beneficiary unless the provider agrees to accept assignment. Carriers have fee schedules based on "usual and customary" charges. "Usual and customary" charges vary from carrier to carrier but often are based on a Resource Based Relative Value System schedule. If the provider charges more than the usual and customary, it is up to the provider to collect the difference from the patient.

Managed Care Organizations (MCO)

A managed care organization is an insurer that provides for both health care services and payment for services, or a prepaid group practice plan. Managed care organization is an umbrella term that includes Health Maintenance Organizations (HMO), provider-sponsored organizations (PSO), or physician-hospital organizations (PHO). These terms are explained in Dunham-Taylor and Pinczuk (2005) *Health Care Financial Management for Nurse Managers: Merging the Heart with the Dollar.*

Conclusion

This chapter covered the reimbursement process in ambulatory settings—community health centers, rural health centers, or private practice settings—where the nurse practitioner is either employed or self-employed. There are helpful "tools" given to both understand billing and coding as well as to more effectively address reimbursement issues.

References

American Medical Association. (2003). *Physicians' Current Procedural Terminology CPT '03.* Chicago: American Medical Association.

Buppert, C. (1999). *Nurse Practitioner's Business Practice & Legal Guide.* Gaithersburg, MD: Aspen.

Davis, James B. (1996). *Reimbursement Manual for the Medical Office : A Comprehensive Guide to Coding, Billing & Fee Management* (3rd edition). Los Angeles, California: Practice Management Information Corporation.

Dunham-Taylor, J., & Pinczuk, J. (2006). *Health Care Financial Management for Nurse Managers: Merging the Heart with the Dollar.* Sudbury, MA: Jones and Bartlett.

Lucas, G. (2001). RBRVS for fee analysis and fee structuring. *New Orleans Medical Business and Conference.*

Medical Learning, Inc. (1997). *Nurse Practitioners-Evaluation & Management Coding.* St. Paul, MN: Medical Learning, Inc.

Practice Management Information Corporation (2000). *The Coder's Handbook.* Los Angeles, California: Practice Management Information Corporation.

Travers, K., Ellis, R., and Dartt, L.A. (Revised July 1995). *Comparison of the Rural Health Clinic and Federally Qualified Health Center Programs.* Washington, DC: A report of the Office of Rural Health Policy by the National Association of Community Health Centers.

World Health Organization. (2003). *International Classification of Diseases 9th Revision, Clinical Modification,* Los Angeles, California: Practice Management Information Corporation

Appendix A

SAMPLE CONTRACT BETWEEN
SHERIFF'S DEPARTMENT
COUNTY, TENNESSEE
and
NAMED STATE UNIVERSITY
COLLEGE OF NURSING

This agreement is entered into on _____ by and between Sheriff's Department, County, herein after referred to as the AGENCY, and State University, College of Nursing, herein after referred to as the CONTRACTOR.

NOW THEREFORE: In consideration of the mutual agreement contained herein, the parties have agreed and do hereby enter into this contract according to the provisions set out herein:

I. The Contractor agrees to:

Provide clinical services at the County jail within the scope of a family nurse practitioner and registered nurse. Services will include but not be limited to:

1. Admission physicals by nurse practitioner, once a week.
2. Sick call performed by registered nurse to see any inmate who has filed a "Request for Medical Attention." RN will triage, according to RN protocols, regarding the need for NP services at the next visit.
3. Women's health exams completed at Contractor's facility.
4. Billing County for services provided.
5. Consultation/guidance for inmate health care.

II. The Agency agrees to:

A. Reimburse the Contractor according to the agency approved budget (Attachment A) upon receipt of monthly invoices documenting non-reimbursable charges, which reflect salary and benefits in the project by Contractor personnel.

B. Provide space, utilities, equipment (blood pressure cuff, digital thermometer and probe cover, stethoscope, reflex hammer, otoscope, opthalmoscope, glucometer (with strips) and supplies) necessary for the nurse practitioner and registered nurse while providing care at the County Jail.

C. Provide chaperone services for the nurse practitioner/RN at all times when services are not provided at the County jail.

D. County will provide insurance information to the Contractor, including a copy of the insurance card, if available.

III. The parties further agree that the following shall be essential terms and conditions of this agreement:

A. Each party assures that it will not discriminate in the performance of this agreement on the grounds of race, creed, color, sex, religion, age, national origin, disabilities, or veteran status.

B. The term of this contract shall be for a period of one (1) year, from August 1, 2003, through July 31, 2004. After the initial one (1) year period, this agreement is renewable for successive one (1) year periods for a maximum of (4) four additional years.

C. This agreement may be terminated, for cause, by either party by giving written notice to the other at least thirty (30) days before the effective date of termination. After the initial one (1) year period, this agreement may be terminated upon thirty (30) days notice for any reason.

D. Any and all claims against the contractor for personal injury and/or property damage resulting from the negligence of the contractor in performing any responsibility specifically required under the terms of the agreement shall be submitted to the Board of Claims or the Claims Commission for the State of Tennessee. Damages recoverable against the institution shall be expressly limited to claims paid by the Board of Claims or Claims Commission pursuant to T.C.A. Section 9-8-301 et. seq.

E. This contract shall not be binding until it is signed by all parties.

SHERIFF'S DEPARTMENT
COUNTY, TENNESSEE

_____

Sheriff
County, Tennessee

STATE UNIVERSITY
COLLEGE OF NURSING

_____

Dean, College of Nursing

_____

Vice President for Health Affairs

ATTACHMENT A

**SHERIFF'S DEPARTMENT
COUNTY, TENNESSEE**

Nurse Practitioner Contract

August 1, 2003 – July 31, 2004

Nurse Practitioner @ $40.00/hr
Registered Nurse @ $25.00/hr

Appendix B

New Provider Credentialing Process

Name: _____

Specialty: _____

Location: _____

Start Date: _____

DOB: _____

County of Birth: _____

Company	Date Prepared/ Signed	Date Sent	Approved	Expiration
Certificate of Fitness				
Health-Related Boards				
Preceptor letter updated				
Blue Products pre-app				
Blue Contracts				
John Deere Pre-Assessment				
John Deere Contracts				
PHP/Cariten Contract				
Medicare				
VA Medicaid				
NC Medicaid				
Mountain States				

Appendix C-1

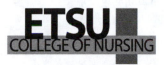

FOR OFFICE USE ONLY
Chart # _____

NEW PATIENT DATE	UPDATES		

PATIENT INFORMATION   Race: **Asian/Pacif**   **Black**   **Caucasian (White)**   **Hispanic**
American Indian   **Other**   *(Optional)*   **1**
2   3   4   5   9

Legal Name _____
Sex_____   Marital Status S   M   W   D

Mailing
Address_____
_____
          (Street)   (City)
(State)   (Zip)

Birthdate_____ Social Security # _____-____-_____ Home Phone
_____
                                                                (Area Code)

Emergency Contact (other than spouse if married)   Name
_____
              (other than parents if a child)   Relationship
_____ Phone _____

EMPLOYMENT INFORMATION

Patients employer
_____
_____
          (Name)   (Address)   (City)
(State)   (Zip)

Business Phone _____   Position
_____

Spouse s Name _____   Employer
_____

Business Phone _____
Position_____

INSURANCE INFORMATION *(Please present all insurance information upon arrival to the clinic)*

Primary Insurance
Company Name_____

Secondary Insurance
Company

Name_____

Claims Address _____

Claims Address

_____

_____

_____

Policy Holder_____

Policy

Holder_____

Holder s SS#_____ Date of Birth_____

Holder s

SS#_____ Date of Birth_____

AUTHORIZATION AND RELEASE

I authorize the Health Center to examine and treat me and or my child or ward. I authorize the Health Center to release any and all clinical information necessary in order to submit my insurance claims to my insurance companies. I also request that my insurance companies pay benefits directly to the Health Center for services rendered. I understand that the Health Center will refund any overpayments on my account. For the purpose of health care education, I consent to the admittance of observers to the examination rooms.

My right to prepare advance directives about what medical treatment I may want to receive if I became physically or mentally unable to communicate my wishes has been explained to me.

Signature of patient or parent (if minor): _____*Witness*

_____

*Date:*_____

_____

Appendix C-2

Sample Consent Agreement

Consent to the Use and Disclosure of Health Information for Treatment, Payment, or Healthcare Operations

I, (PATIENT'S NAME), understand that as part of my healthcare, this Medical office originates and maintains health records describing my health history, symptoms, examination and test results, diagnoses, treatment, and any plans for future care or treatment. I understand that this information serves as:

- A basis for planning my care and treatment

- A means of communication among the many health professionals who contribute to my care

- A source of information for applying my diagnosis and surgical information to my bill

- A means by which a third-party payer can verify that services billed were actually provided, and

- A tool for routine healthcare operations such as assessing quality and reviewing the competence of healthcare professionals

I understand and have been provided with a Notice of Information Practices that provides a more complete description of information uses and disclosures. I understand that I have the right to review the notice prior to signing this consent. I understand that the organization reserves the right to change their notice and practices and prior to implementation will mail a copy of any revised notice to the address I've provided. I understand that I have the right to object to the use of my health information for directory purposes. I understand that I have the right to request restrictions as to how my health information may be used or disclosed to carry out treatment, payment, or healthcare operations and that the organization is not required to agree to the restrictions requested. I understand that I may revoke this consent in writing, except to the extent that the organization has already taken action in reliance thereon.

I wish to have the following restrictions to the use or disclosure of my health-information:

I fully understand and accept/decline the terms of this consent.

_____

(SIGNATURE)

_____

(DATE)

Appendix C-3

AUTHORIZATION FOR DISCLOSURE OF HEALTH INFORMATION

separate authorization, as defined by HIPAA, must be used if the authorization is for ychotherapy notes.]

_____   _____
Name of Patient   Birth Date

_____   _____
Street Address   City, State, Zip

AUTHORIZES: **3. RELEASE PROTECTED HEALTH INFORMATION TO:**

_____   _____
me of Health Care Provider/Plan/Other   Name of Health Care Provider/Plan/Other

_____   _____
eet Address   Street Address

_____   _____
y, State, Zip Code   City, State, Zip Code

INFORMATION TO BE RELEASED:

_ Medical History, Examination, Reports   ___ Surgical Reports
_ Treatment or Tests   ___ Hospital Records Including Reports
_ Immunizations   ___ Allergy Records
_ X-ray Reports   ___ Prescriptions
_ Laboratory Reports   ___ Consultations
_ Entire Record   ___ Other (Specify):_____

r the reasons below which require special permission to release otherwise privileged information, ase release records pertaining to:

_ Mental Health   ___ Developmental Disabilities
_ Alcoholism   ___ Drug Abuse
_ HIV (AIDS)   ___ Sexually Transmitted Diseases
_ Other (Specify): _____

)R THE FOLLOWING DATE(S): _____

PURPOSE FOR NEED OF DISCLOSURE: (Check applicable categories)

_ Further Medical Care   ___ Personal
_ Insurance Eligibility/Benefits   ___ Changing Physicians
_ Legal Investigation or Action   ___ Other (Specify): _____
_____

I understand that if the person(s) and/or organization(s) listed above are not health care providers, health plans or health care clearinghouses, who must follow the federal privacy standards, the health information disclosed as a result of this authorization may no longer be protected by the federal privacy standards and my health information may be redisclosed without obtaining my authorization.

Your Rights with Respect to This Authorization

- **Right to Receive Copy of This Authorization -** I understand that if I agree to sign this authorization, which I am not required to do, I must be provided with a signed copy of the form.

- **Right to Refuse to Sign This Authorization -** I understand that I am under no obligation to sign this form and that the person(s) and/or organization(s) listed above who I am authorizing to use and/or disclose my information may not condition treatment, payment, enrollment in a health plan or eligibility for health care benefits on my decision to sign this authorization. *[As a provider or Health Plan, the rule permits you to condition treatment, payment, enrollment in a health plan or eligibility for health care benefits on the signing of this authorization in the following circumstances:*
  (a) a health care provider may condition the provision of research-related treatment on the provision of an authorization to use and/or disclose an individual s health information for such research;
  (b) a health plan may condition enrollment in the health plan or eligibility for benefits on the provision of an authorization required prior to enrollment in a health plan, if:
    (i) the authorization is for the health plan s eligibility or enrollment determinations or for its underwriting or risk rating determination and
    (ii) the authorization is not for the use and/or disclosure of psychotherapy notes;
  (c) an entity subject to the Rule may condition the provision of health care that is solely for the purpose of creating health information for disclosure to a third party on the provision of an authorization for the disclosure of the health information to such third party.
  If you wish to make such conditions, you must include a description of these circumstances upon signing of this authorization.]

- **Right to Withdraw This Authorization -** I understand written notification is necessary to cancel this authorization. To obtain information on how to withdraw my authorization or to receive a copy of my withdrawal, I may contact:_____. I am aware that my withdrawal will not be effective as to uses and/or disclosures of my health information that the person(s) and or organization(s) listed above have already made in reference to this authorization.

Disclosure of Direct or Indirect Payment Received by Any Person or Organization Authorized to Use or Disclose my Health Information - I understand that the following person(s) and/or organization(s):___
_____
_____

(If no direct or indirect payment will be received, no one may be inserted in the blank above.)

___ will not be receiving any direct or indirect payment in connection with the use or disclosure of my health information.

___ will be receiving payment, as described below, in connection with the use or disclosure of my health information (describe amount or nature of any direct or indirect payment):_____

_____

Expiration Date: This authorization is good until the following date(s) _____ or

ent(s) (specify event) _____
   (An expiration date is not required if the authorization is for research purposes.)

ave had an opportunity to review and understand the content of this authorization form. By signing this
   authorization, I am confirming that it accurately reflects my wishes.

. **Signature of Patient:** _____   Date: _____
   (If signed by person other than patient, state relationship and authority to do so.)

tient is: Minor   Incompetent   Disabled   Deceased

gal Authority: Custodial Parent   Legal Guardian   Executor of Estate of Deceased
                    Power of Attorney for Healthcare   Authorized Legal Representative

Appendix C-4

ETSU
COLLEGE OF NURSING

Name and Address of Medical Facility

	OFFICE VISITS		FEE	X	CODE	INJECTIONS	FEE	X	CODE	IMMUNIZATIONS	FEE
X	CODE	**NEW PATIENT**			95115	ALLERGY, ONE			90647	HIB (3 dose schedule) V03.81	
	99201	PF/STRTFWD			95117	ALLERGY, MULTI # _____			90657	FLU (6-35 mos) V04.8	
	99202	EXPANDED PF/STRTFWD			J1100	DECADRON _____ MG			90658	FLU (> 3 yrs) V04.8	
	99203	DETAILED / LOW			J1055	DEPO PROVERA 150 MG			90669	PNEUMOCOCCAL V03.82	
	99204	COMPREH / MODERATE			J0570	LA BICILLIN 900,000-1.2 MIL UN			90700	DtaP V06.1	
	99205	COMPREH / HIGH			J2550	PHENERGAN			90718	Td V06.5 (adult)	
	90862	PHARM. MAINT.			J0696	ROCEPHIN _____ MG			90707	MMR V06.4	
X	CODE	**ESTAB. PATIENT**			86580	TB SKIN TEST			90713	IPV V04.0	
	99211	NURSE VISIT			J1885	TORADOL _____ MG			90716	VARICELLA V05.4	
	99212	PF/STRTFWD				**OTHER** _____				HEP B (Ped/Adol.) **V05.3**	
	99213	EXPANDED PF / LOW			CODE	ADMINISTRATION			90746	HEPATITIS (Adult) V05.3	
	99214	DETAILED / MOD			90788	ANTIBIOTIC ADMINISTRATION					
	99215	COMPREH / HIGH			90782	OTHER ADMINISTRATION		X		VFC ADMINISTRATION	

	PREVENTIVE MEDICINE			X	CODE	PROCEDURES/ TREATMENTS			90471	SINGLE DOSE	
									90472	TWO OR MORE	
	EST	Pt. Age			92552	AUDIOMETRY			CODE	**IN HOUSE LABS**	
99381	99391	<1 YEAR			92567	TYMPANOMETRY			82947	GLUCOSE FINGER STICK	
99382	99392	1-4 YRS			99173	VISION SCREEN W/PE (NC) W/O —PE			82270	HEMOCCULT	
99383	9393	5-11 YRS			69210	CERUMEN REMOVAL			85018	HGB FINGER STICK	
99384	99394	12-17 YRS			69200	FB REMOVAL EAR			81025	URINE PREGNANCY TEST	
99385	99395	18-39 YRS			65205	FB REMOVAL EXTERNAL EYE			81002	URINE DIP	
99386	99396	40-64 YRS			30300	FB REMOVAL NOSE			87210	WET MOUNT	
99387	99397	65 & OVER			94664	AEROSOL TX. INITIAL			9000	HANDLING FEE RSS	
					94665	AEROSOL TX. SUBSEQUENT			99000	HANDLING FEE URINE C&S	
	OB/GYN VISITS				94150	PEAK FLOW **(NO CHARGE)**			99000	HANDLING FEE WOUND	
					94760	**PULSE OXIMETRY** (NO CHG)			82951	GLUCOSE TOLERENCE TEST	
X	CODE	TYPE			16000	INITIAL BURN TREATMENT				OTHER:	
59426NC	GLOBAL PREGNANCY NO CHARGE VISIT				16020	SUBSEQUENT BURN TX					
					17110	LESION DESTRUCTION (1-14)			CODE	SUPPLIES	
594____	ACCUMLATIVE PRENATAL #VISITS____				17111	LESION DESTRUCTION (15 & >)					
59430	POSTPARTUM VISIT				93005	EKG			A6263	ACE WRAP BANDAGE	
Q0091	PAP SMEAR					Other:			A4565	ARM SLING	

Demographic and insurance information produced from a computerized medical office software system would appear here and would include current balance due.

Note: As CPT codes change annually, use this form for reference only!

Appendix C-5

Patient s Name: Medicare # (HICN):

Advance Beneficiary Notice (ABN)

NOTE: You need to make a choice about receiving these health care items or services. We expect that Medicare will not pay for the item(s) or service(s) that are described below. Medicare does not pay for all of your health care costs. Medicare only pays for covered items and services when Medicare rules are met. The fact that Medicare may not pay for a particular item or services does not mean that you should not receive it. There may be a good reason your doctor recommended it. Right now, in your case, **Medicare probably will not pay for —**

Items or Services:

Because:

The purpose of this form is to help you make an informed choice about whether or not you want to receive these items or services, knowing that you might have to pay for them yourself. Before you make a decision about your options, you should **read this entire notice carefully.**

- Ask us to explain, if you don t understand why Medicare probably won t pay.
- Ask us how much these items or services will cost you (Estimated Cost: $_____).

PLEASE CHOOSE **ONE** OPTION. CHECK **ONE** BOX. **SIGN & DATE** YOUR CHOICE.

_ **Option 1. YES. I want to receive these items or services.**

I understand that Medicare will not decide whether to pay unless I receive these items or services. Please submit my claim to Medicare. I understand that you may bill me for items or services and that I may to pay the bill while Medicare is making its decision. If Medicare does pay, you will refund to me any payments I made to you that are due to me. If Medicare denies payment, I agree to be personally and fully responsible for payment. That is, I will pay personally, either out of pocket or through any other insurance that I have. I understand I can appeal Medicare s decision

_ **Option 2. NO. I have decided not to receive these items or services.**

I will not receive these items or services. I understand that you will not be able to submit a claim to Medicare and that I will not be able to appeal your opinion that Medicare won t pay.

_____   _____
     Date   **Signature of patient or person acting on patient s behalf**

NOTE: Your health information will be kept confidential. Any information that we collect about you on this form will be kept confidential in our offices. If a claim is submitted to Medicare, your health information on this form may be shared with Medicare. Your health information which Medicare sees till be kept confidential by Medicare.

OMB Approval No. 0938-0566   Form No. CMS-R-131-G   (June 2002)

Appendix D

CMS 1500

PLEASE
DO NOT
STAPLE
IN THIS
AREA

HEALTH INSURANCE CLAIM FORM

| | PICA | | | | | | | PICA | | |

1. MEDICARE (Medicare #)   MEDICAID (Medicaid #)   CHAMPUS (Sponsor's SSN)   CHAMPVA (VA File #)   GROUP HEALTH PLAN (SSN or ID)   FECA BLK LUNG (SSN)   OTHER (ID)   1a. INSURED'S I.D. NUMBER   (FOR PROGRAM IN ITEM 1)

2. PATIENT'S NAME (Last Name, First Name, Middle Initial)

3. PATIENT'S BIRTH DATE   MM   DD   YY   SEX   M   F

4. INSURED'S NAME (Last Name, First Name, Middle Initial)

5. PATIENT'S ADDRESS (No., Street)

6. PATIENT RELATIONSHIP TO INSURED   Self   Spouse   Child   Other

7. INSURED'S ADDRESS (No., Street)

CITY   STATE

8. PATIENT STATUS   Single   Married   Other   Employed   Full-Time Student   Part-Time Student

CITY   STATE

ZIP CODE   TELEPHONE (Include Area Code)   ( )

ZIP CODE   TELEPHONE (INCLUDE AREA CODE)   ( )

9. OTHER INSURED'S NAME (Last Name, First Name, Middle Initial)

10. IS PATIENT'S CONDITION RELATED TO:

11. INSURED'S POLICY GROUP OR FECA NUMBER

a. OTHER INSURED'S POLICY OR GROUP NUMBER

a. EMPLOYMENT? (CURRENT OR PREVIOUS)   YES   NO

a. INSURED'S DATE OF BIRTH   MM   DD   YY   SEX   M   F

b. OTHER INSURED'S DATE OF BIRTH   MM   DD   YY   SEX   M   F

b. AUTO ACCIDENT?   PLACE (State)   YES   NO

b. EMPLOYER'S NAME OR SCHOOL NAME

c. EMPLOYER'S NAME OR SCHOOL NAME

c. OTHER ACCIDENT?   YES   NO

c. INSURANCE PLAN NAME OR PROGRAM NAME

d. INSURANCE PLAN NAME OR PROGRAM NAME

10d. RESERVED FOR LOCAL USE

d. IS THERE ANOTHER HEALTH BENEFIT PLAN?   YES   NO   *If yes,* return to and complete item 9 a-d.

READ BACK OF FORM BEFORE COMPLETING & SIGNING THIS FORM.

12. PATIENT'S OR AUTHORIZED PERSON'S SIGNATURE I authorize the release of any medical or other information necessary to process this claim. I also request payment of government benefits either to myself or to the party who accepts assignment below.

SIGNED ____ DATE ____

13. INSURED'S OR AUTHORIZED PERSON'S SIGNATURE I authorize payment of medical benefits to the undersigned physician or supplier for services described below.

SIGNED ____

14. DATE OF CURRENT: MM   DD   YY   ILLNESS (First symptom) OR INJURY (Accident) OR PREGNANCY(LMP)

15. IF PATIENT HAS HAD SAME OR SIMILAR ILLNESS. GIVE FIRST DATE   MM   DD   YY

16. DATES PATIENT UNABLE TO WORK IN CURRENT OCCUPATION   MM   DD   YY   FROM   TO   MM   DD   YY

17. NAME OF REFERRING PHYSICIAN OR OTHER SOURCE

17a. I.D. NUMBER OF REFERRING PHYSICIAN

18. HOSPITALIZATION DATES RELATED TO CURRENT SERVICES   MM   DD   YY   FROM   TO   MM   DD   YY

19. RESERVED FOR LOCAL USE

20. OUTSIDE LAB?   YES   NO $ CHARGES

21. DIAGNOSIS OR NATURE OF ILLNESS OR INJURY. (RELATE ITEMS 1,2,3 OR 4 TO ITEM 24E BY LINE)

1. ____   3. ____
2. ____   4. ____

22. MEDICAID RESUBMISSION CODE   ORIGINAL REF. NO.

23. PRIOR AUTHORIZATION NUMBER

24. A. DATE(S) OF SERVICE From MM DD YY To MM DD YY	B. Place of Service	C. Type of Service	D. PROCEDURES, SERVICES, OR SUPPLIES (Explain Unusual Circumstances) CPT/HCPCS | MODIFIER	E. DIAGNOSIS CODE	F. $ CHARGES	G. DAYS OR UNITS	H. EPSDT Family Plan	I. EMG	J. COB	K. RESERVED FOR LOCAL USE
1										
2										
3										
4										
5										
6										

25. FEDERAL TAX I.D. NUMBER   SSN   EIN

26. PATIENT'S ACCOUNT NO.

27. ACCEPT ASSIGNMENT? (For govt. claims, see back)   YES   NO

28. TOTAL CHARGE $

29. AMOUNT PAID $

30. BALANCE DUE $

31. SIGNATURE OF PHYSICIAN OR SUPPLIER INCLUDING DEGREES OR CREDENTIALS (I certify that the statements on the reverse apply to this bill and are made a part thereof.)

SIGNED ____ DATE ____

32. NAME AND ADDRESS OF FACILITY WHERE SERVICES WERE RENDERED (If other than home or office)

33. PHYSICIAN'S, SUPPLIER'S BILLING NAME, ADDRESS, ZIP CODE & PHONE #

PIN#   GRP#

(APPROVED BY AMA COUNCIL ON MEDICAL SERVICE 8/88)   **PLEASE PRINT OR TYPE**   APPROVED OMB-0938-0008 FORM CMS-1500 (12/90), FORM RRB-1500, APPROVED OMB-1215-0055 FORM OWCP-1500. APPROVED OMB-0720-0001 (CHAMPUS

UB92

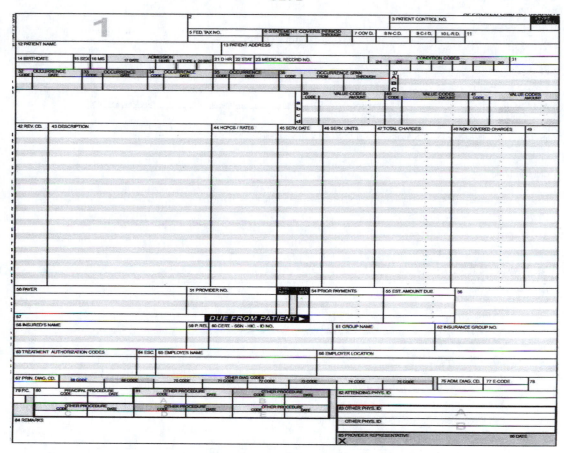

Appendix E

Health Center

Time Arrived _____

MCO:_____

Name: Date:DOB: Age:Chart#:_____

ALLERGIES: Appt time: Time seen:_____   Time finished:_____   ?>50% counseling Y N

LMP_____   T   P   R   BP   HT   WT_____   HC_____
Imm UTD: Y NHealth Hx reviewed: Y N Tobacco use Y N ETOH use Y N Passive smoke Y N
Current Medications:(see med list for chronic meds

Chief complaint:

History of Present Illness: (4+ elements for 99203/99214 or update of 3 or more chronic problems)

Previous Problem Resolved? Y or N Comments:

Family/social history:

ROS (99201/99212=none, 99202/99213=pertinent to CC, 99203/99214=2-9 systems, 99204/99205/99215=complete — at least 10)

PHYSICAL EXAM: (99201/99212=1-5 bullets 99202/99213=6 bullets; 99203/99214=12 bullets; 99204/99205/99215=At least 9 areas, 2 bullets each) *=bullet
Constitutional: (* 3= vital signs *general appearance)

SKIN: (*inspection *palpation)
WNL N/A

EYES: (*insp conjunctiva/lids *exam pupil/iris *fundoscopic exam)
WNL N/A

EN: (*insp E/N *otoscopic exam * hearing * insp nasal mucosa/septum/turbinates)
WNL N/A

MOUTH/NECK: (*exam of neck *exam of thyroid * lymph nodes *exam oropharynx *insp lips teeth gums)
WNL N/A

CV: (*palp *auscultation, exam of *carotids *abd aorta *femoral *pedal *extremities for edema/varicosities)
WNL N/A

LUNGS: (*resp effort *percussion *palpation *auscultation)
WNL N/A

BREASTS: (*insp breasts *palpation of breasts/axilla)
WNL N/A

ABD/GI: (*exam for masses/tenderness *exam liver/spleen *hernia check *rectal exam *stool for occult blood
WNL N/A

GU:Male: (*scrotal contents *penis *digital prostate exam)
WNL N/A

GU: Female: (pelvic exam-*ext genitalia/vagina/ urethra *bladder *cervix *uterus *adnexa)
WNL N/A

LYMPH: (palp of *axillae *groin *other)
WNL N/A

MSK: (*gait/station *insp/& or palp digits/nails *insp/palp joint/bone/muscle for general defects *ROM *stability *muscle strength /tone
WNL N/A

NEURO: (*Cranial nerves *DTRS *Sensation)
WNL N/A

PSYCH: (*description of judgement/insight *brief MSE)
WNL N/A

ASSESSMENT:
1. _____New Stable Ongoing Worsening
2. _____New Stable Ongoing Worsening
3. _____New Stable Ongoing Worsening
4. _____New Stable Ongoing Worsening
Other:_____
PLAN:

Next Visit:

Patient instructions : Verbal Y Written Y Both Y

Testing ordered (all):

1. _____Matched to Dx.#_____ 4._____Matched to Dx.#_____
2. _____Matched to Dx. #_____ 5._____Matched to Dx.#_____
3. _____Matched to Dx. #_____ 6._____Matched to Dx.#_____
Medicare Waiver signed Y N NA TN care lab _____JCH lab_____ EHHC lab_____ Other lab_____
Test results:

Referral/Consultation_____

Signature:_____
**Preventive visit scheduled: Y N Work/School excuse given Y N Date of Return_____
Decision making:
Level of Decision Making Number of dx/options Amt of Data to review Risk Code

Straightforward Minimal Minimal or None Minimal 99202/99212

Low complexity Limited Limited Low 99203/99213
Moderate complexity Multiple Moderate/Complex Moderate 99204/99214
High complexity Extensive Extensive/Complex High 99205/99215
Notes:

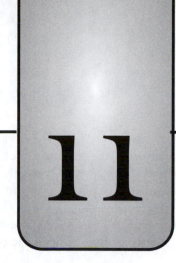

Managing Resources/Budgeting in Ambulatory Care

Beth A. Cherry, MSN, RN, CNA, CMPE

Introduction

In today's health care world, a positive cash flow and expenses kept within defined limits is crucial to the future of the organization. Ambulatory care provides an environment that lends itself to unique opportunities for creativity in reducing expenditures and enhancing revenue.

In the role of a nurse manager in Ambulatory care, it is likely that input related to the budget will focus on patient care equipment and staffing needs of the unit. However, the nurse manager must never lose sight of the importance of the nursing staff to increase the revenue flow to the organization. For example, it is important to assure that all procedures that the nurse performs are documented, including injections, blood draws, and medication usage, could represent potential revenue to an organization. Collection of required co-payments by the receptionist at the time of service is another way to ensure revenue coming in to the organization. Over time, and depending on the size of the setting, this can add up to a large amount of money that is due to the organization.

This chapter provides the tools for understanding the budget, along with the components necessary for preparation of both the operating and capital budgets.

Preparing the Capital Budget

The *capital budget* refers to equipment or services that are forecasted for the upcoming year. These are larger expenditures, generally $1,000 and over. Your organization can define the minimum cost of an item or service to be part of the capital budget for the upcoming year. Additionally, your organization may separate major and minor capital requests. For example, minor capital may be within the price ranges of $1,000–$49,000, whereas major capital may be any item or service over $50,000. Again, this is individually defined by the organization. Major capital requests often require more information and justification in the budgeting process. Items under $1,000 are usually placed in the operating budget.

Capital dollars are generally the first to be budgeted. It is a good idea to keep information about capital item requests throughout the year. When asked for input related to needed equipment and services for the upcoming year, an assessment can be made as to the current and future needs of the unit. Once the capital needs are well-defined, obtain quotes for equipment and services from the vendors, and rank the requests in order of importance. Then, the financial staff who make the decisions for capital expenditures can have an idea of the unit's primary needs. Exhibit 11-1 is an example of an annual capital request, placed in order of identified needs for the unit.

It is often helpful to include a justification for the request along with the dollar quote.

Preparing the Operating Budget

The *operating budget* consists of many components, all of which are discussed in this chapter. Barnett and Mayer (1992) describe a budget as "a plan or schedule adjusting expenses during a certain period to the estimated or fixed income for that period" (p. 184). In other words, an operating budget is a plan or operating tool for income (revenue) and expenditures (expenses) within a defined period of time, usually a calendar or academic year. Flexibility in adjusting expenses based on income throughout the year is important in

Exhibit 11-1   A Prioritized Capital Equipment Request

HOSPITAL XYZ
2004 Capital

MEDICAL EQUIPMENT

VENDOR	EQUIPMENT	PRICE
	Humphrey Visual Field, Model 750 with Table and Printer	$23,400
	Delphi-C Bone Densitometer	$59,525
	Mac 8 EKG Machine	$3,800
	Cordless Oscillating Saw and Blades	$1,190
	Automatic Blood Pressure Machine	$2,400
Total		**$90,315**

IT

VENDOR	EQUIPMENT	PRICE
	Healthquest computer/monitor for Surgical Specialties	$3,500
	Three computer/monitors (Orthopedics, Primary Care, and Ophthalmology)	$3,000
	EMR Rollout: 63 computers/monitors	$88,200
	19 printers	$7,600
Total		**$102,300**

BUILDING

VENDOR	EQUIPMENT	PRICE
	Two American flags with lights	$6,000
	Water softener for building	$28,000
Total		**$34,000**

managing the operations of the unit. Therefore, the nurse manager needs to understand the budgeting process as well as the ongoing reports that may be provided regarding revenue and expenses. The nurse manager who manages several different specialties or product lines may be responsible for overseeing multiple cost centers within the operating budget. There are several types of budgets, including:

- *Zero-based budgets*—Preparing a zero-based budget refers to "starting from scratch." If one can imagine starting fresh with a new unit and being charged with preparing a document that includes expenses related to staffing, equipment, supplies, and services, along with projections for revenue, one would understand a zero-based budget. (These components will be discussed later in the chapter.)

- *Historical-based budget*—Historical budgets are based on prior information that is available to the nurse manager. In looking at expenses for the previous year, the nurse manager may be asked to cut dollars from the budget, yet deal with the inflation that generally occurs related to salaries and supplies. There are two ways in which this can be handled. The first is to simply cut expenses for staffing and supplies. However, this may not be realistic given the needs of the unit and the volume of patients that come to the unit. The second method is to look at prior revenues and find creative ways to enhance it so that a balanced budget can be formulated.

Components of a Budget

Revenue

Revenue refers to the income of a particular unit and is generated by patient charges. In the Ambulatory setting, charges can be broken out into several categories, including professional clinic and hospital charges, hospital outpatient, pharmacy, and miscellaneous revenue. The organization defines these categories. The total of all charges for a particular cost center are referred to as the *gross charges*. Hospitals and Ambulatory care centers have contracts with many insurance companies, including Medicare/Medicaid, commercial payers, and managed care organizations. Additionally, they often provide charity discounts, courtesy discounts, and make provisions for uncollected debt. The formula for the contractual discounts along with uncollected money will vary based on the terms of the insurance companies' contracts with the organization, location, and patient population of the institution. Once these projected figures are calculated into the gross revenue, the nurse manager has a better picture of what the true projected income is for the cost center.

Expenses: Salaries and Benefits

Now we must look at the expense side of the budget—the money going out of the organization. The salaries and benefits paid to employees constitutes the largest amount of the operating budget. Understanding the staffing needs of a unit is crucial when determining the budget.

First, determine the duties of the nursing and reception staff, and the level of educational preparation needed for the role. It is important to remember that there is more flexibility in the use of different levels of staffing in the Ambulatory setting. In looking at the entire salary and benefit budget for a particular unit (or cost center), the physician or ancillary patient care providers will need to be included. The nurse manager may only be responsible for providing input on what the nursing and reception staff salaries will be.

Once staffing is determined, the nurse manager must cost out the actual salary, allowing for raises. This should include benefit costs. The nurse manager most likely has a combination of part-time and full-time employees. The following example shows how to determine annual salaries. To calculate this, it is important to understand that a 0.1 FTE refers to four hours of work.

> 0.1 FTE = 4 hours of work

So, an *hourly* employee who works three full days (or 24 hours per week) would be considered a 0.6 FTE. (24 hours ÷ 4 hours × 0.1 FTE = 0.6 FTE.) An hourly employee who works five days per week (or 40 hours) would be a 1.0 FTE.

> **Full Time Equivalent (FTE)**
>
> 40 hours/week x 52 weeks = 2,080 hours/year

The example above illustrates how hours per year for a full-time employee are determined. A part-time employee who works less than 40 hours per week can also be determined as a percent of FTE by the explanation above. For example, an employee who works two days per week would be considered a 0.4 FTE and works 832 hours per year. The calculation is as follows:

> 2 days (8 hours per day) = 16 hours of work
> 16 hours of work (0.1 FTE is 4 hours of work) = 0.4 FTE
> 2,080 hours per year x 0.4 = 832 hours per year

Now, the missing piece needed in order to budget the salary expense is the hourly rate of pay. If an employee earns $15.00 per hour, the annual budgeted salary expense would be $12,480. The calculation is as follows:

$15.00/hour x 832 hours/year = $12,480

This calculation is made for each employee, as salaries within the same job will vary.

Next, the expense for employee benefits needs to be determined. Generally, the organization defines a percentage of the salary to use as a guideline for determining benefit expense. The higher the benefit package for the employee (such as more vacation time, more sick time, or benefits due the employee related to travel expenditures for work-related responsibilities or conferences), the higher the percentage for benefit costs. For example, physicians that receive 20 days of vacation and $5,000 per year in travel expenditure costs the organization more in benefit coverage than a Medical Assistant who receives a lower salary, 10 vacation days, and no travel benefits. As a general rule, benefit expenses are 18–20 percent of the salary expense. Nurse managers should verify this percentage with the financial or budget office within their own organization.

The following is an example of the annual salary we calculated above ($12,480) with a benefit package of 18 percent:

$12,480 x 0.18 = $2,246.40/year for benefits
$12,480 + $2,246.40 = $14,726.40/year for salary and benefits
Or
Knowing that 100% (1.0) of the salary amount is $12,480,
$12,480 x 1.18 = $14,726.40/year for salary and benefits

Therefore, the total cost of the employees' salary and benefits is $14,726.40.

Now, let's try an example of a 40-hour/week employee who earns $22.00/hour and has a benefit package at 20 percent. What would the annual salary be? Cost of benefits? Total salary and benefit package?

40 hours/week = 1.0 FTE
40 hours/week = 2,080 hours/year
2,080 hours x $22.00/hour = $45,760 annual salary
$45,760 x 0.20 = $9,152 cost of benefits
$45,760 + $9,152 = $54,912 total annual salary and benefits
Or
$45,760 x 1.20 = $54,912 total annual salary and benefits

Expenses: Supplies and Equipment

Supplies and equipment are the items necessary to take care of patients on a daily basis. Expenses for supplies and equipment are often broken into categories referred to as *line items*. Properly used, line items help both the nurse manager and the financial office to determine what expenses may not be in line with the budgeted figures that were projected for the year (over or under budget). This allows the nurse manager to make adjustments throughout the year and to control expenses before they get out of hand.

Using an historical budget model, some information can be gathered looking at the expense trends for a particular line item based on what the expenses were in years past and at what rate they have grown. Budgeting for supplies and equipment is also based on a second component—*volume projections* (discussed later in this chapter). Medical supplies include items used in patient care such as drugs, IV solutions, sutures, implants, etc. Non-medical supplies can include line items such as forms, office supplies, minor equipment, books and publications, food and catering expenses, uniforms, and other supplies. These items must not be forgotten when preparing the budget. Exhibit 11-2 is an example of medical and non-medical supply and equipment expenses.

Your organization most likely has a template in place to define the line items and what should be included. Be sure to budget for yearly inflation of costs, which usually are around three percent. Again, the financial office of your organization determines what the projected inflation rate will be for the upcoming year.

Expenses: Indirect Costs

Indirect costs are those expenses carried by the organization but allocated and used by the unit. These are usually related to the expenses of the facility or property. Examples can include utility charges (telephone, pagers, gas, water, and electric), linen/laundry, rental of space or equipment, maintenance contracts, repairs of equipment or property, depreciation of equipment and buildings, landscaping, and snow removal. Again, these represent separate line items in the expense budget. The percentage of allocation to a specific unit is determined by the finance office, but is often based on the size and income of a particular cost center. Exhibit 11-3 gives an example of line items to be included in the indirect budget expenses.

Contribution Margins

Contribution margin refers to the amount of charges a unit has billed (gross revenue) minus the expenses it has incurred for salaries and benefits, supplies and

Exhibit 11-2   Hospital XYZ

Internal Medicine Department
Budget 2004

	Actual 2003	Budget 2004	YTD-Aug 2004	Annualized 2004	Budget 2005	Total New 2005	Budget 2005
Medical/Surgical Supplies							
Medical/Surgical Supplies	1,803	7,245	1,523	3,046	3,500		3,500
Rebates							
Central Supply							
PT Education Supp.							
Drugs	7,894	86,697	39,463	78,926	81,300		81,300
IV Solutions							
Implants							
Blood Products							
Instruments							
Reagents & Consumables	273	4,183	2,379	4,758	4,800		4,800
Film							
Contrast Media							
Sutures							
Disposables							
Oxygen & Gases							
Inventory Var.							
Med/Surg Other							
Medical/Surgical Supplies Total	9,970	98,125	43,365	86,730	89,600	—	89,600

Exhibit 11-2 Hospital XYZ *(continued)*

	Actual 2003	Budget 2004	YTD-Aug 2004	Annualized 2004	Budget 2005	Total New 2005	Budget 2005
Non-Medical Supplies							
Forms							
Minor Equipment	258		791	1,582	2,039		2,039
Office Supplies	2,476	9,162	1,271	2,542	2,700		2,700
Books & Publications	283	1,471					
Purchased Food & Supp.			93	186	240		240
Catering Expenses							
Uniforms	183	157	(30)	(60)	(78)		(77)
Linen							
Supplies Others	114	872	423	846	1,090		1,090
Non-Medical Supplies Total	**3,314**	**11,662**	**2,548**	**5,096**	**5,991**	**—**	**5,992**
Medical Services							
Purchased Medic.	—						
Medical Services Total	**—**	**—**	**—**	**—**	**—**	**—**	**—**
Non-Medical Services							
Purchased Services	5,934	10,304	14,868	29,736	38,320		38,320
Purch Non-Medic Svcs							
Parking Services	131						
Advertising/Marketing							
Community Support							
Corporate Membership							
Recruitment							
Search Fees							
Processing Fees							

Exhibit 11-2 Hospital XYZ *(continued)*

	Actual 2003	Budget 2004	YTD-Aug 2004	Annualized 2004	Budget 2005	Total New 2005	Budget 2005
Software Maintenance							
Freight/Courier							
Postage							
Printing	2,246	5,071	1,622	3,244	4,180		4,180
Laundry							
Joint Commission							
Purch Service Other							
Non-Medical Services Total	**8,311**	**15,375**	**16,490**	**32,980**	**42,500**	**—**	**42,500**
Consulting-Prof Services							
Consulting Fees							
Legal Fees							
Mgt Company Fees							
Prof Svc Other							
Consulting-Prof Services Total	**—**	**—**	**—**	**—**	**—**	**—**	**—**
Travel & Education							
Travel	3,211	5,875	2,549	5,098	6,000		6,000
Dues & Licenses	2,910	2,000	1,615	3,230	3,300		3,300
Staff Prof. Dues	2,260	4,147	2,325	4,650	4,700		4,700
Registrations	3,663	4,100	1,485	2,970	3,100		3,100
Business Meetings							
Local Mileage Reimb.	450	569	628	1,256	1,300		1,300
Accreditation							
T&E Other	361	1,808	22	44	57		57
Travel & Education Total	**12,855**	**18,499**	**8,624**	**17,248**	**18,457**	**—**	**18,457**

Exhibit 11-3 Hospital XYZ

Internal Medicine Department
Budget 2004

	Actual 2003	Budget 2004	YTD-Aug 2004	Annualized 2004	Budget 2005	Total New 2005	Budget 2005
Property							
Rent/Lease Space							
Rent/Lease Equip.							
Mtce Contracts							
Repair-Bldg & FX							
Repair-Equip.			225	450	580		580
Veh. Mtce							
Prop. Taxes & Asses.							
Utilities-Gas							
Utilities-Telephone							
Utilities-Pagers	259	823	257	514	662		662
Utilities-Long Distance							
Utilities-Cellular	192	521	234	468	603		603
Utilities-Cable							
Property Total	**451**	**1,344**	**716**	**1,432**	**1,845**	**—**	**1,845**
Depreciation							
Building							
Fixed Equip.							
Major Moveable	5,000						
Depreciation Total	**5,000**	**—**	**—**	**—**	**—**	**—**	**—**
Administrative Expenses							
Chargebacks	24,552	71,694	27,194	54,388	76,289		76,289
Chargeback-CCHS							
Administrative Expenses Total	**24,552**	**71,694**	**27,194**	**54,388**	**76,289**	**—**	**76,289**

equipment, and other expenses. These are the direct expenses; contribution margins do not include indirect expenses.

> Gross charges − Expenses = Contribution Margin

Net Income

Net income refers to the contribution margin minus the indirect expenses, and includes such things as the building costs, electricity, and gas costs.

> Contribution Margin − Indirect Costs = Net Income

The following section provides formulas and examples of what is described above.

Volume Projections

Volume projections by product line (i.e., orthopedics, cardiology) are crucial to the preparation of a budget for Ambulatory care. In fact, volume of visits and procedures for a particular product line help to determine the gross charges for the cost center.

Visits

When determining visit volume, it is important to understand who will be providing the service. For example, many organizations use physicians as well as nurse practitioners, physician assistants, and residents to provide direct care. These services need to be billed. Services performed by resident physicians are billed under the attending or teaching physician, and must be included in the attending or teaching physician's volume figures. Depending on the laws of the state, nurse practitioners may be included in the attending physician's billings or their services may be billed separately on their own. Either way, accurate visit and procedure volumes must be budgeted so gross charges can be budgeted and a realistic expense budget can be determined.

The first step in the process is to accurately determine how much of the provider time will be spent doing direct patient care that can be billed. This amount can include not only actual clinic visits and procedures, but also any professional charges that are incurred from rounding on admitted patients in the hospital, long-term nursing facilities, or other off-site facilities. In general, it is important to determine ways to either increase payments, or increase visit volume, to make up for the annual inflation costs as discussed earlier in this chapter.

Once the FTEs of specific providers are determined, the schedule of patient appointment slots for that provider will need to be determined. There are benchmarks available for ambulatory care which outline, by specialty or product line, the median visit volume and the 80th percentile for visit volume. One resource is the McGladrey and Pullen benchmarks. Further explanation of the McGladrey and Pullen benchmarks can be found in the resource area of the Medical Group Management Association website (www.mgma.com). These benchmarks, based on percentage of provider FTE, can be used as a guide to determine appropriate volume projections.

Of course, it is always necessary to assure that the provider is able to attain these projections, and that the schedule of patients works in tandem to reflect a volume that matches the projections. Exhibit 11-4 provides an example of a report by Worked RVUs for a Primary Care, Internal Medicine practice. Exhibit 11-5 is another example of Worked RVUs for a Medical Specialty Practice.

Procedures and Surgeries

The volume projections must also include a product line that provides office procedures and minor surgeries. Generally, these types of visits are reimbursed at a higher rate than office visits.

Determining Reimbursement Rates

To prepare a budget that reflects the estimated revenue that will be generated and paid, it is important to determine as accurately as possible the volume of visits and procedures that the provider will have in the upcoming year. In addition, the reimbursement rate, by product line and type of visit or procedure, will need to be determined. As discussed earlier in this chapter, one must understand the payer mix for the patient population that is served by the ambulatory clinic. Payer mixes can be determined by calculating the number of visits that are billed under a certain carrier (commercial, managed care, Medicare/Medicaid, etc.), and by determining a percentage of volume that carrier covers compared to the total visits.

Let's look at an example of a practice that has a total visit volume of 125,000 visits annually. The commercial payers account for 50,000 visits, Medicare/Medicaid for 43,750 visits, Managed Care for 25,000 visits, and Self Pay patients for 6,250 visits. What are the percentages of payer mixes? The formula is given below:

Commercial Insurance: 50,000 visits/125,000 annual visits = 0.40 or 40% of the payer mix.

Medicare/Medicaid: 43,750 visits/125,000 annual visits = 0.35 or 35% of the payer mix.

Managed Care: 25,000 visits/125,000 annual visits = 0.20 or 20% of the payer mix.

Self Pay: 6,250 visits/125,000 annual visits = 0.05 or 5% of the payer mix.

Tracking and understanding the break out of payer mix along with the average rate of payment, or reimbursement, is necessary to complete the budgeting process for revenue or, more simply stated, payments. For example, if you *earn* $900 per week but after taxes and deductions you are *paid* $650 per week, you would not want to spend the $900 earned amount. This is true when preparing a budget. Accurate determinations of what the clinic will be paid is necessary in order prepare the expense side of the budget.

Exhibit 11-4   Performance Indicators

Primary Care, Internal Medicine
Benchmark Based on McGladrey & Pullen
June 2004

Physician	%FTE	Jan 04	Feb 04	Mar 04	Apr 04	May 04	Jun 04	Totals
A	100%	652	655	517	707	437	718	**3,686**
B	100%	566	538	485	359	517	540	**3,005**
C	100%	526	439	498	432	483	372	**2,750**
D	100%	625	77	574	565	387	458	**2,686**
E	100%	392	546	478	441	438	344	**2,639**
F	100%	404	461	488	331	486	422	**2,592**
G	100%	316	523	333	452	462	459	**2,545**
H	100%	395	375	462	446	324	425	**2,427**
I	100%	433	311	517	328	385	437	**2,411**
J	100%	315	473	362	383	390	453	**2,376**
K	100%	386	344	405	449	317	350	**2,251**
L	100%	528	271	376	353	265	436	**2,229**
M	100%	276	353	420	438	435	293	**2,215**
N	100%	351	306	381	437	369	369	**2,213**
O	100%	375	365	491	266	210	498	**2,205**
P	100%	334	277	489	372	324	402	**2,198**
Q	100%	428	324	378	285	361	408	**2,184**
R	100%	356	302	453	279	378	407	**2,175**
S	100%	304	308	459	374	191	510	**2,146**
T	100%	391	356	272	452	229	441	**2,141**
McGladrey & Pullen 80 Percentile		347	347	347	347	347	347	2,082
Department Average		332	307	368	334	312	372	2,025

Exhibit 11-5   Performance Indicators

Medical Specialty
Benchmark Based on McGladrey & Pullen
June 2004

Physician	%FTE	Jan 04	Feb 04	Mar 04	Apr 04	May 04	Jun 04	Totals
AA	100%	780	629	692	615	649	580	3,945
BB	100%	431	517	695	766	395	664	3,468
CC	100%	443	602	532	670	547	366	3,160
DD	100%	565	365	613	498	300	501	2,842
EE	100%	518	374	477	472	447	510	2,798
FF	100%	371	248	335	335	424	339	2,052
GG	100%	323	314	256	388	276	414	1,971
McGladrey & Pullen 80 Percentile		347	347	347	347	347	347	2,082
McGladrey & Pullen Median		582	492	581	604	490	544	
Department Averages		553	492	581	604	490	544	

Exhibit 11-6 provides an example of a worksheet that can be used to set up the budget for volume projections.

The best and most accurate way to determine the percentage of charges that will be paid is to use historical data from your own organization. Keep in mind however, that ambulatory satellite locations may have different reimbursement rates than the main hospital ambulatory center. To further explain, if the organization is located in a large metropolitan area versus the satellite location in the suburbs, the payer mix may differ based on a higher amount of commercial payers in the suburbs. The worksheet shown in the previous exhibit illustrates revenue from procedures by multiplying the number of estimated procedures by the average dollars that are paid for the procedure. Keep in mind that the worksheet is separated out by product line or specialty, and the procedures for your organization can be streamlined as to what is most often performed. The nurse manager is in an excellent position to help provide this information, especially if there is no historical data available through the financial data-reporting systems of the organization.

The next section of the exhibit outlines *visit volume for new and established patients*. Again, these types of visits are reimbursed at a different rate. An

Exhibit 11-6 Hospital XYZ

Internal Medicine Department
Budget 2004

FTEs		Actual 2003	Budget 2004	YTD-Aug 2004	Annualized 2004	Budget 2005	Total New 2005	Budget 2005
Staff								
Exempt		2.62	5.45	5.82	5.82	6.85		6.85
Hourly		4.37	12.37	12.47	12.47	13.2		13.2
Agency								
Total FTEs		6.99	17.82	18.29	18.29	20.05		20.05
Activities								
Providers	**% Effort**							
Dr. B	0.60			1,039	2,076	2,100		2,100
Dr. C	0.80			1,857	3,714	3,600		3,600
Dr. D	1.00			2,674	5,348	5,000		5,000
Dr. E	1.00			347	694	3,600		3,600
Dr. F	0.90			593	1,186	4,050		4,050
Dr. G	0.65			1,539	3,078	2,000		2,000
Dr. H	1.00			1,954	3,908	3,600		3,600
Dr. I	0.85					1,080		1,080
Total Activities	6.80			10,003	20,004	25,030		25,030
Total RVUs				8,721	17,442			

understanding of the ambulatory location and practice, along with the patient population within the location, is important to prepare this information. Is this a new location? Is this a new specialty in the location? Are the practices well established and limiting new patients? New physicians or established practices that are trying to build their client base tend to have a higher percentage of "new" patients over an established practice that may not be accepting many new patients. Again, information on the percentage rate of reimbursement of charges is necessary.

The next line illustrates what is referred to as *off-site encounters*. These are visits the provider may make to nursing homes and assisted living facilities, and hospital inpatient professional charges.

The last line, *other activity*, refers to any other income where reimbursement can be planned. For example, perhaps the provider works as the city medical director and is paid on a regular basis for his/her time. This money would be deposited to the clinic, while the clinic pays the provider's salary.

Regardless of where the visit revenue is generated, the use of certified coders can assure that all possible billings are being captured and billed at the appropriate visit level. Coders can provide billing audits of billed charges compared to physician documentation to assure physicians are billing at the appropriate level for optimal reimbursement and that they are not under- or over-coding.

Now that you have learned about all of the components to be included in the budget worksheet, Exhibit 11-7 is an example of a complete budget worksheet.

Charges and Costing Out of Services

When a new service or procedure is offered in the ambulatory setting, or if it is necessary to raise charges, a systematic way to determine the charge must exist. First, let's discuss raising charges. Often, these determinations are made by the organization's financial office. On average, the organization looks at the competition within the market area, current insurance reimbursement rates, inflation, and how the organization performed financially over the past year. Generally, the national inflation rate is three percent. You may refer to Chapter 11 on "Budget Development and Evaluation" in the book, *Health Care Financial Management for Nurse Managers: Merging the Heart with the Dollar*, by Dunham-Taylor and Pinczuk, which discusses the market basket index, a method finance departments use to determine inflation rates.

Now suppose that the clinic has decided to add a new service. As the nurse manager you are asked to provide information as to the cost to the clinic to perform the procedure. In other words, you are asked to *cost out the service*. Considerations need to be given to staffing, medical equipment and supplies, non-medical supplies, depreciation, and any other overhead cost related to the service.

Exhibit 11-7   Hospital XYZ *(continues)*

Internal Medicine Department
Budget 2004

FTEs	% Effort	Actual 2003	Budget 2004	YTD-Aug 2004	Annualized 2004	Budget 2005	Total New 2005	Budget 2005
Staff		2.62	5.45	5.82	5.82	6.85		6.85
Exempt								
Hourly		4.37	12.37	12.47	12.47	13.2		13.2
Agency								
Total FTEs		6.99	17.82	18.29	18.29	20.05		20.05
Activities Providers								
Dr. B	0.60			1,039	2,076	2,100		2,100
Dr. C	0.80			1,857	3,714	3,600		3,600
Dr. D	1.00			2,674	5,348	5,000		5,000
Dr. E	1.00			347	694	3,600		3,600
Dr. F	0.90			593	1,186	4,050		4,050
Dr. G	0.65			1,539	3,078	2,000		2,000
Dr. H	1.00			1,954	3,908	3,600		3,600
Dr. I	0.85					1,080		1,080
Total Activities	6.80			10,003	20,004	25,030		25,030
Total RVUs				8,721	17,442			

Exhibit 11-7 Hospital XYZ *(continues)*

	Actual 2003	Budget 2004	YTD-Aug 2004	Annualized 2004	Budget 2005	Total New 2005	Budget 2005
Revenues & Expenses							
Revenues							
New Visits %			9,150	**9.40%**			
New			940	383,442	479,734		479,734
Est Visits %			7,962	**79.60%**			
Estimated			1,007,079	2,014,158	2,519,963		2,519,963
Other Visits %			248	**2.48%**			
Consulting			52,639	106,278	131,716		131,716
				21.58			
Other Activities			215,847	431,694	540,103		540,103
Gross Revenue	1,665,767	3,033,268	1,636,270	3,272,540	3,671,515		3,671,515
Collection Rate	51.38%	45.01%	50.17%	50.17%	50.17%		50.17%
			1,636,269	3,272,539			
Deducts	(809,963)	(1,668,097)	(815,278)	(1,630,556)	(1,829,347)		(1,829,347)
Net Revenue	**855,804**	**1,365,171**	**820,992**	**1,641,984**	**1,842,168**		**1,842,168**
Net Revenue Per Visit			82	82	74		74
Other Revenues							
Other Revenues	1,770	64	1,150	2,300			
Prof Revenue							
Other Revenue Total	**1,770**	**64**	**1,150**	**2,300**			
Total Net Revenue	857,574	1,365,235	822,142	1,644,284	1,842,168		1,842,168

Exhibit 11-7 Hospital XYZ *(continued)*

	Actual 2003	Budget 2004	YTD-Aug 2004	Annualized 2004	Budget 2005	Total New 2005	Budget 2005
Expenses							
Salary & Benefits							
Staff Salaries	394,594	805,868	370,405	740,810	704,729		704,729
Exempt Salaries							
Hourly Salaries	142,975	425,826	218,004	436,008	308,421		308,421
Agency Salaries							
Other Salaries	(775)		(1,650)	(3,300)			
Salaries Total	536,794	1,231,694	586,759	1,173,518	1,013,150		1,013,150
Benefits	120,492	250,335	143,233	286,466	222,893		222,893
Benefits Total							
Salaries & Benefits	657,286	1,482,029	729,992	1,459,984	1,236,043		1,236,043
Medical/Surgical Supplies							
Medical/Surgical Supplies	1,803	7,245	1,523	3,046	3,500		3,500
Rebates							
Central Supply							
PT Education Supp.							
Drugs							
IV Solutions	7,894	86,697	39,463	78,926	81,300		81,300
Implants							
Blood Products							
Instruments							
Reagents & Consumables	273	4,183	2,379	4,758	4,800		4,800
Film							

Exhibit 11-7   Hospital XYZ (*continued*)

	Actual 2003	Budget 2004	YTD-Aug 2004	Annualized 2004	Budget 2005	Total New 2005	Budget 2005
Medical/Surgical Supplies (*cont.*)							
Contrast Media							
Sutures							
Disposables							
Oxygen & Gases							
Inventory Var.							
Med/Surg Other							
Medical/Surgical Supplies Total	**9,970**	**98,125**	**43,365**	**86,730**	**89,600**		**89,600**
Non-Medical Supplies							
Forms							
Minor Equipment	258		791	1,582	2,039		2,039
Office Supplies	2,476	9,162	1,271	2,542	2,700		2,700
Books & Publications	283	1,471					
Purchased Food & Supp.			93	186	240		240
Catering Expenses							
Uniforms	183	157	(30)	(60)	(78)		(77)
Linen							
Supplies Others	114	872	423	846	1,090		1,090
Non-Medical Supplies Total	**3,314**	**11,662**	**2,548**	**5,096**	**5,991**		**5,992**
Medical Services							
Purchased Medic.							
Medical Services Total							

Exhibit 11-7 Hospital XYZ *(continued)*

	Actual 2003	Budget 2004	YTD-Aug 2004	Annualized 2004	Budget 2005	Total New 2005	Budget 2005
Non-Medical Services							
Purchased Services	5,934	10,304	14,868	29,736	38,320		38,320
Purch Non-Medic Svcs	131						
Parking Services							
Advertising/Marketing							
Community Support							
Corporate Membership							
Recruitment							
Search Fees							
Processing Fees							
Software Maintenance							
Freight/Courier							
Postage							
Printing	2,246	5,071	1,622	3,244	4,180		4,180
Laundry							
Joint Commission							
Purch Service Other							
Non-Medical Services Total	8,311	15,375	16,490	32,980	42,500		42,500
Consulting-Prof Services							
Consulting Fees							
Legal Fees							
Mgt Company Fees							
Prof Svc Other							
Consulting-Prof Services Total							

Exhibit 11-7 Hospital XYZ *(continued)*

	Actual 2003	Budget 2004	YTD-Aug 2004	Annualized 2004	Budget 2005	Total New 2005	Budget 2005
Travel & Education							
Travel	3,211	5,875	2,549	5,098	6,000		6,000
Dues & Licenses	2,910	2,000	1,615	3,230	3,300		3,300
Staff Prof. Dues	2,260	4,147	2,325	4,650	4,700		4,700
Registrations	3,663	4,100	1,485	2,970	3,100		3,100
Business Meetings							
Local Mileage Reimb.	450	569	628	1,256	1,300		1,300
Accreditation							
T&E Other	361	1,808	22	44	57		57
Travel & Education Total	12,855	18,499	8,624	17,248	18,457		18,457
Property							
Rent/Lease Space							
Rent/Lease Equip.							
Mtce Contracts							
Repair-Bldg & FX							
Repair-Equip.			225	450	580		580
Veh. Mtce							
Prop. Taxes & Asses.							
Utilities-Gas							
Utilities-Telephone							
Utilities-Pagers	259	823	257	514	662		662
Utilities-Long Distance							
Utilities-Cellular	192	521	234	468	603		603
Utilities-Cable							
Property Total	451	1,344	716	1,432	1,845		1,845

Exhibit 11-7   Hospital XYZ *(continued)*

	Actual 2003	Budget 2004	YTD-Aug 2004	Annualized 2004	Budget 2005	Total New 2005	Budget 2005
Depreciation							
Building							
Fixed Equip.							
Major Moveable	5,000						
Depreciation Total	5,000						
Total Other Expenses	39,901	145,005	71,743	143,486	158,393		158,394
Total Expenses	697,187	1,627,034	801,735	1,603,470	1,394,436		1,394,437
CONTRIBUTION MARGIN	160,387	(261,799)	20,407	40,814	447,732		447,731
Administrative Expenses							
Chargebacks	24,552	71,694	27,194	54,388	76,289		76,289
Chargeback-CCHS							
Administrative Expenses Total	24,552	71,694	27,194	54,388	76,289		76,289
Net Contribution Margin	135,835	(333,493)	(6,787)	(13,574)	371,443		371,442

As discussed in the preceding section on components of a budget, the nurse manager must look at salaries and benefits, supplies and equipment, and other expenses that may be associated with the new service. The nurse manager must first determine what equipment and supplies are necessary to perform the service. Vendors will need to be contacted if the equipment is to be purchased, and a quote will need to be obtained. Many supplies may already be standard within the existing clinic services, but any new supplies must have a price attached as well. Volume projections will need to be determined to predict how much supply is needed (as well as to assist in determining revenue).

Understanding the Budget Sheet

In preparing the budget, and subsequently analyzing it, it is important to understand not only the budget components, but also the different format and styles for communicating budget information. One must understand that organizations use different methods to communicate this information to the management staff. As previously discussed in this chapter, volume projections and actual volume of visits are crucial to understanding how to prepare a budget. In addition, volumes assist the nurse manager in understanding why a budget may not meet projected revenue.

The budget sheet in Exhibit 11-8 shows revenue and expense items by line (often referred to as *line items*) along the left margin. Across the top are the line items by month and year-to-date. In this particular example, the year-to-date information is for a half year, or January through June. The monthly reporting is for the month of June only.

For each of the monthly and year-to-date reporting sections at the top, there are three areas to evaluate: that of budget, actual, and variance figures. Let us look at each component separately:

- **Budget**—Budget refers to the original budget preparation that was done, or the *plan* that was presented the prior year for the upcoming year. In looking at the current budget, it gives the nurse manager a reminder of what revenue and expenses had been planned on both a monthly and yearly basis. The year-to-date shows how the present situation compares with what was planned.

- **Actual**—The dollar amounts listed here refer to the actual money spent (expenses) and the money billed out and/or collected (revenue).

- **Variance**—The variance refers to the difference between the budget estimate and the actual activity, and can be either positive or negative. In this example, the variance is illustrated as the difference between the actual column and the budget column. You may notice on some reports that a negative balance is indicated by either a minus sign or with the numbers in

Exhibit 11-8 Hospital XYZ

Original Budgets vs Actuals
JAN 04 TO JUN 04

	Budget	Actual	Variance	Pct	Budget	Actual	Variance	Pct
Revenues								
Professional-Clinic	$4,763,400	$4,714,000	$(49,400)	-0.01	$34,512,000	$36,900,000	$2,388,000	0.07
Professional-Hospital	$1,605,000	$1,463,000	$(142,000)	-0.09	$11,390,000	$10,701,000	$(689,000)	-0.06
Hospital-Inpatient	$100	$20	$(80)	-0.80	$400	$150	$(250)	-0.63
Hospital-Outpatient	$430,000	$435,000	$5,000	0.01	$3,309,000	$3,741,000	$432,000	0.13
Gross Revenue	**$6,798,500**	**$6,612,020**	**$(186,480)**	**-0.03**	**$49,211,400**	**$51,342,150**	**$2,130,750**	**0.04**
Contractual Discounts	$(3,885,000)	$(3,820,000)	$65,000	-0.02	$(28,050,000)	$(29,900,000)	$(1,850,000)	0.07
Other Discounts	$(75,000)	$(72,000)	$3,000	-0.04	$(540,000)	$(565,000)	$(25,000)	0.05
Uncollectibles	$(125,000)	$112,000	$237,000	-1.90	$(870,000)	$(910,000)	$(40,000)	0.05
Total Deducts	$(4,085,000)	$(3,780,000)	$305,000	-0.07	$(29,460,000)	$(31,375,000)	$(1,915,000)	0.07
Total Net Revenue	**$2,713,500**	**$2,832,020**	**$118,520**	**0.04**	**$19,751,400**	**$19,967,150**	**$215,750**	**0.01**
Expenses								
Physician Salaries	$595,000	$586,634	$(8,366)	-0.01	$4,480,000	$4,360,000	$(120,000)	-0.03
Employee Salaries	$479,000	$438,000	$(41,000)	-0.09	$3,730,000	$3,486,000	$(244,000)	-0.07
Salary Expense	**$1,074,000**	**$1,024,634**	**$(49,366)**	**-0.05**	**$8,210,000**	**$7,846,000**	**$(364,000)**	**-0.04**
Employee Benefits	$220,000	$201,500	$(18,500)	-0.08	$1,745,000	$1,680,000	$(65,000)	-0.04
Salary/Benefits	$1,294,000	$1,226,134	$(67,866)	-0.05	$9,955,000	$9,526,000	$(429,000)	-0.04
Med/Surg Supplies								
Supplies	$38,800	$7,887	$(30,913)	-0.80	$285,000	$238,000	$(47,000)	-0.16
Drugs	$580,000	$608,000	$28,000	0.05	$4,290,000	$4,675,000	$385,000	0.09

Exhibit 11-8 Hospital XYZ (*continued*)

	Budget	Actual	Variance	Pct	Budget	Actual	Variance	Pct
Med/Surg Supplies (*cont.*)								
IV Solutions	$1,300	$2,200	$900	0.69	$10,000	$12,000	$2,000	0.20
Instruments	$500	$100	$(400)	-0.80	$5,000	$4,500	$(500)	-0.10
Sutures	$50	$55	$5	0.10	$100	$500	$400	4.00
Other	$29,350	$6,758	$(22,592)	-0.77	$249,900	$180,000	$(69,900)	-0.28
Total	**$650,000**	**$625,000**	**$(25,000)**	**-0.04**	**$4,840,000**	**$5,110,000**	**$270,000**	**0.06**
Non-Medical Supplies	$19,500	$12,750	$(6,750)	-0.35	$141,500	$125,000	$(16,500)	-0.12
Non-Medical Services								
Freight/Courier	$650	$800	$150	0.23	$4,500	$5,300	$800	0.18
Postage	$200	$250	$50	0.25	$750	$800	$50	0.07
Printing	$3,800	$3,675	$(125)	-0.03	$27,500	$30,000	$2,500	0.09
Laundry	$2,500	$2,950	$450	0.18	$16,500	$18,486	$1,986	0.12
Other	$12,850	$27,325	$14,475	1.13	$95,750	$295,414	$199,664	2.09
Total	**$20,000**	**$35,000**	**$15,000**	**0.75**	**$145,000**	**$350,000**	**$205,000**	**1.41**
Travel/Education	$18,500	$9,250	$(9,250)	-0.50	$135,000	$80,000	$(55,000)	-0.41
Property	$41,300	$39,500	$(1,800)	-0.04	$305,100	$266,000	$(39,100)	-0.13
Depreciation	$28,500	$28,500		0.00	$211,200	$211,200		0.00
Other Expenses	$777,800	$750,000	$(27,800)	-0.04	$5,777,800	$6,142,200	$364,400	0.06
Total Expenses	**$2,071,800**	**$1,976,134**	**$(95,666)**	**-0.05**	**$15,732,800**	**$15,668,200**	**$(64,600)**	**-0.00**
Contribution Margin	$641,700	$855,886	$214,186	0.33	$4,018,600	$4,298,950	$280,350	0.07
Indirect Cost Expense	$830,000	$889,000	$59,000	0.07	$6,550,000	$6,850,000	$300,000	0.05
Net Income	$(188,300)	$(33,114)	$155,186	-0.82	$(2,531,400)	$(2,551,050)	$(19,650)	0.01

brackets or parens. In this example, the negative variance is shown with a minus sign. As the nurse manager, you will be able to readily tell those areas that are not performing according to the budgeted plan.

Understanding Relative Value Units (RVU)

The *relative value unit (RVU)* is "a unit of measure designed to permit comparison between the amounts of resource required to perform" a service. A *weight* or value is assigned to "factors such as personnel time, level of skill, stress level, and sophistication of [the] equipment required to render a service. The [Centers for Medicare and Medicaid (CMS)] requires that the three major components of an ambulatory service or procedure provided under Medicare have RVUs assigned to them [for] physician work, practice expense, and malpractice expense" (JCAHO, 1994) (www.aacap.org/clinical/cptgloss.htm).

The *Resource Based Relative Value Scale* is the prevailing model used today to describe, quantify, and reimburse physician services. For example, a routine office visit for an established adult patient credits the physician with anywhere from 0.17 to 1.77 RVUs, depending on the level of visit charged. A Diagnostic Colonoscopy procedure is worth 3.69 RVUs for the physician. For further information on the Resource Based Relative Value Scale (RBRVS) for procedure and visit information, refer to the CMS website at www.cms.hhs.gov.

Patient Satisfaction and Impact on the Budget

The patient's opinion of his/her health care experience and an organization's ability to monitor and measure patient satisfaction are imperative to the successful long-term financial future for an outpatient practice. It is important to realize that health care is a service industry that affords patients many choices of where to receive care. Competition for business is increasing among health care providers. Patients often make judgments about not only their one-on-one visit with the provider but the entire experience from the time they check in to the time they leave. Building loyalty among patients is imperative to gaining market share in the community.

Quality is a term we often hear, but it can sometimes be difficult to define and show in an objective way. Organizations measure quality by looking at topics such as pediatric immunization rates, eye examinations, Hemoglobin A1C rates in diabetic patients, mammogram rates, bone density screenings, rates of colonoscopy, and so forth. These quality measures are required by many regulatory agencies and most recently, by some insurance companies for payment of services.

Measuring the patient's opinion is difficult and subjective, and therefore the results may be perceived as not believable. Some organizations have created their own patient opinion or satisfaction surveys. If prepared and collected properly, this system can give the needed results. Protecting patient privacy while at the same time convincing patients that their opinions need to be honest and straightforward can be challenging. The survey will need to be distributed and collected in a consistent fashion or reliability can be a concern of the provider or outpatient practice being surveyed.

Additionally, the survey should test the entire patient experience. Though more costly, outside agencies that have no connection to the organization can provide a more reliable and inclusive result. These agencies can survey patients in a variety of ways such as via computer, phone, written feedback, and mystery shopping.

No matter what method you choose to evaluate the patient experience, it is important to pay attention to what the patient wants and values. Those are the topics you should be measuring. Patients pass on their experiences by word of mouth to others in the community. If the patient does not return, your financial bottom line is affected.

Conclusion

This chapter reviewed the main points on how to prepare a budget, and has given several examples of how the numbers work in relation to the practical aspects of everyday management. However, the nurse manager responsibilities should not be taken out of context. The nurse manager must continue to pay attention to the quality of patient care being rendered and the patient safety standards that are so important in providing quality, safe care. Every management decision you make has financial implications that affect the overall practice success. Making sure that you are always mindful to make choices that are best for the patient will ensure that success.

References

American Academy of Child & Adolescent Psychiatry. 222.aacap.org

Barnett, A., & Mayer, G. (1992). *Ambulatory Care Management and Practice*. Gaithersburg, MD: Aspen.

Dunham-Taylor, J., & Pinczuk, J. (2006). *Health care financial management for nurse managers: Merging the heart with the dollar*. Sudbury, MA: Jones and Bartlett.

Joint Commission on Accreditation of Healthcare Organizations. (1994). Lexikon: Dictionary of Health Care Terms, Organizations, and Acronyms for the Era of Reform.

Index

Page numbers in italics denote table and figure references.